American Medicine in Transition, 1840–1910

American Medicine in Transition
1840–1910

by JOHN S. HALLER, Jr.

University of Illinois Press

URBANA

CHICAGO

LONDON

FOR ROBIN

© *1981 by the Board of Trustees of the University of Illinois*
Manufactured in the United States of America

Library of Congress Cataloging in Publication Data

Haller, John S
    American medicine in transition, 1840–1910

    Bibliography: p.
    Includes index.
    1. Medicine—History—19th century.   I. Title. [DNLM: 1. History of
medicine, 19th century.   wz60 H185m]
R149.H25   610′.9′034   80-14546
ISBN 0-252-00806-5

Contents

Illustrations

Introduction

UNLIKE ATHENA WHO SPRANG full grown from the head of Zeus, nineteenth-century medicine evolved from a murky antiquity, with traces of its often faulty parentage embarrassingly evident. Generations of medical practices clung tenaciously as physicians sought extensions to the boundaries of ancient knowledge. New theories and old habits jostled uncomfortably in the same medical handbags. As a result, doctors were bedeviled with endless disputes over the consequences of treatment and found themselves forced into organizing and reorganizing their observations, and pronouncing judgments on the claims of the past and the counterclaims of their own present. This confusion, so central to the life of medicine in the nineteenth century, also became a catalyst to the threatened disintegration of authority which the profession had so long cultivated. Victorian medicine provided a twisted image of itself that was self-conscious and dogmatic, critical and gullible, materialistic and self-denying. At its best, nineteenth-century medicine was imperfect, ancient, honorable, and humane, and was ministered by those whose aims were unselfish. At its worst, it was destructive and dishonest, with doctors passing on to suffering patients the mistakes of the past.

Nowhere was the feeling of dissatisfaction more apparent than in the candid remarks of physicians as they viewed the chaos of their generation's medical practices.

Paul-Joseph Barthez (1743–1806): "We are blind men, hitting with a stick at disease or at the patient; so much the better for the patient if we strike the disease."

Benjamin Rush (1745–1813): "What mischiefs have we

done, under the belief of false facts and false theories! We have assisted in multiplying diseases; we have done more, we have increased their mortality."

François J. V. Broussais (1772–1838): "Medical practice is only the art of indulging the patient's vain hopes."

John Godman (1794–1830): "Medicine is at least two centuries behind the point we should have reached if physicians had only kept to the path of pathologic research inaugurated during the Renaissance."

Worthington Hooker (1806–1865): "The science of patient-getting is often more assiduously studied than of patient-curing. Real success is not so much desired as the mere appearance of it."

Nineteenth century society was by no means ignorant of the dissatisfaction which doctors voiced in themselves and in the state of their art. The public's sense of medical dismay, when combined with its own faith in the common man and an almost chiliastic belief in the body politic, culminated in peculiar forms of sectarianism and quackery that challenged medical science to listen without indignation to claims of ready cure. Those enamored with the century's material achievements could choose from an almost endless variety of medicines and patented devices that promised health and happiness. Others who spurned materialism and looked instead to the world of faith and mind cure—Christian Science, Dowieism, Homeopathy, and assorted visionaries—accepted promises that seemed as reassuring as the Mississippi Bubble stock or Elisha Perkins's metallic tractors of an earlier era. The promises put forward by sectarianism and quackery were as much a commentary on the internal problems of medicine in the throes of self-doubt as they were a flourishing of eschatological hope amid the uncertainties of an increasingly secular age.

Furthermore, the personal relationship between physician and patient underwent a major transformation in the nineteenth century. In large part, this personal relationship was a function of community and the manner in which community structure either strengthened or deteriorated amid the complexities of new environments. In rural areas, doctors continued to maintain close contact with generations of patients. In towns and cities the situation changed, particularly with the impact of transportation conveniences that set the walking city into perpetual motion. The coach, tramway, elevated, and other forms of mass transportation combined with immigration, industrialization, and poverty to transpose medical care into a relationship of stranger treating stranger. There was a shifting of both diagnosis and treatment from the home environment, where physicians analyzed patients against the background of family and class setting, to an office, hospital, or dispensary, where anonymity prevailed. Asked to give instant diagnosis of persons who appeared as largely unknown quantities, the "art" of medicine was forced to take a backseat to the "science" of medicine and a host of new influences, including germ theory, medical gadgetry, specificity of disease and preventive medicine.

By the latter decades of the nineteenth century, medicine had undergone major changes both in the United States and abroad. Innovations in surgery, the growth of specialism, and the impact of germ theory had made the changes of previous periods look almost cosmetic by comparison; nevertheless, the day-to-day practice of medicine moved at a snail's pace. One could still see evidence of drastic purging and bleeding, even though the numerical method of Louis and the scientific achievements of Koch, Pasteur, and Lister could no longer be ignored. Doctors who left their apprenticeships or graduated from medical schools in the latter half of the century often went into practice without observing a delivery or once having used a microscope, and faced a culture whose ignorance of asepsis was appalling. While country people insisted on applying hot poultices of cow manure to cuts, many doctors were themselves without the training to do more than lance abscesses, administer age-old remedies, set fractures, or sew up cuts. In more serious cases, they either left the results to Providence or sent patients with acute appendicitis, malignancies, prolapsed uterus or prostatic obstructions by train or buggy to Baltimore, Philadelphia, or other large urban centers for treatment.

Medical science had grown by leaps and bounds over the course of the century; and while some doctors had accommodated to change, others stood like oracles in every branch of medical knowledge, justifying what was not always intelligently understood and seeking assurances from an adulating public rather than from peers. This latter group of doctors, Edward Waldo Emerson, M.D., son of the New England transcendentalist, remarked, could be likened to "a general atlas, which, from the necessities of the case, must show in some sort the whole world, and so has to have large yellow spaces, like the old maps of Africa with perhaps some 'Mountains of the Moon,' or 'Country of the Ethiopians,' or even, as in the oldest maps, representations of monstrous beasts or anthropophagi to fill up with." As a group, these doctors felt comfortable with authority and persisted in treating patients from the judgments of past science and learning, content to finish out their years of practice in the backwaters of intellectual change. Calomel, antimony, bloodletting, whiskey, and opium continued to be the mainstay of their cures; and their patients insisted on dying of acute indigestion, locked bowels, brain fever, ground itch, dew poison, diarrhea, decay, and summer complaints.

Others, captivated by the novelty of change, were disposed to try any new departure in therapeutic practice despite doubtful evidence and false claims. For them change was more a way of life than a reasoned shift in thinking or in theory. Boasting a pliant rationalism in both medicine and economics, they offered a cheery optimism that was more pretense than common sense. Using a new medicine that promised cure was the same as curing. They tried to be not only all ages at once, but also all sides to every issue. This combination of energy and cheapened sophistry produced a medicine that was false—which is not to say it failed to leave its mark.

The majority of doctors, preferring compromise to continued conflict, accepted innovations in theory and practice without changing their values and beliefs. They were content to remain in the comfort of those ideas which supported the structure of their education—ideas or truths which, over time, took on greater importance. Not that each truth had to be tenaciously defended, since few truths could boast immortality. Rather, in their totality, those ideas represented a way of thinking and acting which each doctor integrated into his life's practice. Like those Emerson described as oracles or general atlases, this group of doctors remained unaware of the complexity—and ambiguity—of their medical thinking. Secure in themselves and in the state of their art, they were unwilling to give up a theory under the shock of a fact. Yet, clearly, while they continued to use the doctrines of the past, the meaning and substance had changed. Their public acceptance of traditional dogmas remained at variance with their practice. Dogmatic statements became looser and more metaphorical, as doctors did not intend them to convey the truth. Like a clergy who spoke of miracles from habit rather than intellect, they succeeded in accommodating to new scientific discoveries by allowing progress to prevail without having to show evidence of a personal conversion. They were disposed by temperament to accept change not only as something inevitable but, on occasion, as a substitute for genuine inquiry.

If anything, doctors in the period from 1840 to 1910 were profoundly self-conscious about themselves and their profession. This uneasy self-consciousness was a fundamental reality of the age and reflected the bifurcated nature of their business and ethics, their hatred for and absorption of sectarian ideas, their clinging to old drug theories and their uneasy marriage with modern science. In an age when change was rapid, profound, and unanticipated in its consequences, doctors found themselves committed without fully knowing why or how it had all taken place. What occurred in medicine was no different from what prevailed in the greater culture, for a combination of forces made possible the emergence of modern society and the acceptance of change and even unexpected contradictions as no more than a natural progression of events. The Flexner Report of 1910 ushered in the modern age of institutional medicine in America, while the impact of Darwin's *Origin of Species* (1859) officially sanctioned a change in medical thinking from philosophical rationalism to inductive reasoning. Both these events pronounced an end to medical dogmas and the triumphant ratiocinations of past system-builders. Although each served the needs of a new generation of doctors and laid the foundations of health care during the first half of the twentieth century, each also sowed the seeds of discontent that must await new judgment from a present generation of doctors.

I wish to express my special thanks to librarians Betty Shaw and Susan Thompson whose contributions in all aspects of the researching of this book are warmly appreciated.

I am also grateful to Richard Reich, Mike Abaray, Paul Bastyr, Betty Roeske, Johnnie Taylor, Madlyn Adams, Sue Komara, and Silquia Otero of the Indiana University Northwest Library; to Jim Self, Larry Fortado, Rhonda Nathan, Theresa Rohrabaugh, Sally Hager, and Nancy Vossmeyer of the Indiana University library system; to Dorothy T. Hanks, Lucy Keister, and Otis A. Parman of the National Library of Medicine; to my colleagues Paul Kern, Marion J. Mochon, James Lane, Fred Chary, Ronald Cohen, Rhiman Rotz, William Neil, and James Newman; and to Frank O. Williams and Rita P. Zelewsky of the University of Illinois Press. I also appreciate the courtesies extended by the librarians and staff of the Midwest Regional Medical Library, John Crerar Library, Library of Congress, Vanderbilt University Medical Library, Regenstein and Billings Libraries at the University of Chicago, Purdue University Library, New York Academy of Medicine Library, Iowa State University Library, St. Louis Public Library, Rudolph Matas Medical Library of Tulane University, University of Missouri Library, College of Physicians of Philadelphia Library, Yale Medical Library, University of British Columbia Library, the Bio-Medical Library of the University of Minnesota, Stanford University Library, Rutgers University Library, Archibald Church Medical School Library, Enoch Pratt Free Library of Baltimore, University of Michigan Library, Oberlin College Library, Boston Public Library, McGill University Library, Northwestern University Medical School Library, University of Wisconsin Library, St. Louis Medical School Library, Tennessee State Library and Archives, University of Illinois Library of the Health Sciences, Duke University Medical Center Library, University of Kansas Medical Center, Michigan State Library, University of Nebraska Library, University of Cincinnati Library, Emory University Medical Library, and Louisville Free Public Library. Most important, I wish to thank Indiana University, its faculty and staff, for the many services which facilitated the progress of this book.

American Medicine in Transition, 1840–1910

1

*Every Man in His Humor**

CONSTITUTIONAL PATHOLOGY has dominated medical and psychological thought from antiquity into modern times. From the cosmological theories of the Pythagoreans or the mechanistic theories of Hermann Boerhaave (1668–1738), to the physio-chemical pathology of Claude Bernard (1813–1878), the anthropometric measurements made in New York's Presbyterian Hospital in the 1920s and the more recent ideas in somatotyping, constitutional pathology withstood the changing character of medical etiology and therapeutics. Constructed from the earliest observations of human character, it served as ballast amid the chaos of pills, powders, schisms, and heroic therapeutics that so disrupted medicine's coming of age. Even after the decline of humoral theory, the long tradition of constitutional pathology proved a conservative counterforce to the near deluge of eclectic ideas that threatened to overrun medical practice in the eighteenth and nineteenth centuries. Through the humors and the theory of temperaments, constitutional pathology also served to demonstrate the manner in which medical systems both fed and reflected social attitudes. The theory lent to social thought a vocabulary that became a source of metaphor, if it did not actually dictate social values—many of which filtered easily from philosophers to medical men, social scientists, and the popular culture, and provided a uniquely creative force in the history of ideas.

*Portions of this chapter were presented in a paper entitled "A Constitutional Approach to Pathology and the Sciences of Man" delivered before the American Association of Physical Anthropologists in Toronto, April 1978.

Early History of the Humors

Like so much of Western civilization's science and philosophy, constitutional pathology in the form of humoral theory emerged from Greek thought, which in its turn had absorbed elements of Indian and Far Eastern philosophies. The first direct knowledge of humoral theory originated among the Pythagoreans and Empedocles of Akargas (500–430 B.C.), who taught that primal matter consisted of four elements: earth, air, fire, and water. According to the Pythagoreans, each of the four elements manifested a corresponding dryness, coldness, heat, and moistness; and these qualities either singly or in combination formed the humors or radical fluids (blood, phlegm, yellow bile, and black bile) in the animal frame. In effect, the humors were to man (microcosm) what the elements were to the world (macrocosm).[1]

Aristotle's pupil Theophrastus further refined the theory by making a connection between the radical fluids and individual typology, believing the peculiar combination of primary elements manifested in each individual influenced both physique and personality. The basis of the *sanguine* constitution was air (hot and moist) with a temperament characterized by hilarity, mirth, and imagination. Known for a surplus of rich red blood, the sanguine constitution depended upon the secretory actions of the heart. The *phlegmatic* constitution had its basis in water (cold and moist) which Theophrastus identified by the surplus of fine watery fluid, for which the nose and eyes were the natural outlets. He based the *bilious* or *choleric* constitution on fire (hot and dry), inasmuch as its predominant characteristics were excitement, passion, and the "heat of temper." This constitution, caused by a surplus of yellow bile, depended on the action of the liver. Finally, the *melancholic* had his basis in earth (cold and dry), with the eyes usually "directed to the ground," epitomizing interest in difficult problems and mysteries—the scholar's plight. Successive generations of physicians identified this constitution by the surplus of black bile, or dark venous blood produced by the secretory action of the spleen. Clearly, then, constitution and temperament grew from an assortment of philosophical, mathematical, and cultural influences—observations of man, a conception of the radical

PRIME MATTER	QUALITIES	HUMOR	ORGAN	TEMPERAMENT	SEASON	ASTRAL INFLUENCE
Fire	Hot & Dry	Yellow bile	Liver	Bilious or Choleric	Summer	Sun (Mars)
Air	Hot & Moist	Blood	Heart & Lungs	Sanguineous	Spring	Jupiter
Earth	Cold & Dry	Black bile	Spleen	Melancholic	Autumn	Saturn
Water	Cold & Moist	Phlegm	Brain, Lung & Kidneys	Phlegmatic or Lymphatic	Winter	Venus (Moon)

fluids in the animal frame, and an understanding of the elementary principles of matter.[2]

Humoral theory and the temperaments colored all aspects of man, including disease. In his treatise *On the Nature of Man*, Polybus, the son-in-law of Hippocrates, interpreted health as an equilibrium of the four elements in the human constitution. While a specific humor might predominate, giving an individual a peculiar temperament, there was nevertheless a satisfactory mixture (*eucrasia, euexia, euchymia,* or *crasis*) of the remaining humors. When, on the other hand, there developed a morbid predominance of one or more of the humors, the abnormal mixture (*dyscrasia*) turned to disease, with corresponding psychological changes or manifestations. Greek physicians believed that whatever the actual cause for the morbid change in the humors, the body had the innate capacity (*vis medicatrix naturae*) to restore a proper balance. This natural healing process occurred during the "crisis" stage (*coction*) of illness and manifested itself in a drop in the body's temperature, a humoral discharge in the form of urine, stools, sputum, pus, or a combination of factors. Since disease was a morbid alteration in the humors, doctors felt they could hasten the return to natural harmony through a process of purging, cooling, and heating of the body. Thickened by cold and expanded by heat, the humors became the focus of remedial efforts. Solvent remedies were thought to dissolve the humors, while sleep thickened them, narcotics divided and attenuated them, and the lancet removed or diverted the engorged or diseased parts.[3]

Constitutional Typology

The ancient use of the term *humor*, basic to the earliest theories of constitutional pathology, became a "mythical, potent, and subtile fluid, mingling with the bodily substance, and rising, exhalation-like, into the brain, obscuring, revealing, exalting, and depressing the operations of the mind according as it is acting well or ill." Just as in some individuals the blood vessels were full and prominent while in others they were concealed, or in some the skin was florid while in others there was a pale hue, so certain individuals were more capable of exercising judgment and still others were distinguished by their imagination. Traits of indolence, talent, stupidity, passion, kindness, irksomeness, playfulness, and wit were all aspects of humoral influence, and were reflected not only in the physical characteristics of each individual but also in a different degree of health and heredity. Humors and their corresponding temperaments expressed a condition, quality, trait, or peculiarity observable in the physical constitution. They also affected the particular way an individual felt, thought, and acted by marking a predilection in mental and moral habits, tastes, and tendencies. Having a certain humor or temperament was more than simply the outgrowth of a peculiar physical organization. It was the result of both heredity and environment; although the predominant influence remained unsolved and successive changes in man's thinking did little to draw a definitive line between the Scholastic's *materia prima* and *form*.[4]

The *sanguine* constitution, associated with spring and adolescence and noted principally for its life and vitality, was distinguished by certain external signs, including an animated countenance, soft hair with little curl, smooth skin supplied with ample amounts of blood, ruddy complexion, red lips, strong teeth, flushing cheeks, blue eyes, and a soft and plump body which would sweat with even moderate exercise. Sanguineous women had a distinct tendency to voluptuousness. Rarely were persons of sanguine constitution gloomy or morose; rather they showed the best harmony of organs and tissues for health and happiness. Sanguine persons were full of life and, although seldom profound in their thoughts, they were never wholly dull. "They are pleasant companions," one practitioner wrote, "but are better fitted to accompany, or follow and execute, than to lead and command." While lacking in mental daring, depth of feeling, self-denial, and perseverance, they nonetheless evidenced a liberality of sentiment and were too vivacious to brood over the past. Although affectionate in their manner they were inconstant in their loves and friendships. Prompt to take offense, they were seldom anxious to forgive or forget. Similarly, they excelled in ingenuity but disliked profound meditation. Sanguine constitutions were known to be easily affected by external impressions—the memory was tenacious, the perception prompt, the imagination lively. Physicians referred to the statues of Antinous and Apollo Belvedere as best displaying the external marks of this temperament but applied the characteristics also to Mark Anthony, Alcibiades, Richard Coeur de Lion, Prince Rupert, Cardinal Richelieu, Shakespeare's Hotspur, Romeo, and Brutus, Homer's Ajax, the Frenchman Marat, and the boxer John L. Sullivan. The sanguine temperament was predominant in the female sex as well as among ballet dancers and trapeze performers.[5]

In the *bilious* or *choleric* constitution, associated with summer and adulthood, the subcutaneous veins were easily visible and the pulse strong and hard. The bilious person had a dark or sallow complexion, firm muscular movement, a strong appetite, dark sparkling eyes, strong teeth, hard and curled black hair, and a moderately fleshy body. Individuals with this constitution were strikingly masculine, displaying sternness, strength, and quickness of perception. They were abrupt, stubborn, impetuous, suspicious, dogmatic, generous, ambitious, violent, and inflexible in pursuing their goals. Those possessing this particular constitution had seized governments, and through their courage and audacity, carried out the greatest triumphs—and the most heinous crimes—in history. The heroes, martyrs, and tyrants of the ages—men like Achilles, Alexander, Caesar, Mohammed, Attila, Luther, Cromwell, Washington, Shakespeare's Cassius, Napoleon, Lee, Booth, Stonewall Jackson, and Ulysses Grant—were among those most frequently cited as examples of the bilious temperament.[6]

When individuals contained an excessive proportion of liquids over solids, giving the body an increased bulk, a fleshy appearance, dull countenance; weak and slow pulse, pale skin and light hair, the constitution was known as *lymphatic* or *phlegmatic* (sometimes called *leuco-phlegmatic*), associated with autumn and middle age. For these types, the vital functions were languid, the memory spotty, and the attention wavering. By the eighteenth century doctors had begun using the term *lymphatic* to designate this constitution, believing that the secretory system (lymphatic and absorbents) did not act thoroughly enough to prevent the cellular tissues from filling. As a consequence, lymphatic persons were rarely tall or athletic; instead they had a light complexion, which indicated a deficiency of red corpuscles, and their languid nature reflected the poor circulation of blood through the system. Phlegmatic persons were seldom achievers, as they lacked the drive necessary for either mental vivacity or power. They were most easily identified by a heavy, rounded head, thick lips and cheeks, short nose, blue eyes, good teeth, and deficient muscle tone. Although often possessed of great intellectual capacity, their lack of strength prevented them from turning that faculty to good use. Instead, intellectual labor, along with indulgences in the passions, tended to undermine their health. While conversant, trustful, and successful in business, they had little ambition or enthusiasm. They were good-natured, plodding in their work, logical and sound in their conclusions, apt to be dull companions but constant friends, and short-lived. Examples of this type included Henry VIII, Shakespeare's Falstaff and Benvolio, Louis XVI of France, and Edward the Confessor.[7]

Physicians like Galen, William Cullen, and Laurent Clerc associated the *melancholic* constitution with winter and old age and considered it less a natural condition than a morbid affection, where the black bile prevailed because of derangements in the spleen (usually assumed from observations of vomit, urine, or stools). While occurring naturally in some individuals, the melancholic constitution also appeared abnormally ("melancholy adust") from excessive burning or "adustion" (from Latin *adurere*, "to burn") of one or more of the humors.[8] Brought on by both physical causes (food, climate, lack of sleep and exercise) and psychological agents (immoderate passions and intellectual exhaustion), the melancholic temperament manifested itself in anxiety, insomnia, irritability, peevishness, fears, and a variety of complaints that fell into the category of neuroses. Doctors considered the neurotic manifestations of this humor difficult to treat, let alone cure, with many of its stages degenerating into deep depression and sometimes even madness. Thomas Willis (1622–75), for example, believed that madness and melancholy were "so-much akin, that these Distempers often change, and pass from one into the other."[9] Doctors pointed to Tiberius, Tasso, Pascal, Cowper, Mrs. Browning, and even Shakespeare's Hamlet (who, although considered naturally sanguine, was changed by stress and misfortune to melancholic) and King Lear (originally choleric) as examples of the melancholic constitution and temperament.[10] The classic description of this constitution exists in Robert Burton's *The Anatomy of Melancholy* (1621), a popular book that went through hundreds of editions in Europe and America and articulated the polymorphous nature of this "English malady." Following Burton's intellectual odyssey, melancholy became a fashionable state of mind, as well as a psychological and medical condition, which rivaled hysteria, hypochondriasis, and neurasthenia in appealing to status-conscious neurotics.[11]

The four constitutions played an important role in early English literature, with writers such as Shakespeare and Ben Jonson focusing entire plays on temperamental peculiarities. British novelists like Fielding, Scott, Dickens, and George Eliot gave strict attendance to the temperaments, which provided a convenient literary mechanism for observant readers to discern the strengths and weaknesses of their heroes and villains. The concept of foreordination that so pervaded Calvinistic thinking in the seventeenth century carried over into eighteenth and early nineteenth century novels with plots that rested firmly on the constitutional determinism of leading characters.[12]

Besides the four constitutions designated by the ancients, Edinburgh's James Gregory (1753–1821) pointed to yet another type, which he identified as *nervous* because of the susceptibility of so many individuals to nervous disorders. Like the melancholic, the nervous constitution was not so much a natural condition as an acquired one—created by the sedentary nature of urban living, the studious or fashionable life, lack of physical exercise, improper habits of parents, romantic literature, dress, diet, climate, and generally intemperate habits. Marked by small, soft, and wasted muscles, a slender form, soft complexion, trepidation, anxiety, and irritability, persons of nervous constitution were predisposed to delicate work rather than to tasks requiring muscular activity. Nervous temperaments gave "to the artisan delicacy and beauty of touch and finish; to the professional man feeling, sympathy, and susceptibility; to the poet restlessness, intensity, and brilliancy; and to the orator vividness, splendor, and refinement of thought, word and gesture." Examples include Voltaire, American financier Jay Gould, Edgar Allen Poe, and the poet Shelley. One physician writing in 1866 even suggested that the "high nervous temperament of the southern people," most notably Jefferson Davis, had actually precipitated the Civil War.[13]

The nervous constitution received special notoriety in the nineteenth century, as doctors theorized that nervous energy (or its absence) more adequately reflected the constitution of the urban middle class. In the United States, the New York neurologist George M. Beard coined the term *neurasthenia* to explain the nervous exhaustion or nervelessness affecting the intellectual classes of industrial society. Before long, neurasthenia had become the harbinger disease of America—both a disease and an object of social value, since suffering from neurasthenia classified the individual as one of the brain-workers of advanced civilization. As a substitute for Burton's melancholia, neurasthenia became not only an inevitable prospect facing society's business and scholarly leaders, but also an index against which to measure America's claim to superiority in the nineteenth century.[14]

Etiological Continuity

The third century Roman physician Galen, as medical historian Esmond Long accurately observed, "out humored the most extravagant humoralists of the school of Cos" by adding five more divisions or genera to the four of Hippocrates. In doing so, Galen made medical pathology in the succeeding centuries a paean to Greek medicine. Galen also developed an extensive pharmacological system by ranking medicines according to their supposed qualities of heat, moistness, cold, and dryness, and prescribing them in proportion to their capacity for returning the body's radical fluids to normal. Roman physicians treated the morbid conditions of the black bile or melancholic humor by prescribing strong doses of mandragora and hellebore because of their reputed ability to provoke a dark form of diarrhea colored with blood. They also eliminated the toxic effects of the humor through bleeding piles, phlebotomy, purging, and even suggested masturbation and sexual intercourse as an alternative means of correcting its melancholic depressions.[15]

Galenic pathology ruled supreme for nearly fifteen centuries. One exception was Paracelsus (1493–1541) whose ontological bias caused him to regard disease as an entity having existence apart from the patient. Rather than the individual's humor determining the cause and nature of disease, he held that it was "the individual disease that conditions the patient and manifests itself in a characteristic picture."[16] Despite the views of Paracelsus and the later theories of Jean Baptist van Helmont (1577–1644), whose treatise *De Humoribus Galeni* (1648) substituted a theoretical system based upon chemical principles, humoral pathology received the serious attention of medical men until the flourishing of scientific ideas in the seventeenth century, when the theory underwent a series of reinterpretations that took into account newer ideas in physics and philosophy. One such innovator was Hermann Boerhaave of Leyden (1668–1738) who taught that the living body consisted of two principal elements: fluids and solids. Although Boerhaave accepted the constitutional basis of disease, his observations into the nature of blood caused him to replace the humoral theory of the Greek school with the suggestion that the four radical fluids were simply constituent parts of the blood, differentiated by the diameters of the body's circulatory channels, which permitted only certain of the particles to flow. The diversity of body fluids—sweat, milk, semen, urine, mucus, etc.—resulted from the action of the solids upon the principal humors of the blood. Boerhaave never clarified the precise manner in which this action took place except that good health resulted from a balanced interaction between solids and fluids. In this sense, a proper pathological analysis of health and disease depended upon a study of both solids and fluids in the body and not just the radical humors.[17]

The German physician and chemist, Georg Ernst Stahl (1660–1734) accepted the constitutional theory of disease but challenged the interpretations of Galen and Boerhaave by substituting a vitalistic system more in keeping with his own philosophical beliefs. In his *Theoria Medica Vera* (1708), Stahl noted that the condition of the mind and not the fluids (or solids and fluids) caused the morbid changes in the body. The mind or *anima* acted upon the fluids to produce the particular temperaments. Stahl based his variation of constitutional pathology on the discovery of a new principle in matter that he called "phlogiston" or the matter of fire that existed in all bodies. Although Stahl repudiated humoral pathology, he nevertheless retained the temperaments to delineate the constitutional types created by the anima. Accordingly, there was the thin-blooded phlegmatic, the thick-blooded melancholic, the hot-blooded sanguine, and the sour-acrid blood of the bilious or choleric constitution.[18]

Albrecht von Haller (1708–77), the Swiss physician and disciple of Boerhaave, was yet another innovator in medicine who built his own particular arrangement of the temperaments on the theory of irritability of the solid fiber or what he preferred to call the "vital actions of the system." Like the constitutional theorists before him, he maintained the validity of the temperaments but arrived at their definition from yet another source. In his *Elementa Physiologiae Corporis Humani* (1759), Haller placed the temperaments on a strictly physiological basis. When the fiber was firm and irritable, the body was considered bilious; when firm but less irritable, it was sanguine; when very lax and irritable, it was melancholic; and when poor in both tone and irritability, the result was phlegmatic. Erasmus Darwin, the English physician, philosopher, and poet of Derby, accepted Haller's derivation of the temperaments on the basis of the vital power; but he replaced the ancient terminology with the words *irritative, sensitive, voluntary* and *associate*, or, as he preferred to designate them, "the temperament of diseased irritability, the temperament of sensibility, the temperament of diseased voluntary, and the temperament of increased association."[19]

The French anatomist and vitalist Marie François Xavier

Bichat (1771–1802) constructed his own division of the temperaments on what he felt were eight distinct organic arrangements of the body—membranous, vascular, glandular, ligamentous, osseous, cartilaginous, muscular, and medullary or nervous. "Life," he wrote, "rests upon a tripod made up of respiration, circulation, and nervation." They, in turn, were sustained by the brain, spinal cord, heart, lungs, arteries, veins, nerves, glands, and intestines, all of which had specific functions. The predominance or deficiency of any one or combination of these organs or functions stamped the individual with peculiar physical and mental characteristics. Moreover, since tissues were the sustainers of the vital functions, each with its own characteristic property, they were consequently the seat of disease and not the organ. François J. V. Broussais (1772–1838), in his turn, constructed a set of six temperaments based upon the functional development, which he identified as gastric, bilious, sanguineous, lymphatico-sanguineous, anemic, and nervous. Like Bichat, he insisted that it was not the organ but the tissues ("gastro-enteritis") which were the seat of disease. Although destructive in their antiphlogistic extremes, the contributions of Broussais and Bichat provided a bridge to the cellular pathology of Theodor Schwann in the 1830s and to the later work of Rudolph Virchow, who was able to assert that "there are no general diseases. From now on we shall recognize only diseases of organs and cells." Ultimately, it was Virchow's *Cellular Pathology* (1858) that put an end to the last vestiges of humoralism. In doing so, however, Virchow undermined the foundations of constitutional pathology by arguing that, for the future, pathology must abandon all prior theories founded upon diathesis and dyscrasis and, instead, rely on histology.[20]

Phrenology and the Temperaments

While constitutional pathology faced an uncertain future in the corridors of traditional medicine, it nonetheless received vocal support from the new science of phrenology, introduced by the Vienna-educated physician and neuroanatomist Franz Joseph Gall (1758–1828) and his pupil and co-worker Johann Gaspar Spurzheim (1776–1832), who had set out to establish a psychology of man based on anatomy and physiology. In effect, phrenology encouraged the study of human nature to move from the citadels of philosophy and logic and center in the physical sciences. Gall's science of "organology" evolved from the earlier work of the Swiss-German John Kaspar Lavater (1741–1801), a theologian and physiognomist, whose early interest in "magnetic trance" had led him to studies involving the interaction of the mind and body. In his *Physiognomische Fragmente* (1775), Lavater believed it possible to construct a "frontometer," whereby the state of the mind (i.e., temperament) could be obtained by gauging the varying temperatures of certain parts of the body. In similar fashion, phrenology taught that the brain consisted of some twenty-seven (Gall) to thirty-five (Spurzheim) independent faculties (calculation, memory, ideality, amativeness, etc.) discernible in different locations of the brain and which scientists, through precise measurement of the cranium, could calculate with a high degree of precision.

Gall maintained a conservative professional practice, limited principally to an upper class clientele; and support for his theories came from such prestigious figures as Broussais, Corvisart, Goethe, Blumenbach, Hufeland, and Geoffroy Saint-Hilaire. His disciples, on the other hand, had all the attributes of eschatological zealots who carried the truths of the materialistic science of the mind to all classes and applied its doctrines to virtually every phase of culture—from religion and therapeutics to education and penal reform. Four years after Gall's death in 1828, Spurzheim visited the United States and began a lecture tour which proved so successful that eminent individuals like Nathaniel Bowditch, Joseph Storey, and President Josiah Quincy of Harvard were sufficiently impressed with the theory to treat it seriously. Both the Boston Medical Association and the editors of the *American Journal of Medicine* found the science similarly appealing.[21]

Interest in this new variation of constitutional pathology continued to grow during the 1830s; and with the visit of the Scottish disciple George Combe (1788–1858) in 1838–1840, notable converts appeared among doctors, preachers, and the social elite. Boston surgeon John Charles Warren, Dr. Samuel Gridley Howe, and Dr. Fuller of the Hartford Retreat for the Insane were among the noted converts to the science of bumps. Physician Charles Caldwell of Transylvania University, one of phrenology's more bombastic champions, spurred interest in the new science during the early decades of the century. Known by both friends and enemies as "the American Spurzheim," the Louisville doctor became the leading proselytizer of phrenology in the Midwest. Other advocates included Henry Schoolcraft, Horace Greeley, Henry Ward Beecher, Horace Mann, Theodore Dwight Weld, and Clara Barton. American writers such as Twain, Poe, Simms, Holmes, Stowe, Bryant, Melville, and Whitman went so far as to incorporate the pseudo-science in their literary works as a means of further exemplifying character roles. European writers, including Balzac, George Sand, Baudelaire, Thomas Carlyle, and Flaubert, did the same.[22]

The widely divergent views held by phrenologists regarding the applicability of their new doctrine caused the pseudoscience to degenerate eventually into a spirited heterodoxy that simply mirrored the growing sectarianism in the psychologies of man. By the 1860s and 1870s phrenology was left to writers like Orson and Lorenzo Fowler, who entertained the public with their eclectic's love of mental gymnastics. Through their efforts, phrenology became an immensely marketable science—a layman's guide to self-knowledge.[23] Yet, the constitutional assumptions of phrenology, aided by the inferences drawn from the publication of Thomas Laycock's *Lectures on the Physiognomy of Disease* (1862), Charles Darwin's *The Expression of the Emotions in Man and Animals* (1872), and Francis Galton's *Inquiries into Human Faculty and Its Development* (1883) inspired the founders of psychology to initiate investigations into personality, brain functioning, sentiments, propensities, and skull configurations. Despite faulty assumptions, Gall had forged an important link in the chain of intellectual currents that united men like Thomas Willis, Hughlings Jackson, Paul Broca, and James Prichard to the idea of cordical parcellation and localization.[24]

Race and Nationality

From the earliest times, philosophers, naturalists, and preacademic anthropologists had employed constitutional pathology to define the character of nations and individuals.

Geography, nutrition, and environment affected the radical humors and their combinations in the body to produce a preponderant temperament for a given nation or people. The Swedish botanist, Carl von Linnaeus (1707–78) not only originated binomial nomenclature, but applied specific temperaments to each of the four families of man. These portraits were handed down through successive generations of naturalists and contributed to the stereotypes so frequently invoked by nineteenth century scientists and social scientists in their efforts to delineate racial differences and construct a hierarchical scale among the known peoples of the world. Eventually the hierarchy became justification in itself for political legislation relegating the so-called "inferior races" to subordinate roles in the social structure.[25]

Just as phrenology provided an early bridge between the strictly physical aspects of biology and the generalizations made from sociology, so it also offered an easy transition from biology to the classification of the races of mankind. Nineteenth century scientists and social scientists, for example, elaborated on the mental characteristics of each race by combining phrenology with Frederick Blumenbach's (1752–1840) divisions of the races into Mongolian, Caucasian, Ethiopian, Malayan, and American. In their analysis, the Mongolian, whose head was smaller than the Caucasian's, with a larger proportion of its bulk behind the ear and with a less prominent forehead, evidenced such tendencies as combativeness, destructiveness, acquisitiveness, secretiveness, cautiousness and imitation; likewise, the Mongolian was deficient in ideality, causality, and mirthfulness. The Malayan race was active, enterprising, subtle, crafty, unprincipled, treacherous, cruel, and subject to frequent fits of "ungovernable passion, brought on by the use of alcoholic liquors, opium and bang (smoking hemp), in which he seemed to thirst for blood and to be utterly insensible to either fear or bodily pain." The American Indian, on the other hand, had a mental character that expressed energy, persistence, firmness, dignity, bravery, cunning, and cruelty. The Ethiopian's mental temperament was more difficult to determine than the others. Although lively, amiable, excitable, and impulsive, there was also evidence of a "slow, steady energy and patient endurance. . . . With all his amiability, sympathy, and real kindness of heart, the Negro can be guilty of the greatest cunning, ferocity, and cruelty."[26]

Before phrenology died a pauper's death in the corridors of science, it served as midwife to craniometry, whose spokesman, Paul Broca (1824–80), introduced the stereograph, craniograph, goniometer (which measured the facial angle) and various other instruments used to derive statistical generalities from the evidence of skull differences among the races. No sooner were the instruments employed, however, than racial enthusiasts sought to use their measurements as indicators of moral character, intelligence, and social tendencies. Indeed, before the century was over, physical anthropology had absorbed so many of the inferences drawn from phrenology and the theory of temperaments that thoroughly proper race studies appeared sidetracked for want of instruments that had not already prejudged the inferiority of the "lesser races." Presumptive inferiority was at the very foundation of early anthropology and, remaining there, rose to the pinnacle of truth with the myth of scientific certainty.[27]

Constitutional Theory and Disease

Throughout the ages, physicians taught that an accurate assessment of constitution and temperament would aid in the proper diagnosis and prognosis of disease. Knowledge of the predispositions and tendencies of the temperaments allowed the careful surgeon to correctly evaluate a patient's susceptibility to disease, the amount of assurance needed by each patient, and the patient's ability to follow instructions. Some physicians considered the temperaments so essential to medical science that Patrick Black (1813–79), for example, arranged his outpatients at St. Bartholomew's Hospital on seats according to their physiognomy. From this practice, he was supposedly able to discover the presence and disposition of disease in patients and also to help lay the foundation for proper prognosis.[28] Similarly, J. Nicolas Corvisart (1755–1821), Joseph Skoda (1805–81), Ferdinand von Hebra (1816–80), Joseph Bell (1837–1911), and Jacob M. DaCosta (1833–1900) were known to "ticket off the occupations as well as the diseases of their patients at a glance."[29]

Even the American Medical Association's 1847 *Code of Eth-*

ics urged patients to confide in only one physician; "for a
medical man who has become acquainted with the peculiarities of *constitution, habits,* and *predispositions,* of those he
attends, is more likely to be successful in his treatment than
one who does not possess that knowledge" (italics mine).[30]
Through proper understanding of the constitution, a physician could recognize the recuperative powers along with the
degree of shock a person could sustain in operative work.
"In anesthesia, it will indicate the element best calculated to
support the patient during the trying ordeal, and which of
the anesthetics offer the best results." Knowledge of the constitution and temperament was also an aid in analyzing possible complications, and particularly in treating the very
young. It likewise enabled the obstetrician to guide, by suggestion and encouragement, the mother's energies in controlling the expulsive efforts of childbirth.[31] In this regard,
lymphatic patients had a greater endurance and insensibility
to pain due primarily to the coarser organization of the
nerve, "in respect to their ultimate molecules, whereby they
do not so quickly or so powerfully respond, as in the other
temperaments." In contrast, the nervous temperament had
little power to endure pain.[32]

Out of these assessments, doctors concluded that sanguine
persons were generally healthy, but that when disease did
occur, it affected the heart and arteries, producing plethora, apoplexy, pneumonia, pleurisy, acute fever, and hemorrhages which required antiphlogistic remedies, especially
venesection. Persons of sanguine constitution were also more
prone to venereal disease. This susceptibility, doctors argued, was primarily due to a moral weakness—the sanguine
temperament being more reckless and passionate in nature.
Similarly, sanguineous individuals suffered from a dispro-
portionate arthritic diathesis because of moral and dietetic
failings. With respect to diabetes, one doctor wrote that
"spirit-drinking is an important predisposing cause of this
obscure disease" and there, again, the sanguine temperament was the most susceptible. Mania and madness were
likewise peculiar to persons of sanguine (and choleric) constitutions, as were skin diseases such as lupus, erysipelas,
psoriasis, eczema, and pemphigus; some even suggested that
spedalkshed and pellagra were constitutional hazards.[33]

Diseases in the sanguine constitution and temperament derived from the declining use of the vital fluid after maturity. In other words, most of the blood was expended in the early years for the nourishment and growth of the body; with the arrival of maturity, the vital fluid tended to accumulate and produce congestions. For that reason, doctors thought sanguine persons "seldom lived to old age, being cut off by their own imprudence, or by the turbulence of their passions, in the vigor of manhood." Remedies administered to patients of sanguine constitution included cardiac stimulants to enhance peripheral circulation, depressants in active disease conditions, and alteratives after inflammation. Frequently, doctors reported that sanguineous patients suffered sudden losses of body fluids followed by either rapid recovery or a hurried collapse of the system. Those who understood the peculiarities of this constitution seldom interfered with the evacuations, since they understood them to be nature's method of throwing off the disease.[34]

The liver, or bile-making organ, considered by doctors to be overactive in the bilious temperament, possessed enormous energy at the expense of the cellular and lymphatic systems. The pulse remained strong, hard, and frequent. Not surprisingly, bilious persons were most prone to diseases of the hepatic organs and biliary secretions—congestion, inflammation, and fluxes, which produced indigestion as well as mental depression. Those with a decidedly bilious habit succumbed to sadness, melancholy, hypochondriasis, or depression. Doctors suspected that insanity was far more pronounced in the bilious temperament and could be transmitted by heredity. The most commonly used medications included the active evacuants, particularly purgatives and emetics. Bilious constitutions tolerated antispasmodics, motor depressants, and arterial sedatives; but motor excitants were contraindicated.[35] Bilious persons of dark complexion could bear mercurial treatment well and, in fact, required larger doses than those of fair complexion. "Many persons of the dark complexion not only bear mercury well," Jonathan Hutchinson observed in 1882, "but enjoy better health whilst taking it, and are not unfrequently much and permanently benefited by a long course."[36]

The lymphatic constitution, with its tendency to obesity

and a "sensual and grovelling mind," was exceedingly pre-disposed to gout, watery fluxes, rheumatism, apoplexy, chol-era, cancer, typhoid fever, diphtheria, scarlatina, and tuber-culosis. Lymphatic persons were often depicted as having a scrofulous diathesis and, although able to sustain pain, were considered poor health risks who lacked the vitality to resist disease. In cases of cholera and typhoid fever, one physician wrote in the 1860s, "I never look for the patient's recovery, if he be a subject of the lymphatic temperament; in [diphtheria and scarlatina] they may sometimes, but I never make a favor-able prognosis." Doctors favored cathartics to relieve portal congestion, and cerebral stimulants, particularly strychnine, to support the cardiac and respiratory apparatus in the lym-phatic constitutions.[37]

The frequency of sudden infant death caused many physi-cians to direct their attention to the temperaments for a pos-sible solution to the vexing problem. In 1826 Alexander Hood noted five cases of sudden death associated with en-larged thymus. John Heinrich Kopp, writing in the 1830s, designated the disease as thymic asthma, and blamed death on hyperplasia of the thymus gland which caused mechanical pressure on the trachea. Although Virchow supported Kopp's theory in the 1860s, subsequent doctors considered thymic asthma identical to laryngismus stridulus and reasoned that the enlarged thymus only rarely caused an obstruction of the larynx. This interpretation held until 1888, when Paul Gra-witz reopened the issue by reporting several cases of sudden infant death in which autopsy indicated an enlarged thymus and again questioned whether or not the deaths were caused by mechanical pressure upon the air passages, nerves, or ves-sels. In 1889 the Vienna physician Arnold Paltauf published a collection of 127 case histories of infant death during the first year of life and demonstrated that there was an unusual enlargement of the lymphatic glands; the victims also had a pasty complexion, an enlarged spleen, and organs filled with blood. By the turn of the twentieth century, doctors were still blaming the lymphatic constitution for crib death and even for epilepsy and rachitis.[38]

Persons of nervous constitution were thought to be suscep-tible to more illnesses than those of any other type. Because of their more rapid heart beat and unequal blood distribution, they suffered from liver complaints, indigestion, explosive temper, undue sexual emotions, neuralgia, epilepsy, and insomnia. Because they were petulant, petty, and rankled by the slightest passion, they were liable to convulsive difficulties, particularly hysteria. The nervous temperament was highly susceptible to the immoderate use of stimulants and narcotics; and because doctors commonly treated nervous or neurasthenic patients with opiates and alcoholic draughts, diseases attributed to the nervous temperament were actually traceable to drug overuse. Not surprisingly, delirium tremens, chronic alcoholism, apoplexy, paralysis, and insanity were frequent occurrences among those with nervous temperaments.[39]

One mark of the extensive use given to constitutional pathology in the nineteenth century was in the policy of life insurance companies to request a person's temperament on application forms. Medical men had advised companies to account for temperament in the belief that differences in disease and death rate among the various constitutions would eventually lead to more correct actuarial tables and perhaps even to revised premium rates.[40] Insurance companies underwrote a large portion of the Sanitary Commission's expenses during the Civil War convinced that meaningful information would be gained from statistics on the physical condition of the northern soldier.[41] While doctors had long studied the relation of the temperaments to disease, little had been done to relate the temperaments to vital capacity. Nor, for that matter, was there any large body of data demonstrating these relationships. Advocates for the study argued that anthropometric tabulations collected from soldiers during the war years would provide sufficient raw data from which considerable information could be drawn, including the marked tendency or immunity of the constitutions to disease. Support also came from Charles Darwin, who in 1862 had expressed interest in the relationship between hair, skin complexion, and disease and had sought permission from the United States Army to obtain the information during the course of the Civil War. Darwin wrote:

> In the spring of 1862 I obtained permission from the Director-General of the Medical Department of the Army to transmit to the surgeons . . . a blank table, with the following ap-

pended remarks, but I have received no returns. "As several well-marked cases have been recorded with our domestic animals of a relation between the colour of the dermal appendages and the constitution; and it being notorious that there is some limited degree of relation between the colour of the races of man and the climate inhabited by them; the following investigation seems worth consideration. Namely, whether there is any relation in Europeans between the colour of their hair, and their liability to the diseases of tropical countries. If the surgeons of the several regiments, when stationed in unhealthy tropical districts, would be so good as first to count, as a standard of comparison, how many men, in the force whence the sick are drawn, have dark and light-coloured hair, and hair of intermediate or doubtful tints; and if a similar account were kept by the same medical gentlemen, of all the men who suffered from malarious and yellow fevers, or from dysentery, it would soon be apparent, after some thousand cases had been tabulated, whether there exists any relation between the colour of the hair and constitutional liability to tropical diseases. Perhaps no such relation would be discovered, but the investigation is well worth making. In case any positive result were obtained, it might be of some practical use in selecting men for any particular service. Theoretically the result would be of high interest, as indicating one means by which a race of men inhabiting from a remote period an unhealthy tropical climate, might have become dark-coloured by the better preservation of dark-haired or dark-complexioned individuals during a long succession of generations." [42]

Although Darwin was unable to obtain a response to his request, the Provost-Marshal-General's bureau tabulated more than a million examinations of men in the Union Army, and from those statistics, physician Ely Van de Warker (1841–1910), one of the founders of the American Gynecological Society, constructed tables designed to improve the diagnostic tools of medical science. Van de Warker believed that temperaments had their origin "deep and unchangeably fixed in the organic life of each individual." Drawing from J. H. Baxter's two volumes of statistical tabulations on Union soldiers, he attempted to simplify matters by applying the sanguine and lymphatic temperaments to those recruits with light-colored hair and skin and blue or gray eyes, while designating the bilious and nervous temperaments to those with sallow or dark complexions, black eyes and hair. By indicating vital capacity from a ratio of chest expansion ("a free chest-expansion implies a large consumption of oxygen, and this, in turn, calls for a large demand for food, with a proportional muscular vigor"), he observed that the size and muscular vigor of the sanguine and lymphatic temperaments exceeded those of the bilious and nervous. Similarly, in a study of the ratio of diseases to complexion, he found that the sanguine and lymphatic temperaments had greater predisposition to skin diseases as well as problems of the digestive, circulatory, and locomotor systems. The bilious and nervous temperaments, on the other hand, had about the same frequency of nervous disease as the other two temperaments.[43]

As medical science underwent massive changes during the second half of the nineteenth century, particularly with the work of Rudolph Virchow, Louis Pasteur, and Robert Koch, doctors began to cast aside their earlier generalizations regarding the constitution and to think more in terms of cellular pathology with specific diseases and specific morbific causation. The research of French chemist Louis-René Le-Canu (1800–1871) nevertheless marked a continued effort to reinstate constitutional pathology by analyzing the ratio of water, albumen, and red globules in the blood.

RATIO OF WATER, ALBUMEN, AND RED BLOOD GLOBULES
IN THE BLOOD OF DIFFERENT TEMPERAMENTS

	SANGUINE	LYMPHATIC	DIFFERENCE
	Water	Water	
Females	793.007	803.710	10.703
Males	786.584	800.566	13.982
	Albumen	Albumen	
Females	71.264	68.660	2.604
Males	65.85	71.701	5.851
	Red Globules	Red Globules	
Females	126.990	117.300	8.874
Males	136.497	110.667	19.830

According to LeCanu, water, plasmic material, and red blood globules traveled to the brain in proportions fixed by the peculiar temperaments; thus differences were not only discernible but sufficiently so to determine an individual's vigor, tenacity, and mental breadth.[44]

Late in the nineteenth century, the Viennese physician Karl Rokitansky (1804–78), a professor of pathology who performed thousands of postmortem examinations, developed a theory of "crases" and "stases" in which the blood became the habitat of disease. One medical historian suggested that Rokitansky's theory was "an altogether misguided, if courageous, attempt to restore humoral pathology, which has been steadily losing ground since Vesalius first took issue with Galen." Rokitansky's quixotic efforts fell before the harsh criticism of Rudolph Virchow and his cellular pathology, but the constitutional aspects of his theory continued in use through the physio-chemical pathology of Claude Bernard, Harvey Cushing, Arthur Biedl, and Wilhelm Falta, whose research on the internal secretion of organs (*milieu de l'intérieur*) gave new life to the old humoralism. According to Bernard, who was once a student of François Magendie at Hôtel Dieu, a vital link existed between the body fluids and temperament (i.e., psychological characteristics), with disease indicating a breakdown of the body's homeostatic mechanism that kept the two factors in harmonious accord. While Bernard recognized the importance of discovering the disease agent through advances in bacteriology, he considered it just as crucial to understand why the body's homeostatic mechanism was not functioning properly.[45] In other words, the answer to the problem of causality depended not only on a thorough understanding of specific infection but on the general condition or *cachexis* of the host, since the body fluids formed an internal environment that provided the particular conditions of existence for the cell. The debate between proponents of the "soil" and "seed" theories continued through the turn of the century, even though it appeared that bacteriology all but dominated physiology. Nevertheless, the development of serology and endocrinology provided a continual challenge to specificity of disease and the advances of bacteriology.[46]

By the late nineteenth century, it was apparent to many in the medical profession that the term *constitutional pathology* had been too generally applied and that, as with the terms *chorea, hysteria, dyspepsia,* and *vapors,* doctors either had to redefine the term or abandon it altogether. In an effort to resolve the confusion, medical men began to supplement the doctrine through the addition of words such as *predisposition, idiosyncracy,* and *diathesis*—terms which related to specific diseases and morbific causes. While using the word *temperament* to denote the sum of the physical peculiarities of an individual, they employed the term *diathesis* to refer to the body's proclivity to suffer from a particular type of disease. In this more refined approach, temperament did not denote disease or even the predeliction to disease; diathesis, on the other hand, did suggest either a hereditary or recurrent susceptibility or special proneness to disease. In other words, temperament became a matter of physiology, while diathesis became a matter of disease.[47] As physician F. B. Stephenson remarked in 1888, "diathesis may be looked upon as a soil in relation to the production of disorder; and temperament comparable with atmospheric conditions, considered the means through which exciting causes act, or gain access—it is the proper physiognomy of each person."[48] Only through a proper understanding of the temperaments and diathesis would diagnosis, prognosis, and treatment of disease become more accurate. There was, it appeared, merit in the view that "we are killed not so much by diseases as by diathesis."[49]

Jonathan Hutchinson (1828–1913), senior surgeon of the London Hospital, reflected a genuine concern for proper application of terminology when he suggested the following definitions.

> *Temperament*—a term applicable to the sum of all the physical peculiarities of an individual, exclusive of all definite tendencies to disease. . . . Temperament concerns the original inherited organization of the individual, and does not include anything which is the result of the influences to which his life has exposed him. That which has accrued to him during life goes to produce or aggravate diathesis, but can do nothing in modification of temperament.
>
> *Diathesis*—any bodily condition, however induced, in vir-

tue of which the individual is, through a long period, or usually through the whole life prone to suffer from some peculiar type of disease . . . may be acquired as well as inherited.

Idiosyncracy—applicable to any definite peculiarity of organization of which the consequences may occur unexpectedly and otherwise inexplicably. It does not . . . imply any special proneness to disease, only that under certain well known circumstances, results which are peculiar to the individual will certainly occur.[50]

Hutchinson, who authored *The Pedigree of Disease* (1884), which he dedicated to Darwin, considered it important to ascertain the external influences affecting the peculiarities of disease, and urged physicians to take a life history of their patients from infancy onward so as to become better acquainted with their idiosyncrasies. Diagnostic capability was enhanced as much by the state of the parasitic host as it was by a thorough understanding of the science of bacteriology, which was able to isolate and identify organisms of disease. Knowing a patient's medical portrait prevented subsequent errors in treatment; it also increased medical knowledge into the real nature of disease. "It is not only as regards the prescription of many drugs that a knowledge of our patient's peculiarities become important to us in practice," Hutchinson wrote, "but the advice we have to give in respect to places of residence, mode of life, and general management are often of far more importance than the medicine prescribed, and its wisdom or the reverse may depend on the knowledge or the ignorance of the individual peculiarities, and those peculiarities frequently do not display themselves in any of the symptoms, and can be recognized and revealed only by a correctly-kept history." If physicians made an honest effort to discover the general constitution, disposition, and idiosyncrasies of their patients, so as to determine the state, probability, and predisposition of a patient to disease, the study of disease would demonstrate neither a recent origin nor even a dependence on existing influences but the product of "long descent" through hereditary transmission.[51] Darwin called this phenomenon "a permanent abiding predisposition to certain classes of disease."[52]

Knud Faber, in his *Nosography in Internal Medicine* (1923), considered the matter of constitutional pathology crucial to the future of medicine. While he thought it important not to take from Pasteur and Koch the revolutionary implications that specific diseases and specific morbific causes would have on future medical pursuits, nevertheless he thought it equally important to consider constitution and constitutional diseases as having significant bearing on any diagnostic work. "No one knows better than the physician," he argued, "that human beings are not 'born alike,' but already at birth differ in 'constitution,' both as regards build and organic functions. As is generally recognized, there is no hard and fast line between the normal and abnormal, but medically speaking one would be inclined to demand a certain unfitness, a lowering of efficiency of the individual or organ concerned in order to speak of a constitutional anomaly, a constitutional disease."[53] Max H. Lewandowsky, in his work on nervous diseases published in 1912, reiterated the same attitude when he wrote: "We now conceive of each of the pathological processes as a single, gradually developing phenomenon resulting from the action of the specific etiologic agent, though with variations depending on individual circumstances or external conditions."[54]

Through the development of serology and endocrinology, the consideration given by doctors to the patient's constitution continued to rival the advance of bacteriology. For those who viewed health and disease as a diathesis of the growing human organism, medicine also became a branch of anthropometry, which sought to determine through careful measurements an outward and visible sign of the body's internal secretionary system. In 1857 the anatomist Benedict Auguste Morel (1809–73) related cranial morphology with pathological characteristics. Later, during the 1880s, doctors employed specimens of blended portraits (using Galton's stereograph) to elicit the physiognomy of disease by establishing diathetic types such as phthisis, strumous, rheumatic, gouty, and nervous. Other examples of anatomical diagnosis included the efforts of Friedrich W. Beneke in 1878 and Frederick Kraus during the 1890s. Beneke made extensive postmortem measurements of body organs in an effort to estimate their functional power; while Kraus and his disciples established an anthropological clinic at Charité in Berlin, where, through anthropometric measurements, they attempted to correlate abnormal differences in heart, lungs, liver, kidneys, etc., with functional disturbances. These efforts marked the culmination of work begun earlier by the French materialists, most notably F. Thomas de Troisvèvre, who in 1821 taught that the proportional dimensions of the abdomen, chest, and head could determine which of seven temperaments a person manifested. Intending to take the guesswork out of diagnosis, he sought an arithmetic gauge of the temperaments. Assuming that those with the largest heads were the most intelligent, and those with the largest abdominal cavities were the biggest eaters, and so on, he theorized that the size of an organ would always denote its functional capacity and body temperament.[55]

In an endeavor to seek the genotype by way of the phenotype, physician George Draper, associate in medicine at Columbia University in New York, combined anthropometry, hormonal theory (the machinery which gives the human body its shape, texture, and constitution) and disease. Draper first took notice of measurements and morphological descriptions when he discovered a similarity in appearance among those afflicted with acute poliomyelitis during an epidemic in 1916.[56] Recognizing inadequacies in existing observational and descriptive procedures, he called on the services of David Seegal of the department of anthropology of Harvard University, and together they proceeded to establish anthropometric techniques which became the basis of his work in the Constitutional Clinic at New York's Presbyterian Hospital. The anthropometry employed by Draper and Seegal was based largely on the work of Aleš Hrdlička, H. H. Wilder, Quételet, Paul Broca, Giuseppe Sergi, Paul Topinard, Sir Arthur Keith, and Achille deGiovanni. Believing that most doctors in his own day were "better students of disease than of its subjects," Draper urged the application of "old school" pathology, which endocrinology had reintroduced into medical science by giving it a new rational basis for belief.[57] Draper's work in constitutional pathology also derived from the earlier endeavors of Thomas Addison, Thomas Laycock, and Jonathan Hutchinson, all of whom had agreed that the "habitus or physical form of the individual bears an important relationship to disease."[58] He took issue with the Italian clinician deGiovanni of Padua and his followers, who insisted that morphology actually determined disease. "Rather does it appear," Draper argued, "that the anatomic features of an individual form one of a set of basic unit characters, predetermined by heredity, and influenced to some extent by environment, which together make up the constitution."[59]

Draper was not alone in his efforts to reestablish a constitional basis for disease in the early decades of the twentieth century. The development of Mendelian genetics and endocrinology gave added impetus to the work of Raymond Pearl in constructing life-tables (1919–27), Karl Pearson's *Relationship of Health to the Psychical and Physical Characters in School Children* (1923), Frances G. Crookshank's studies on epidemic constitutions (1926), and Julius Bauer's *Constitutional Principles in Clinical Medicine* (1934). All were examples of continuing research on pathology. Advances in statistical methodology, along with the labors of Darwin and Galton on inheritance, combined to carry the ancient doctrine of the humors into the modern age. For its own part, physical anthropology not only absorbed the same philosophical assumptions of the constitutional school of medicine, but provided an inestimable contribution to physiology and pathology through its measurement of constitutional types.[60]

Criminal Anthropology

Constitutional pathology also played a supportive role in the development of criminal anthropology. The founder of the anthropological school of criminal law, Cesare Lombroso (1835–1909), paid special attention to the cephalic index and to photography in differentiating between the casual offender and the hereditary and pathological criminal. The work of Lombroso, a professor of forensic medicine in Turin, Italy, along with the investigations of Giuseppe Sergi, Enrico Ferri, Raffaelle Garofalo, and Moritz Benedikt, relied heavily on the phrenological theories devised earlier by Gall, Spurzheim, and George Combe, the twenty-eight volumes of Jean-Martin Charcot's *Iconographie* (1888–1918), the anthropometrical techniques of Paul Broca, and the earlier inferences drawn from the theory of temperaments. As biological determinists, the Lombrosians accounted for the personality

of the criminal in their conviction that heredity—in the form
of certain identifiable characteristics and pathological influences—was the major factor in criminal behavior. In doing
so, they placed criminal responsibility directly on the shoulders of the individual rather than blaming society or other
environmental influences. They claimed that upward of
forty percent of the total number of criminals were identifiable from birth—the results of atavism, degeneration, or im-
becility that had roots in racial ancestry—and distinguishable
by certain measurable physiognomical peculiarities.[61]

The Lombrosian school reached its peak notoriety in the
1880s when its methodological and naturalistic claims placed
it in the forefront of the century's sciences. As first generation social Darwinists, the Lombrosians insisted that notions
of humanitarianism and free will were outmoded sentiments
that had little bearing on a proper science of man and society.
In effect, criminals formed a variety within the human family
that could be distinguished by a low type of physique, an anatomical and physiological standard of brain, body, and mind
that fell short of the typical man. By identifying as criminal
certain anatomical characteristics, the anthropological school
of criminal law relegated the social environment to insignificance. Not until Gabriel Tarde, Paul Topinard, Léonce Man-
ouvrier, W. R. Mc Donell, and Charles Goring (known as the
"acclaimed destroyer of Lombrosian theories") challenged
biological determinism with more appealing sociological and
environmental explanations did the Italian school face an
equally "scientific" alternative.[62]

Besides the criminal anthropometry of Lombroso, constitutional pathology continued to make inroads with the help
of Darwin's *Origin of Species* (1859) and *Descent of Man* (1871),
with the translation of J. G. Mendel's monograph in 1902,
and the setting up by Sir Francis Galton of his anthropometric laboratory in 1884. Galton, for example, experimented in the 1870s with "composite portraiture" of the
criminal class. Using a stereoscope, a machine which created
a composite portrait by optically superimposing two portraits
and blending the two, he was able to use the collection of
criminal photographs in the possession of Sir Emund Du-
Cane, Director General of Prisons, and arrive at what Huxley
called "generic" portraits, or which Quételet would have

identified as "typical" or "averages." These efforts, along with the pioneering studies of Ignaz P. Semmelweis (1818–65) and Pierre Charles Alexandre Louis (1787–1872), became landmarks in statistical quantification and biometry.[63] The application of statistics to the study of man came to fruition in 1901 with the establishment of the journal *Biometrika,* edited in consultation with Francis Galton by W. F. R. Weldon, Karl Pearson, and C. B. Davenport. As Galton explained it, biometry had an element in common with mathematics, anthropology, zoology, botany, and economic statistics. The objective of biometry was to "afford material which shall be exact enough for the discovery of incipient changes in evolution which are too small to be otherwise apparent."[64] Pearson also urged the creation of a National Institute for Anthropology to study the cranial, anthropometric, and physical characters of man, to identify general degeneracy through the study of insane, tubercular, epileptic, idiot, hysteric and mental defectives, and to improve the national race through stringent selection for parenthood.[65]

The later works of Earnest A. Hooton and Sheldon and Eleanor Glueck in the 1930s and 40s were indicative of concerns which Lombroso, Galton, and Pearson had earlier voiced. Hooton resounded with bitterness against the American environmental credo, which had all but condemned any effort to understand hereditary factors in human behavior. Allowing for the importance of human variation and differentiating environmental factors, he nevertheless firmly insisted "that different physical racial types of man will display mental and emotional qualities diverging from one another, in conformity to their respective peculiarities of physical organization which are of hereditary origin."[66] He urged physical anthropologists to look beyond the failures of Gall, Lavater, and other "misguided seekers of anatomical shortcuts." With more accurate classification of physical human types, Hooton believed that psychologists, psychiatrists, and sociologists could "then proceed to the study of mental processes and social conduct in groups and individuals without having the additional complicating factors of racial, physical heterogeneity to confuse . . . psychological and sociological issues."[67] Both he and the Gluecks pointed to physical traits and characteristics common among criminals (cranial capacity, cranial and facial asymmetry, etc.) which indicated that criminals were "physically differentiated according to the types of offense which they commit and . . . are biologically as inferior to humble but lawabiding citizens as they are sociologically."[68]

Behavioral Sciences

Constitutional pathology and psychology of individual differences as pointed out in phrenology and in the temperaments underlined themes in the works of Benjamin Rush and C. Van Diik on insanity and hypochondriasis, the positivist theories of August Comte, the early writings of the American Psychiatric Association, and the writings of William James.[69] Professor J. McKeen Cattell and Dr. Livingston Farrand required examiners who carried out physical and mental measurements of one hundred students of Columbia University in 1894–95 and 1895–96 to discern the temperament (choleric, sanguine, melancholic, and phlegmatic) from the bearing, the address, the "tout ensemble" of each student in the study. In 1912 both Auguste Chaillou and Léon MacAuliffe sought to establish norms of congenital physical constitutions for military purposes that corresponded strikingly with the sanguine, bilious, lymphatic, and nervous temperaments.[70]

In similar fashion, Ernst Kretschmer's *Physique and Character* (1925) used psychiatric data and profiles to correlate constitution and mentality. According to Kretschmer, it was possible to ascertain the boundaries between sickness and health in the human frame. Psychic disorders were not simply brain disorders which Gall and his disciples described by transforming craniometry into a scientific speciality. "We see beside the brain, the whole complex of ductless glands (the ultimate stronghold of the chemistry of the body), which . . . has the profoundest influence on the psychic development."[71] Physique was not a symptom of the psychosis; nevertheless, "physique and psychosis, bodily function, and internal diseases, health personality and heredity are each, separately, part-symptoms of the constitutional basis which lies at the bottom of the whole."[72] Medical examination of cretinism, myxoedema, cachexia strumipriva and exophthalmic goitre were clear indications of the influences of the thyroid gland. Kretschmer wrote that it was not a great step from the influence of the thyroid to suggest "that the chief normal types of temperament, cyclothymes and schizothymes are determined, with regard to their physical correlates, by similar parallel activity on the part of the secretions, by which we naturally do not mean merely the internal secretions in the narrow sense, but the whole chemistry of the blood, in as much as it is also conditioned to a very important degree, e.g., by the great intestinal glands, and ultimately by every tissue of the body."[73]

Even Freud stressed constitutional differences among children as narrowing the role of psychiatrists in the use of social or professional (i.e., environmental) corrective therapeutics. "The expectation that we shall be able to cure all neurotic symptoms," he wrote, "is derived from the lay belief that neuroses are entirely superfluous things which have no right whatever to exist. As a matter of fact they are serious, constitutionally determined affections, which are seldom restricted to a few outbreaks, but make themselves felt as a rule over long periods of life, or even throughout its entire extent." Freud was quick to recognize that in their hurry to find the precipitating causes of a given disease or illness, doctors had neglected the constitutional element in therapeutic practice.[74] Over and above the environmentalist position for the causation of psychoses, there were genetic and organic components that invited measurements of individual differences. Constitutional pathology, infused with genetic evolution as a result of the influence of both Darwin and Galton, became an important determinant of behavior and a foundation for psychiatry. Terms such as *character, personality, mind,* and *temperament* remained the unifying components of mind-body relationships, which carried over into the twentieth century.[75]

Exemplary of this position was W. H. Sheldon, whose *Varieties of Human Physique: An Introduction to Constitutional Psychology* (1940) continued into the mid-twentieth century the effort to connect physique and temperament. Sheldon expressed hope that all the various disciplines that at one time had approached the problem of constitution (anatomy, physical anthropology, physiology, physiological chemistry, clinical medicine, pathology, psychology, psychiatry, sociology, and the social sciences) would make a concerted effort to study the psychological aspects of human behavior as related to morphology and physiology.[76] His technique of somatotyping, developed by combining anthroposcopy with anthropometric measurements, owed much to Beneke of Vienna, deGiovanni's school of clinical anthropology in Padua, Viola's designation of three morphological types (microsplanchnic, normosplanchnic, and macrosplanchnic), and Sante Naccarati's work at Columbia University in 1920 on human typology and his use of the correlation coefficient and mental test. Sheldon praised Kretschmer for his emphasis on psychological chemistry, William Osler for his efforts to teach physicians the ability "to diagnose the patient as well as the disease," and George Draper for his delineation of gallbladder and ulcer types of physique.[77] "If human beings can be described in terms of their most deep-seated similiarities and differences," he wrote, "it may prove not impossible to differentiate between heredity and the effects of environment. This differentiation, if achieved, would provide the needed leverage for an attack on many social problems, ranging all the way from vocational guidance and military specialization to the isolation and elimination of cancer."[78]

Retrospect

Like most philosophical dogmas, the elements of constitutional pathology were woven from many fibers; and, whereas they were arranged into new divisions and subdivisions with the divergence of the sciences and social sciences, they not only survived centuries of speculation but also derived support from such diverse fields as photography, anthropometry, endocrinology, and psychiatry. The groundswells of therapeutic reform were unable to dislodge the concept; at best, successive generations of doctors, scientists, social scientists, and faddists could only produce new variations of the original theme. Society still speaks of good and bad humors, employs constitutional words like sthenic, neurasthenic, and hypersthenic, and uses the terms sanguine, choleric, and melancholic in referring to psychological types. "From the cab-driver, who sizes up his customers to be 'sure of his shilling,' to the physician and artist, who study face and figure from a higher specific viewpoint," medical historian Fielding

Garrison remarked, "the estimation of the appearance of the individual with reference to his ultimate character has ever been a matter of intense human interest."[79] The derivation of these constitutional differences, however, like the Indian names of our rivers, are forgotten monuments to an ancient world.

2

When Lancet Was King *

IN THE HISTORY OF MEDICINE, no greater transformation occurred in the management of disease than the general abandonment of bloodletting during the course of the nineteenth century. For more than three thousand years of recorded history and an unknown period of time before that, abstraction of blood as a curative, palliative, and preventive measure had remained paramount in the armory of medical therapeutics. Support for bleeding long predated Hippocrates and continued through the eras of Galen, Sydenham, and Hunter. The nineteenth century saw men like Fordyce Barker, Albrecht von Graefe, Brown-Séquard, and Henry I. Bowditch praise its use; and in another symbolic indication of its popularity, the *Lancet*, founded in 1823, became the Hector of English orthodox medical journals. Even William Osler (1849–1919), whose many editions of *Principles and Practice of Medicine* (1892; 8th ed., 1912) were heavily in use in the early twentieth century, recommended bleeding as a good practice. Despite variations of theory and innovations in science, no other antiphlogistic remedy (with the possible exception of calomel) survived the disputes of empiricism and rationalism, of eclectics, methodists, pneumatists, Galenists, Arabists, Brunonians, Broussaisists, and assorted system-builders. Its application even in the early twentieth century evidenced the singular manner in which bleeding controlled both medical and secular assumptions about disease.

*Portions of this chapter were previously published as "The Glass Leech: Wet and Dry Cupping Practices in the Late Nineteenth Century," *New York State Journal of Medicine*, LXXIII (1973), 583–92.

Early History

Neither Hippocrates nor any of the early Greek physicians spoke of bleeding as a new technique; indeed, the practice of bloodletting was in general use in Egypt, Assyria, Scythia, and elsewhere before being introduced into Greece. "We are thus thrown back to unknown antiquity for the origin of the therapeutic use of blood-letting," G. W. Balfour wrote in 1894, "and there we are baffled by the thick darkness that has settled down upon the doings of these bygone ages."[1] As Hippocrates explained it, the therapeutic use of bleeding derived from the natural and spontaneous occurrence of "critical hemorrhages" that sometimes preceded the crisis stage in acute disease. No doubt some early empiric had noted the sudden change in constitution that followed an accidental evacuation of blood. The relief given to the constitution by perspiration, to headache by epistaxis, to the congested uterus by menstrual flow, or dyspnea by slight haemoptysis, fathered notions that the loss of blood from artificial wounds would prevent or even cure disease. Pliny suggested that mankind first learned of the practice by observing the instinctive actions of the hippopotamus, which regularly relieved its bilious constitution by striking its leg against a sharp reed to open a vein, and eventually stopping the flow by rubbing the wound in mud. Ulloa, who accompanied Pizarro on his conquest of Peru, attributed the practice of bloodletting among the South American Indians to bats, which supposedly bled people from the foot while they slept at night.[2] This combination of chance, folklore, and empiricism convinced early doctors and surgeons that inducing an artificial crisis would hasten the resolution of disease. In any case, the withdrawal of blood from the vein (venesection or phlebotomy) or artery (arteriotomy) to reduce the flow of blood became known as *general* bloodletting, while the abstraction of blood from a part or from the neighborhood of a diseased area through the capillaries by leeches, scarification or cups, was known as *local* bloodletting.

The Greek surgeon Podalirius, a son of Aesculapius, gave the earliest account of bloodletting (1134 B.C.) when he told of being shipwrecked on an island on his return from the Trojan war and there saving King Damaethus's daughter,

Princess Syrna, by bleeding her from both arms. The event also marks the first known instance that a physician was rewarded for his labors with the hand of the patient in marriage.[3] The practice of bloodletting was later employed by Hippocrates, Celsus, Caelius Aurelianus, Aretaeus of Cappadocia, Galen, Paul of Aegina, Alexander of Tralles, Avicenna, and scores of admiring disciples. Asclepiades, a Greek physician who practiced in Rome more than a hundred years before the Christian era, resorted to bleeding, scarification and cupping; and Aretaeus was not only an advocate of bleeding, but was also among the earliest physicians to practice arteriotomy.[4] Asclepiades based his preference for bleeding on the theory that living bodies depended upon the natural motion of corpuscular atoms through the pores. In disease, he argued, the natural motion had stopped; hence, he scarified the surface of the skin and then applied cups. The humoralist Galen (129–200 A.D.) provided the following rules for bleeding, and later physicians departed little from his rationale:

> 1. Treat not the disease but the man; judge the propriety, amount, and necessity for repetition of bloodletting by the individual symptoms exhibited in each case and not by the nomenclature.
> 2. Observe, also, the natural constitution of the patient— e.g., the extremes of life, youth, and old age that cause bloodletting to be badly borne. Certain races, such as the soft-fleshed Celtic nations, do not stand it.
> 3. Take note also of epidemic influences—e.g., do not bleed much in the dog-days and in moist, warm weather, when, of course, septic poisons are most rife.
> 4. Mistake not physiological for morbid changes; such, for example, as the fullness of pulse that accompanies the first stage of digestion for permanent fullness.
> 5. Take blood from vessels that communicate directly with the chief seat of inflammation.
> 6. Often, in spite of apparent or real general debility, it is desirable to take blood, since benefit to the locally affected part, and the consequent benefit to the system, compensates for the depletion.[5]

The general bleeding practices of the early Greeks supported the theory of *revulsion*, which insisted that the most appropriate way to bleed an individual was to "breathe" or "tap" a vein as near to the diseased organ as possible, and to continue bleeding until syncope. In doing so, they sought to remove the bad blood from around the part and draw good blood from other regions of the body. On the other side of the argument were the Arabists who, supporting the theory of *derivation*, opened a vein in the foot and allowed the blood to trickle drop by drop, believing that at the onset of inflammation it was important to remove blood slowly from a distant part of the body, thus coaxing the disease from the inflamed area. Until the beginning of the sixteenth century, European doctors followed the derivation practice set down by Avicenna of pricking a vein in the foot. In 1514, however, Parisian physician Pierre Bissot, who was an admirer of Hippocrates and the older revulsive techniques, advocated bleeding from the arm and on the same side as that of the lesion. In supporting his method during a pleuritic epidemic in Paris, he precipitated a storm of controversy among the medical faculty. After a protracted and vindictive feud, during which the French parliament actually banished Bissot in 1518, the issue took on religious connotations, with Pope Clement VII himself joining in the feud.[6] Charles-Jacques Bouchard (1837–1915) would later demonstrate that the difference between revulsion and derivation was imaginary and futile, since both created a "centre of fluxion which [interrupted] the tendency of the fluids toward a diseased part."[7]

From the twelfth century onward, bloodletting became suffused with astrological overtones that gave clear admonitions on when and how to draw blood. Purgation and bloodletting calendars abounded after the invention of the printing press; and bleeding acquired a prophylactic character, with individuals employing it along with baths and other forms of hygiene. The *Regime sanitatis* or *Code of Health*, written in the twelfth century for King Robert of Normandy, included the following verses:

> In what Months it is Proper, and what Improper to Bleed.
> Called lunar, are September, April, May,
> Because they move beneath the Hydra's sway.
> Two days—September first, May thirty-first—
> For bleeding and for eating goose are cursed.

When blood abounds in full age or in youth,
May'st bleed many lunar months, forsooth;
Bleed freely, if you would prolong life's day.
                    . . .
What Parts Are to Be Depleted and at What Seasons.
In spring and likewise in the summer tide,
Blood should be drawn along from the side.
In autumn sere, or on cold winter's day,
Take from the left in corresponding way.
Four parts distinct we must in turn deplete—
The liver, heart, the head, and last the feet.
In spring the heart—liver when heats abound,
The head or feet, when'er their turn comes round.[8]

In later centuries, society looked upon vernal bleedings as essential to the well-being of every healthy person past the middle period of life. The heavy consumption of meat at every meal, the large draughts of malt liquors and old port, and the lack of physical activity during the winter months combined to produce an engorgement of the secretory and excretory organs. Doctors, barber surgeons, and laymen interpreted the loss of a few ounces of blood as most advantageous in these circumstances—a practice which "could not fail to aid in ridding the body of noxious materials."[9] As one doctor remarked, bleeding "will ameliorate all the symptoms, afford a refreshing sleep, cause the skin to perspire, and the bowels to relax, increase the appetite, and give a feeling of relief and ease which no other remedy or any mode of diet is able to supply."[10]

By bleeding to the marrow cometh heat,
It maketh clean your brain, relieves the eye:
It mends your appetite, restoreth sleep,
Correcting humours that do waking keep
All inward parts, and senses also, clearing—
It mends the voice, touch, smell, and taste and hearing.[11]

The maxim A bleeding in the Spring/Is physic for a King actually applied to both king and subject; and during the seventeenth and eighteenth centuries, prophylactic bleeding became an autumn and spring affair for the listless habits of country and urban populations. Country doctors were vocal supporters of bleeding and, even into the 1880s and 1890s, they justified their sanguinary practices on the basis of the "full-blooded" and "over-fed" constitutions of farmers and their servants.[12] Doctors bled when patients' limbs felt heavy, when urine was thick, and when the pulse was fast and strong—depending, of course, on whether the season was too hot or too cold, or if the moon was too old or too new.[13]

Although the Greeks had employed venesection to artificially induce an early crisis in disease, later physicians discovered that bleeding reduced the body's heat and so prescribed it as a curative agent in most cases of fever. They likewise used it to restore equilibrium to the body following general or local tension, to reduce congestion of the visceral organs, to reduce general or local pain, to restore the motion of the blood following concussion or obstructions of the heart, in relief of convulsions, and in certain acute cases of hemorrhage in order to create a diversion.[14] In general, diminishing the quantity of blood in the capillaries of the inflamed part remained the basis of thinking throughout the history of bloodletting. One physician in 1871 likened its effects to that of a vacuum pump. "The arteries and veins," he wrote, "are tubes hermetically sealed against the atmospheric air. Draw blood from either an artery or vein, and a vacuum is produced proportionate to the amount abstracted. We infer, then, that the mass of blood rushes forward to fill the vacuum thus created, carrying with it a part, at least, of the engorged blood in the inflamed part. The opening of a vein tends to divert the circulation and draw the current to the orifice from which the stream issues."[15]

Prior to William Harvey's (1578–1657) discovery of the blood's circulation, doctors thought the blood varied in composition in different parts of the body so that while disease might contaminate one part, the rest of the body's blood could remain healthy. Harvey's discovery had little substantive effect on the mode of therapeutic practice; given the new knowledge, doctors merely opened a convenient vein regardless of its proximity to the disease. Before long, indications for bleeding were almost as legion as the known diseases. The Englishman Thomas Sydenham (1624–89) extended bloodletting to everything but diabetes, cholera morbus, dropsy, and suppression of lochial discharges.[16] From Boerhaave's doctrine of plethora to Stahl's phlogiston and the mechanical theories of John Brown and Friedrich Hoffmann, bloodletting remained the principal weapon in medical therapeutics. During the early 1700s, Hoffmann theorized that inflammation resulted from a spasm of the blood vessels and that unless "jugulated" through bleeding, rupture and suppuration of the organ would occur; he sought confirmation for his hypothesis in the appearance of the organs after death. William Cullen and subsequent generations of physicians looked to bloodletting as the principal treatment for inflammation. A bandage and the lancet became the physician's "passport to the confidence of his patients [and] the chief source of emolument to himself." When combined with leeches, cups, and a scarifier, the tools for healing were nearly complete.[17]

Bleeding Techniques

The choice of bleeding technique depended in great measure on the type, duration, and obstinacy of the disease. Light affections yielded easily with simple revulsives such as friction, warm fomentations, leeches (sanguisuction), or cups, while more serious diseases demanded a greater evacuation of blood with free sanguine depletion.[18] The most common operation, that of phlebotomy, required a lancet (the physician's "pocket companion"), a piece of linen, two square bolsters, a vessel to receive the blood, a sponge with warm water, vinegar, and wine or Hungary water to rouse the patient. In order to accelerate the flow of blood, patients coughed or squeezed on a small stick held in the hand. Although nineteenth century physicians preferred to bleed from the arm, they occasionally bled from the ankle or small toe for disorders of the head and breast, as well as for menstrual dysfunction and hemorrhoids. Physicians also bled from the forehead, the temples, and the occipital veins (particularly when there were indications of violent pains, vertigo, delirium, melancholy, and madness), in the belief that bleeding from the vicinity of the brain would more easily evacuate the "offending matter of the disease." Before proceeding, the surgeon would tie a handkerchief tightly around the patient's neck, forcing the veins to protrude. On occasion doctors bled from the jugular vein for madness, ophthalmia, apoplexy, headaches, and general lethargy. They sometimes even bled from the two small veins under the tongue, and from the penis in "inflammatory disorders"

of that member. In arteriotomy, doctors preferred to abstract
from the temporal artery, believing that they could obtain
blood in greater quantity and more promptly than from a
vein. Most doctors, however, were reluctant to attempt arteriotomy even when the symptoms indicated it, since the
effects were not always certain. Specifically, doctors found
that in inflammatory diseases, arteriotomy was not as effective, and inflammatory symptoms recurred more frequently
after arteriotomy than when blood was taken from a vein in
the arm.[19]

Since diseases varied in their degree of tolerance to loss of
blood, doctors employed bloodletting as an added diagnostic
tool. By examining the quantity, tolerance, and speed of the
blood, the physician could distinguish between inflammation
and irritation or irritation and depression. If, for example, a
person showed signs of syncope after the abstraction of a
small quantity (i.e., twelve ounces) of blood, then a doctor
might conclude that the patient was suffering from irritation
rather than inflammation, which would necessitate a reversal
of treatment, including mild purgatives, anodynes, gentle
stimuli, and nutritious diet. Similarly, peritoneal inflammation tolerated large losses of blood, while intestinal irritations
reacted quickly to small losses. Persons suffering from en-
cephalitis exhibited large tolerance to depletion, while those
with headaches were unable to endure the abstraction of too
much blood. By applying the lancet early in the illness to the
standing patient, physicians believed they could quickly determine the manner of disease and the appropriate remedy.[20]

Doctors typically employed local bleeding when local
symptoms alone existed or when symptoms were subdued by
previous general bleeding. When, for example, a person received a blow on the head that created a fever, doctors would
bleed from the arm until the febrile symptoms were subdued. If inflammation continued around the point of injury,
they then applied leeches or cups to the adjacent parts. Doctors estimated the quantity of blood obtained by a good leech
to approximate about one ounce. These invertebrate animals, available from most pharmacies, were applied almost
anywhere on the body—from the stomach or neck to inflamed gums and even the mucous membrane of the vagina.
To avoid having patients see the leeches, doctors placed two
or three in a cup or hollow of an apple which they then held

against the spot designated for the abstraction of blood. Under the influence of François Joseph Victor Broussais (1772–1838), the use of leeches reached unprecedented scale, as some 41,654,300 were imported into France alone in 1833.[21]

Because blood flowed only slightly when leeches were employed in local or topical depletion, doctors frequently resorted to "wet cupping," which consisted of making small incisions or scarifications on the surface of the skin and then increasing the flow of blood by suction. The earliest medical men applied their lips to the surface wound and sucked the blood. Later, in the days of Hippocrates, cuppers employed a small gourd or cucurbit made with two openings. One of the openings was applied to the scarification; the operator sucked the other to create a partial vacuum and then closed it with melted wax. Early cups were constructed of brass, bone, or pottery, while most later instruments were made of blown glass. The professional or amateur cupper normally carried five glasses ranging from an inch in diameter across the mouth and three inches deep, to three inches in diameter and five or six inches deep. While early glasses were crudely built, later cups were graduated with precision to allow the operator to measure the amount of blood abstracted. Doctors could choose from an assortment of glass sizes, shapes, and designs, as well as inventions that combined the scarificator, vacuum process, and glass into one instrument allowing the skin to be raised and scarified and blood abstracted in a single operation. There were also special adapters for the cucurbit that cuppers applied to the nipple for drawing milk or inserted into the throat, vagina, or rectum. In the latter instances, cuppers attached a tube of glass or metal, either straight or curved, to the cucurbit and air syringe. Called at various times the "glass leech" or the "doctor's sucking glass," cups became a standard medical tool during the course of the nineteenth century.[22]

In earlier times cuppers employed a razor, scalpel, or lancet to break the skin. These instruments had many disadvantages, including the painfulness of the puncture wounds, the lack of uniformity in the incisions, and the frequent need to repeat the procedure to obtain the required amount of blood. The spring-box scarificator, which made its appearance in the seventeenth century, was one of the more important innovations in the art of cupping. It consisted of a metal box fitted with two or more rows of spring-mounted lancets shaped in the form of crescents, with five or six lancets in each row, which performed a half-rotary motion on an axis. Instead of requiring the cupper to make punctures or several incisions with a knife or scalpel, the spring-mounted scarificator accomplished the incision instantly and with less pain. The lancets were sprung by a trigger mechanism that released them against the surface of the skin. The depth of the lancet could be regulated by an adjusting screw. The success of the operation depended upon the depth of the lancet setting. Too deep an incision was as ineffective as one that was too superficial. Smaller scarificators of three or four lancets were designed for children and for delicate operations around the temple, neck, and ears. Cuppers were constantly advised to make sure the scarificator remained clean and in excellent working order. Because efforts to procure blood by means of a rusty scarificator often resulted in tearing the tissues, cuppers regularly greased the mechanism by springing it through a piece of mutton fat and tested the sharpness of the blades by springing it once or twice through a roll or piece of new bread.[23]

Prior to the invention of the air syringe, cuppers introduced a flame into the cucurbit moments before applying it to the scarification to exhaust the air and create a vacuum. Along with the torch, they carried a sponge that was used to prevent spillage while they placed strapping over the incision to encourage rapid healing.[24] In general, the steps set down in the *Boston Medical and Surgical Journal* in 1833 were held in common throughout most of the eighteenth and nineteenth centuries and spoke as much for the art of cupping as they did for the procedure.

> First, the glasses to be applied are placed on the fingers and in the palm of the left hand, and all the glasses necessary for the operation, from the number of one to six, may, with a little practice, be held at the same time; the one applied first, is held between the index finger and the thumb, in a perpendicular direction, the glass looking upwards, and then turned down on the part, and each glass in turn is shifted between the index finger and thumb, and held in the same direction, using those on the fingers before that in the palm.

Second, the lighted torch is taken in the right hand, and the glass exhausted over the part intended to be scarified, by introducing the torch into it, and then withdrawing the torch along the rim of the glass quickly, and at the same time the torch is withdrawn the glass should descend on the skin, just as the cotton leaves it. . . . The glass should never be pressed upon the skin by the hand, but should be suffered to descend lightly on the part allotted to it. I suppose that we have in this instance applied three of the eight-ounce glasses on the loins; according to the foregoing rules, by the time the third glass is applied, the first will have acomplished the intention of its application, namely, to induce a determination of blood to the surface, indicated by its purple hue, showing it is time to apply the scarificator. I suppose, also, that the scarificator has been regulated by the screw beneath, to the depth of a quarter of an inch, as previously recommended, where the integuments are thick; and I then come to the . . .

Third step in the operation, which I would recommend should be nearly as follows: the torch is held in and across the palm of the right hand, by the little and ring finger, leaving the thumb, the fore and middle fingers free to hold the scarificator, which may be done by the thumb and fore finger only; the glass is then grasped by the thumb, fore, and middle fingers, of the left hand, leaving the little and ring fingers free; the edge of the glass is then detached from the skin by the middle finger of the right hand; the scarificator being set, care must be taken not to press upon the button with the thumb too quickly; directly the glass comes off, we apply the scarificator, spring it through the integuments, and then placing it between the free little and ring fingers, of the left hand, we apply the torch to the glass, and the glass to the skin over the incisions, as before recommended.[25]

The diseases for which physicians applied cups varied from apoplexy and consumption, to enlarged prostate, epilepsy, gout, measles, intoxication, sore throat, and lunacy. In treating many of these illnesses, doctors applied cups to the back of the neck, where they abstracted ten to twenty ounces using three to five glasses, making the scarification close to the hairline to hide possible scars. Other commonly cupped areas included the shoulders, stomach, spine, chest, loins, and back. Physicians performing autopsies on corpses over the course of the century occasionally remarked on damage caused by the scarificators on the spine and ribs. When cuppers applied glass leeches to the throat, the patient leaned back and a very light incision was made by a small spring scarificator with lancets that projected about one-seventh of an inch. More specialized areas included the elbow (when inflamed and swollen), wrist, knee, ankle, temple, scalp, and behind the ears. Temple cupping was dangerous and required all the doctor's skill to avoid the main branches of the temporal artery. When applying cups to the scalp or behind the ear, the operator shaved the patient to enhance suction and guard against making too deep an incision. The same was true when applying cups to the penis. "I have had a scarificator made with four lancets on each side of the face," one doctor wrote, "leaving a space in the middle which is applied exactly to the urethra, and thus avoiding any danger of wounding this canal, and at the same time enabling me to scarify more deeply, as there is otherwise some difficulty in obtaining a plentiful supply of blood quickly, from a more superficial scarification."[26]

Pleno rivo, ad deliquium

With the possible exception of Thomas Sydenham ("the English Hippocrates"), the seventeenth and eighteenth centuries were without scientific interest in bleeding other than a dogmatic acquiescence in its efficacy for most diseases. Although Sydenham viewed the practice as a sheet-anchor in diseases like pleurisy, he chose to limit its application to those of sanguine temperament and, like Hippocrates, refused to bleed the aged or those invalided for any length of time. Despite his caution, copious bleedings (haematomania) became standard medical treatment, causing van Helmont to complain that "a bloody Moloch presides in the chairs of medicine."[27] Men like Cullen and Gregory in England, Bouillaud and Broussais in France, and Rush in America employed the lancet in almost every stage of disease and in all states of the system. Broussais's pupil Bouillaud, along with Dupuytren and Lisfranc, was said to have drawn more blood than the wars of Napoleon. In accordance with his *coup sur coup*, Bouillaud averaged four to five pounds of blood per patient and, occasionally, upward of ten pounds for prolonged illnesses. His formula for bleeding was simple and direct:

"Bleed in the morning of the first day to sixteen, and in the evening to twelve or sixteen ounces. In the interval, cup to the same amount, or apply thirty leeches. On the second day bleed again, and if pain still continues, cup or leech. The disease, fortunately, for the most part, yields on the third day. If otherwise, don't hesitate, but bleed again. If by a rare chance it should resist to the fourth day, bleed again; but usually it is better to apply a large blister. As a rule you must not give up bleeding until fever, pain, and dyspnoea have almost ceased." For his heroic approach to therapeutics, Bouillaud earned the title of "the most sanguinary physician of Europe."[28]

Physicians Benjamin Rush and Phillip S. Physick influenced the practice of haematomania in America when they reported making single bleedings of one hundred ounces and more during the yellow fever epidemic of 1793, in which one-tenth of the population of Philadelphia died. "The quantity of blood drawn in this fever," reported Rush, "was always in proportion to its violence. I cured by a single bleeding. A few required the loss of a hundred ounces of blood to cure them."[29] Arguing that the standard bleeding practices then employed in Europe were woefully inadequate to subdue the particular harshness of American diseases, he ordered "ten and ten" of calomel and jalap, along with repeated bleedings. In justifying his heroic practice, Rush maintained that blood was quickly manufactured from the patient's body fat and could therefore be abstracted in large amounts without danger. In his "Defense of Bloodletting" in the fourth volume of his *Medical Inquiries and Observations* (1789), Rush insisted that four-fifths of a patient's blood could be abstracted without causing harm. It was for good reason that critics attacked him as the "remorseless Master Bleeder." Rush and Physick were lavish bleeders and their prestige in American medical circles produced many ardent disciples. William P. Dewees (1768–1841) carried the technique of heroic bleeding into obstetric practice, while Nathaniel Chapman (1780–1853), teacher of clinical medicine at the University of Pennsylvania, employed it faithfully in croup by bleeding until syncope.[30] The "sanguinary spirit" of European and American medicine bordered on nihilism, as physicians transferred the applicability of bleeding from one disease to another with an enthusiasm that knew few boundaries. There were cases of patients bled of nearly two and a half gallons within a few days. Unfortunately for most patients, the veins and arteries were forced to pay a heavy price for the profession's errors in pathology.[31] William Cobbett, a pamphleteer and critic, remarked in 1800 that Rush's treatment of yellow fever patients was "one of those great discoveries which are made from time to time for the depopulation of the earth."[32] Indicative of Cobbett's remark was the comment by a doctor reminiscing in the pages of the *St. Louis Medical Journal* in 1859 that he had drawn more than one hundred barrels of blood during his medical career.[33]

Through the early decades of the nineteenth century there was little criticism of bleeding. At most, sentiment concerned bleeding too late, bleeding too infrequently, or too sparingly. Seldom did doctors urge its employment in every case, yet there were few remedies which doctors adopted more frequently and with more satisfaction. Even during surgical operations, doctors viewed bleeding (artificial or hemorrhaging) as beneficial in preventing subsequent febrile symptoms and local inflammations. "Whenever . . . there is any chance of bleeding from the wound, it is of great importance not to be too hasty in dressing it by applying plasters and bandages, so that if any bleeding takes place, all the pain and alarm of undressing the wound is avoided, and the bleeding vessel can be easily secured." In amputations it was common to bleed patients to the extent that the loss of blood would equal the amount estimated to circulate in the limb before the amputation. Unless this was done, patients would be left in a state of plethora that would predispose them to inflammation. The same was considered true of the healthy but plethoric parturient female who was bled so that she might be in the best possible condition for convalescence.[34]

In their normal course of treatment, doctors preferred to bleed prior to all other remedial measures, especially emetics, cathartics, sudorifics, and blisters. And in serious illness, doctors insisted that the remedial effect of bloodletting would be less than satisfactory unless "freely and perseveringly practiced."[35] Gabriel Andral (1797–1876), the eminent French clinical lecturer and pathologist, insisted that in cases of pneumonia, bleeding was most valuable, and "that there is no period of the disease—no condition of the pulse—no ap-

parent debility of the system—no age which forbids its practice."[36] Medical men were fond of comparing bleeding with
the analogy of a carriage stuck in mud; they stressed the importance of removing a portion of the system's burden and
giving the body an opportunity to "rally its forces, repair the
injury," and once again return to normal health.[37] Typical
was the experience, in 1833 at the London Hospital Medical
School, of Sir William Blizard, who treated a man who had
been run over by a chaise and had suffered several broken
ribs. Blizard first purged the patient and then bled him fifteen ounces. The next day he was bled twenty more ounces.
On the third day, twenty leeches were applied to the side
where the patient had suffered the broken ribs, and three
days later Blizard abstracted thirty more ounces of blood. On
the following day he took twenty more ounces, and he followed this in twenty-four hours with more leeches. Between
these heroic procedures Blizard employed blisters, tartar
emetic, and purging; and when last heard of, the victim was
in poor health.[38]

Doctors in the first half of the nineteenth century prescribed bleeding children with as much vigor as adults. Benjamin Rush recalled "many more instances in which bloodletting has snatched from the grave children under three or
four months old, by being used three to five times in the
ordinary course of their acute diseases."[39] Exemplary of this
attitude was Charles C. Hildreth, M.D., of Ohio, who insisted
that the letting of blood from the external jugular was too
often neglected in diseases of children. Although rejecting
the heroic practice so common during the days of Rush, Hildreth and others like him believed that without judicious
use of the lancet, physicians would face "dragging, relapsing
patients" who would allow them no time to eat or sleep. The
child treated for bronchitis with antimony, calomel, squills,
ipecacuanha and blisters instead of bleeding would go
through one relapse after another until the chest began to
rattle. In general, physicians considered bleeding less detrimental to the constitution than protracted medication—an
estimation that, given typical drug dosage, was probably correct.[40] Both William P. Dewees and Hugh L. Hodge, professors of obstetrics at the University of Pennsylvania, taught
the need for bleeding from the cord in certain conditions of

stillborn children, and well into the 1880s, doctors reported having bled children from the arm, foot, and jugular vein in croup, scarlet fever, and various forms of asphyxia. Physicians even employed the lancet as a moral prophylaxis for young boys at the age of puberty. Bleeding was the "best and only remedy for impulsive acts and eccentric emotions"; it removed many evils "both moral and physical, which otherwise might damage the character and health very seriously." [41]

Doctors in mid-century were also concerned with the delicate nature of woman's health, believing her susceptible to complaints during pregnancy that were unknown in previous ages and cultures. Although childbearing was a natural condition for most races and times, Victorian doctors maintained that the Caucasian woman had undergone a degree of "degeneracy" from her use of the corset, the ill effects of education, nervous exhaustion following novel reading, and general lack of exercise. John Vaughan, M.D., of Delaware wrote: "Men, in all countries, and under all circumstances are more or less prompted to exercise by business or pleasure; but the females of civilized nations are generally confined to domestic affairs, the laborious parts of which are performed by servants. Their amusements or pleasurable employments are generally irregular and excessive, much beyond that degree of exercise which promotes a due performance of the animal functions, and gives permanent vigor to the constitution: and an observance of the immediate and progressive symptoms of impregnation, in my opinion, affords demonstrative evidence of *pregnancy being a diseased state*" (italics mine). As a result, doctors interpreted such symptoms as vomiting, capricious appetite, fretfulness, disturbed sleep, sore breasts, and changes in the position of the uterus to be common distresses of the civilized woman. The standard authors who guided obstetric practice in mid-century—men like Denman, Clark, Burns, Hamilton, Gooch, Collins, Ryan, Conquest, Lee, Ramsbotham, Rigby, Gordon, Hay, Armstrong, Velpeau, Francis, and Meigs—typically recommended venesection for problems that occurred during gestation, parturition, and the puerperal state. Venesection brought genuine relief to those irregularities which accompanied pregnancy, since by lessening the volume of the "circulating fluids" it counteracted tendencies to congestion, convulsions, hemorrhage, miscarriage, and rigidity of the uterus, and thereby promoted "the due nourishment and final welfare of the child."[42]

Few writers on the subject of bleeding ever specified the exact amounts to be taken. Instead they employed numerous descriptive terms, such as *laudable, wheyish, buffed, cupped, sizy, spoiled, white scum like cream,* and even *blood of breeding women,* to aid proper diagnosis. Some physicians bled a small quantity of blood and let the "liquid flesh" stand for twelve hours, after which they inspected the content to determine the state of the constitutional diathesis. "If in the blood drawn, the crassamentum is in excess, cleaving to the sides of the basin; or, being in excess, is tough and cupped," one physician remarked, "it is an indication for further bleeding. Should the crassamentum be flat (though buffed), tender, and of but ordinary amount, no further bleeding is indicated."[43] In essence, bleeding required intuitive skills to discern just what amount would suffice, given the constitution of the patient and the nature of the disease. Robley Dunglison (1798–1869), who wrote a variety of medical textbooks, referred to bloodletting as the "discharge of a certain quantity of blood produced by art."[44] As such, bloodletting became the focus of envy of those who admired the professional skills of the practitioner or surgeon. The quick judgment which determined the need for bleeding, the dexterity of the hand in using the lancet and orifice, the amount extracted, the small conversation—here was the medical art at its most exemplary moment.

Anti-Venesectionists

From the beginning, there were physicians who vocally denounced bleeding as needless and destructive. Pythagoras, Empedocles, Chrysippus of Cnidos, and his student Erasistratus of Keos (310–250 B.C.), whose study of the heart came close to discovering the process of circulation, taught that bloodletting was unnecessary. Although opposition to bleeding abated principally as a result of Galen's treatises, Pythagorean and Erasistratian thinking remained alive in medical theory in England and on the continent. The Belgian mystic van Helmont (1577–1644), founder of the iatrochemical school, heeded the warnings of Chrysippus and likewise concluded that venesection was "a pernicious wasting of the treasure of blood and strength."[45] Among medical sectarians, opposition came from homeopathy, whose German founder Samuel Hahnemann theorized that doctors could effectively terminate disease with remedies capable of producing in a healthy person symptoms similar to those of the illness. That homeopathic doctors could prescribe a few decillionths of a grain of phosphorus with as much faith as regulars who emulated the copious bleeding of Rush and Cullen was testimony to the utter confusion that prevailed over orthodox medical practice. Not until Jacob Bigelow of Boston, John Forbes of London, and Joseph Skoda and Joseph Dietl of Vienna demonstrated the self-limiting nature of many diseases and that hay tea (*extractum graminis*) and copious bleeding were extraneous to nature's own process of repair did the profession look beyond the extremes of bloodletting and infinitesimal doses.[46]

Those regular physicians in the early decades of the nineteenth century who refused to bleed usually avoided any direct confrontation with medical orthodoxy. Instead of criticizing accepted theory, they preferred to argue that a change had occurred in mankind's constitution. Exemplary of this thinking was Robert Bentley Todd (1809–60), professor of physiology and general morbid anatomy at King's College in London, who maintained that mankind's power of endurance in health and disease had substantially changed and that stimulants were indicated for the new generation of patients. Todd replaced antiphlogistic and emetic treatment with roast beef, opium, and heroic draughts of brandy, whiskey, wines, and spirits in the belief that these stimulants were necessary to relieve the ravages of pneumonia and other exhausting illnesses.[47] In America, those who found fault with the lancet followed in the footsteps of Todd by attributing the need for therapeutic change to the cholera epidemics of 1832 and 1849 and the subsequent decline in vitality, particularly among the inhabitants of more settled areas of the nation.[48] "The very fact that different periods of time show different characters of disease," Detroit physician Theodore A. McGraw wrote, "should make us critical of all established therapeutics." Remedies that past doctors applied with propriety and benefit in certain diseases might well prove disastrous in the same affections when complicated changes of soil and climate altered the prevailing diathesis.[49]

More critical analysis of bloodletting awaited an article entitled "Researches Principally Relative to the Morbid and Curative Effects of Loss of Blood" published by Marshall Hall, president of the Harveian Society of London and physician to the Nottingham General Hospital. Hall lamented the dearth of diagnostic capability among his colleagues, who ignored the clinical thermometer and gave little value to Laënnec's stethoscope. The laryngoscope, ophthalmoscope, and test glasses for ametropia were unknown to most physicians, and morbid anatomy remained in its infancy despite the pioneering work of Matthew Baillie in the 1790s. In effect, the general practitioner treated symptoms as diseases, and when anything could be labelled as inflammatory, he responded with the inevitable lancet, leech, or cups. If "diagnosis were early and certain," Hall concluded, "perhaps the lancet would never be required."

News of Hall's commentary spread to France, where Pierre C. A. Louis (1787–1872), *chef de clinique* under Chomel in the Hôpital de la Charité, had been experimenting with the effects of bleeding, tartar emetic, and blistering in pneumonia. Louis's experiments were first published in the *Archives Générales de Médecine* for 1828 and afterwards, with the addition of new information gained from research in the Hôpital de la Pitié, assumed the form of a separate work entitled *Recherches sur les effets de la saignée dans plusieurs maladies inflammatoires* (Paris, 1835; Boston, 1836), which he dedicated to Hall. In his study Louis attacked the antiphlogistic regime of the Broussaisists with the precision of statistical evidence, concluding that bleeding had little influence on inflammatory diseases. His insistence that signs and heredity were far more important than symptoms and theories of disease was accepted by Grisolle in 1836 and 1841; by Henry Ingersoll Bowditch (1808–92), who translated the works of Louis into English; by James Jackson, who had made similar studies in Boston on the effects of bleeding; and by a generation of American students who admired Louis as the father of the modern method of notetaking and mathematical accuracy. Understandably then, when Louis finally spoke out against bloodletting after his work at the clinic at La Pitié, the issue became acute; and within a few years bleeding appeared to be on the way to extinction—at least among the newer generation of European educated physicians.[50]

John Hughes Bennett (1812–75), professor of clinical medicine at the University of Edinburgh, who trained in both Paris and Berlin, made a complete break with the past by insisting that doctors place little reliance on the experience of men like Cullen and Gregory, who were "unacquainted with the nature of and the mode of detecting, internal inflammations." Clinical observation based on a more correct diagnosis and pathology, he wrote, had since demonstrated "that artificial nosological groups of symptoms bear no relation whatever to the internal inflammations they were formerly supposed to indicate, and has led to a mass of information connected with internal disease, which, up to this time, has never been correctly systematized." Along with other critics, Bennett insisted that past experiences in treating disease ought not to guide modern physicians, since there was much confusion "resulting from the unacquaintance of the past race of practitioners with diagnosis and pathology." Although the opinions of Cullen, Gregory, Sydenham, Aretaeus, and Hippocrates advanced medicine in their own day, "the principles which guided them ought no more to be considered laws to be followed now by practical physicians, than should the exploded astronomical doctrines of Copernicus and Tycho Brahe be acted on by practical navigators."[51]

Bennett stopped short of repudiating the experiences of the older authorities completely; nevertheless, he thought it dangerous for doctors to rely on their imperfect and vague observations. "Medicine is not a scientific art, which is dependent for its principles on the study of, and commentary on, the older writers." Medicine was not to be read and studied only through the eyes of the ancients; rather, medicine was a modern, advancing scientific art which required constant reinvestigation of existing dogmas. Bennett particularly objected to the argument that the essential nature of inflammation had undergone modification since the days of heroic bleeding. Evidence that heroic bloodletting was little practiced in England and India, for example, while persisting in Italy and Paris (where Bouillaud continued to deplete inflammatory patients in his wards at Hôpital de la Charité), indicated that the character of the therapeutic regime was more the result of individual or theoretical preference than a factor of inflammation or constitution.[52]

In analyzing the available statistical evidence on bleeding in pneumonia in comparison with moderate bleeding and with expectant medicine, Bennett concluded that a greater number of deaths had occurred with heavy bleeding. Specifically, when comparing the mortality rate of Louis and Rasori, who treated pneumonia patients with heroic bleedings and large doses of tartar emetic, with that of Grisolle and Laënnec, who advocated more moderate bleedings, and Skoda, who employed expectant medicine, Bennett discovered the following results:

	DEATHS
Heroic bleeding	1 in 3
Heroic bleeding and tartar emetic	1 in 4½
Moderate bleeding	1 in 10
Expectant medicine	1 in 7¼ [53]

Bennett also noted the statistics of Dietl, who treated 380 cases of pneumonia in Charity Hospital in Vienna. The results were similarly revealing:

	VENESECTION	TARTAR EMETIC	DIET
Cures	68	84	175
Deaths	17	22	14
	85	106	189
Ratio of deaths to cures	1 : 5	1 : 5.22	1 : 13.5

Critics eventually discredited Rasori's curative claims by indicating that of eighty cases treated with bleeding and heroic doses of antimony, all but nine died. According to Strambio and Prato in 1831, Rasori released most of his patients as cured of pneumonia only to have them die shortly afterward of diarrhea. Nevertheless, this Italian innovation influenced Gabriel Andral, Joseph C. A. Récamier, and Armand Trousseau of France, and from there spread to the rest of the continent, the British Isles, and America. René T. H. Laënnec adopted a modified Rasorian method of bleeding from nine to seventeen ounces and then prescribed a grain of tartar emetic every three hours. While the contrastimulant use of antimony was liable to the same destructive effects as heroic bleeding, Grisolle, Bang of Copenhagen, Peschier of Geneva, Trousseau, Thielman, Schmidt and Reuf saw in the innovative approach a potential reason to abandon bleeding altogether by treating patients solely with antimony. Ironically the prudence doctors evidenced in eschewing the lancet did not carry over to their massive doses of quinine, twenty drops of Fowler's solution, and heroic amounts of antimony. None of the theories had much effect on bloodletting, since most practitioners attempted to compromise the issue by prescribing tartar emetic and bleeding on one day and brandy and beef tea to offset any ill effects on the next.[54]

Overall, the application of the numerical method did little to resolve the initial years of debate. Statistical evidence supplied by each physician or tabulated by others seemed merely to confirm what the author intended his figures to show. Although the numerical method constituted no new system of medicine, zealots on all fronts were equal to the task of proving their medical doctrines with statistical material. Initially, the numerical method served only to protract the controversy, since skeptics saw too many areas for differences to exist. Because "no judicious physician ever did, or ever could, treat all his cases of pneumonia alike," it was impossible to judge the mortality of the disease. Rarely did these early statistical summaries take into consideration methods of diagnosis, mode of case selection, season of year, or severity of climate in one year in comparison with others. Moreover, it was apparent that rather than condemning the practice of bleeding outright, the statistical evidence only suggested more moderate and discriminating uses for the lancet.[55] One doctor complained in 1873 that "statisticians rob each case of its individuality and cast it upon the sea of uncertainties pertaining to others of a different character." He continued:

> Thus one series will be all bled, another will receive tartar emetic, and a third will be left to the chances of nature. In the first class some are bled which should have been stimulated; in the second, tartar emetic is administered where bloodletting would have been preferable, and in the third class some are permitted to die from mere overaction. It is evident,

therefore, that a rational treatment must secure to each case its own individuality, and as the shades of difference and the corresponding modifications of treatment can not be expressed in groups, statistics, in this sense, become simply an impossibility. . . . Why may we not retain in practice the depleting process in those cases in which it has been proved to be of service, although the principles upon which depletion was carried to foolish extremes have been proved to be erroneous? And, on the other hand, why may we not continue the system of stimulation in cases in which stimulants are known to be useful?[56]

Despite individual efforts to regard the demise of the lancet as the result of fashionable tastes, the application of the numerical method, a change in the constitution, or the influence of Hahnemann, more astute critics were quick to point out advances in the art and science of medicine which accounted for the changes that took place in medical practice. No one factor but, rather, a combination of forces acted and reacted upon each other to bring about a gradual abandonment of the practice of bleeding. While few "regulars" ventured publicly to condemn the lancet, doctors began speaking of "spoliative bleedings," the dangers connected with anemic constitutions, and the need to recognize all symptoms rather than focus exclusively on a few. From the 1840s onward, Gruelin, Rose, Lehmann, Dumas, Pelouze, and Boussingault made remarkable advances in organic chemistry. Under their seasoned efforts, the body became a living laboratory, and pathology emerged more openly as a field of scientific inquiry. Doctors who had previously speculated over the "buffy coat" of successive bleedings, now made use of the test tube, filter, and microscope in analyzing the constitution of blood and urine.[57]

The thirty years from 1820 to 1850 brought a wave of progress in chemistry, pharmacy (introduction of alkaloids, coal-tar products, and tablet triturates), physiology, and pathology that had the effect of relegating Bouillaud's spoliative syncopal venesection, Broussaisism and Toddism to the backwaters of medical reasoning. Jacob Bigelow's *Discourse upon Self-Limited Diseases* (1835), William J. Walker's treatment for compound and complicated fractures, Worthington Hooker's *Rational Therapeutics* (1857), medical statistics, existing skepticism, the introduction of the hypodermic sy-

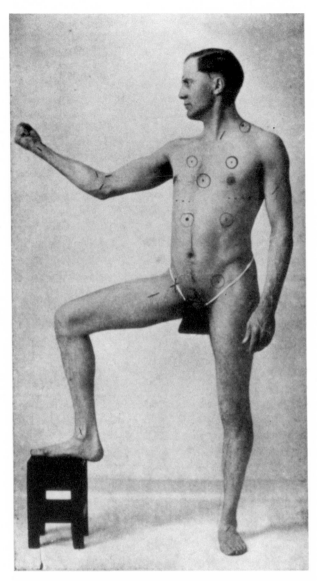

The points marked — represent the locations at which venesection or transfusion may be performed. The points marked ⊙, ..., ..., ⟍, •, /, represent the locations at which wet-cupping, leeching, or scarification may be performed.

Walton Forest Dutton, *Venesection: A Brief Summary of the Practical Value of Venesection in Disease* (Philadelphia: F. A. Davis Co., 1916), opposite p. 64. Courtesy of Indiana University.

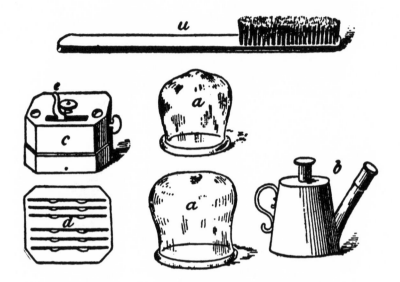

Automatic Scarificator and Accessories

a, Cupping glasses. *b*, Alcohol lamp. *c*, Scarificator. *d*, Capsule or case.
e, Spring set in advance. *u*, Brush for cleaning cupping glasses.

Heinrich Stern, *Theory and Practice of Bloodletting* (New York: Rebman Co., 1915), p. 79. Courtesy of Indiana University.

ringe, and the discovery of drugs such as aconite and veratrum viride combined to scatter the advocates of old-time
medicine. In part, the significance of bleeding lay inversely
with that of pharmacology; bloodletting received its greatest notoriety when the inventory of effective drugs was poor.
The lancet had served in place of heart stimulants, nerve
sedatives, salic of soda, quinine, and chloroform. Nineteenth
century prejudice against bleeding also stemmed from a
change in tempo of the doctor's practice. In this sense, pathology and therapeutics became a function of the changing
relationship between physician and patient. Physicians who
declared themselves against the lancet omitted the procedure partly because bleeding was a lengthy operation that
delayed a busy schedule.[58]

On the whole, those who began their medical practice before the 1830s and 1840s found themselves faced with the
prospect of acknowledging the advances of modern medicine without admitting that those same innovations had
changed their views on bleeding. Advances in pathological
and diagnostic research did little to vary the bleeding practices of such luminaries as Morgagni, Proust, Bichat, Corvisart, Cruveilhier, Bouillaud, and Piorry, who were naturally
reluctant to see their own medical education challenged by a
newer tribe of medical thinkers, however sound their theories might seem. Thus, while critics pointed to breakthroughs
in pathology, chemistry, and diagnostic procedures that
clearly brought into question the profession's continued use
of the lancet, advocates still appealed to medical authorities
for support of bleeding. As W. F. Gairdner of Edinburgh remarked, "the introduction of the stethoscope, so far from
putting an end to abuses, led directly to their extension over
a vast field of hitherto unnoticed diseases. The stethoscope,
in fact, led physicians to discover new diseases, but not to reject old practices." Laënnec's knowledge of morbid anatomy
and diagnosis, Gairdner argued, never led the Frenchman to
bleed patients any less than before.[59]

Who Shall Decide When Doctors Disagree?

As evidence of the tension existing between the old and
new pathology, medical society meetings during the 1860s
continually erupted into debates over the practice of bleed-

ing. Of those who took part in discussions at the meeting of
the New York Academy of Medicine in 1867, only two were
skeptical of its therapeutic use; and even they thought it applicable in certain cases.[60] The members of the St. Louis
Medical Society admitted in 1859 that bleeding no longer answered the needs of western physicians, because inflammation in the Mississippi Valley region became more asthenic
after the Asiatic cholera epidemic in 1832.[61] Nevertheless,
doctors in the region persisted in bleeding patients, believing the lancet would return to its rightful place in the armamentarium through both sound philosophical reasoning and
practical experience. Actually, few doctors insisted that
bloodletting be condemned outright; for most, bleeding simply competed with a newer arsenal of drugs and more conservative therapeutic practices. Doctors insisted on its continued efficacy but in a manner that left sufficient room
for alternative treatments. Oliver Wendell Holmes's remark
in 1861 that venesection had become obsolete in the United
States and Great Britain expressed little more than wish-
ful thinking. As one historian explained, Holmes's remark
was "figuratively too sanguine and literally not sanguine
enough."[62]

As opposition to bloodletting intensified during the 1860s,
Fordyce Barker, who had introduced the hypodermic syringe into American medical practice in 1856, pleaded for
the restoration of the lancet in the management of puerperal
convulsions, insisting that unmistakable clinical evidence favored its employment. Similarly, George T. Elliott of Bellevue Hospital taught that cautious abstraction of blood was
still warranted among plethoric women suffering from early
menopause or suppressed menstruation. In both cases, he
applied leeches to the uterus or epigastrium.[63] Harvey L.
Byrd, professor of obstetrics in Washington University of
Baltimore, remarked in 1872, that "the necessity for the use
of the lancet is as great at the present time as it ever was in
the past."[64] If the physician took proper account of race, age,
sex, and temperament, Byrd felt, there was little reason to
disregard its use. The effects of depletion were unmistakable
in the production of sedative, antiphlogistic, antispasmodic,
and alterative impressions on the system and could bring
about the desired effect more quickly and more efficiently

than any known drug. "Any intelligent physician, who will resort to the lancet in a few cases calling for its use," Byrd concluded, "will not be likely to lay it aside afterwards, though he should encounter . . . prejudice against its use."[65]

Typical of the bleeders in the 1870s was Samuel D. Gross (1805–84) of Jefferson Medical College of Philadelphia, who applied the lancet during the "earlier and gravescent stages" of acute disease. When the morbid effects of disease had already appeared, bleeding not only failed to perform any service, but also robbed the system of the strength needed to maintain the vital processes and ensure cure. "A copious bleeding at the outset of a violent inflammatory disease is gold," Gross commented, "but at its height, lead; or, to express myself more clearly, life in the one case, death in the other." In drawing blood, the Philadelphia surgeon measured the quantity abstracted by the impression it made on the system, which he ascertained by the pallor, the heart's action, abatement of pain, headache, thirst, and restlessness. He thought it essential to look for these signs and to judge them quickly and correctly. "It was also important to draw blood from a large vein, if possible, and at a rate of two to three ounces per minute. In no instance did he think it appropriate to bleed to syncope, "but merely to the approach of this condition." If the symptoms of the disease returned, Gross recommended the resumption of bleeding by either reopening the original orifice or selecting another vein. "Under such circumstances," he cautioned, "the practitioner must, like a wary general, make forced marches, and follow up his successes, not waiting until the enemy has entrenched himself behind his works, but striking heavy blows while he has the opportunity." Nevertheless, he considered all bleeding as spoliative, in that it diminished the quantity of blood both in the part affected and in the system. It weakened the heart's power and prevented it from sending blood "with the same force and velocity into the suffering structures." Bloodletting also unlocked the emunctories, thereby inducing greater secretion; it disgorged the blood vessels at the seat of the disease by encouraging a more balanced circulation. Admitting that remedies such as aconite, gelsemium, veratrum viride, digitalis, mercury, salicylic acid, and tartar emetic performed similar functions on the system, Gross insisted nevertheless that bleeding would work more quickly and with less difficulty.[66]

Though bleeding was decidedly in disfavor during the 1870s, doctors continued to carry lancets. In 1875 W. M. Clarke of the Bristol General Hospital remarked: "No one bleeds, and yet from the way in which I find my friends retain their lancets, and keep them from rusting, I cannot help thinking that they look forward to a time when they will employ them again."[67] Those who continued to practice bleeding were thus pleased to see a renewed plea for its revival in the late 1870s and 1880s. "Although I am not a prophet or the son of a prophet," Gross commented in 1876, "I venture to predict that the day is near at hand, if indeed it has not already arrived, when this important element of treatment, so long and so shamefully neglected, will again become a recognized therapeutic agent, and will thus be instrumental in saving many lives, many an eye, many a lung, many a joint, and many a limb."[68]

From the 1880s and on into the early twentieth century, bloodletting as a curative treatment underwent a brief revival. A doctor writing in the *Iowa Medical Journal* in 1909 claimed to have begun bleeding late in his career, not having heard about the practice during his earlier medical training.[69] Part of the revived interest in bleeding stemmed from evidence that mortality in pneumonia had increased precipitously since the abandonment of the lancet. After reviewing statistical evidence from several cities, Robert Reyburn, M.D., dean of the medical department of Howard University, urged a return to venesection in cases of pneumonia as well as cerebral engorgement and puerperal eclampsia.[70]

Frederick A. Packard, M.D., a resident physician in the Pennsylvania Hospital in the 1880s and 1890s, resorted to bleeding in cases of fever, croupous pneumonia, dyspnea, uremia, aneurism, cerebral apoplexy, and in severe hemoptysis.[71] Even Osler advocated venesection in arteriosclerosis, cerebral hemorrhage, emphysema, heart disease, pneumonia, yellow fever, and sunstroke. In capitalizing on this revival, Doctors Meyer and Manges at the Mount Sinai Hospital in New York invented a more simple procedure to replace the bloody spectacle that so often occurred over bedclothes and towels. With the use of an aspirating needle connected to rubber tubing, they devised an easy and effectual method of puncture without incision, so that the amount of blood could be withdrawn and measured exactly and kept sterile for examination purposes.[72]

Perhaps the realization by some that the newer sciences had done much to improve man's knowledge of morbid processes but little to provide cure led doctors to suggest a return to older forms of treatment. Perhaps, too, they could not accept the assumption that their medical ancestors were all fools. Sydenham, Cullen, the Hunters, Churchill, Denman, and Dewees were careful, observing, and earnest men who could not be accused of perpetuating a delusion so monstrous and injurious. On the whole, however, those doctors who preferred to think in terms of constitutional pathology or the general character of the individual rather than the specificity of disease continued to employ the lancet and urged its greater application. James Rogers, M.D., of Knoxville wrote in 1873: "We feel much inclined to adopt the humoral pathology as taught by Hippocrates, Galen, Celsus, and Sydenham that fever is produced by the presence of noxious substances in the blood; not only in the case of fevers, but in all other diseases, the blood becomes contaminated or depraved, either by the reception of noxious substances from without, or in consequence of changes going on within the body."[73] As Samuel Gross remarked in his work on surgery, "general bleeding may justly be regarded as standing at the head of the list of constitutional remedies . . . as it is at once the most speedy and the most efficient means of relief."[74] Both Gross and Rogers maintained that blood was intimately involved in the chain of pathological processes; however, they tried to explain the process in the simplest way: if the blood was diseased, then part of it must be withdrawn. Modern medicine, on the other hand, recognized the same relationship between blood and body and with a clearer understanding of antiseptics and organo- and sero-therapy applied "blood-cleaning agents" rather than bloodletting.[75]

Those doctors who continued to bleed in the latter decades of the nineteenth century argued that the sufferings of women in menopause had worsened since the profession's restraint on bleeding. Mankind's intentions to the contrary, nature demanded a "substitute for the habitual flux which

has subsided." In similar fashion, young women who suffered menstrual irregularities, dysmenorrhea, or temporary
suspension were no doubt affected more seriously with headaches and throbbing pulse from the lack of moderate bleeding. A doctor observed in 1890 that "an opiate combined with
sedatives and antispasmodics may afford relief, but bleeding
will leave the patient much better during the interval and at
the approach of the next period." Late into the 1890s doctors
were still abstracting blood during puerperal convulsions.
Philadelphia obstetrician Charles D. Meigs took from thirty
to sixty ounces in a single bleeding at the onset of convulsions, claiming that it saved lives.[76]

Even at the turn of the twentieth century, physicians continued to employ bleeding in gynecological cases. Bedford
Fenwick, physician to the Hospital for Women in London,
employed the lancet, cups, and leeches in treatment of more
than a thousand cases of dysmenorrhea, subinvolution, ster-
ility, ovaritis, and cardiac disease. However, he found leeches
awkward to use, since they drew little blood, and left wounds
that were sometimes difficult to heal. Leeches had "a spirit of
intense curiosity," which occasionally caused them to explore
the interior of the uterus, the Fallopian tubes, and even the
abdominal cavity if the physician was not careful in controlling their application. Because of these impediments, Fenwick
preferred scarification of the cervix.

> The patient is laid on her left side, with the hips quite out to
> the edge of the couch, and the knees drawn upwards. A spec-
> ulum, of as large a size as the vagina will permit, is passed, and
> the cervix brought fully in view and cleaned with a mop of
> cotton wool. The best form of scarifier is a sharp-edged,
> lance-shaped knife mounted on a long handle. The operator,
> sitting or kneeling with his head on a level with the speculum,
> steadies this with his left hand while his right, holding the
> knife pen-fashion, passes the blade up the passage and punc-
> tures the cervix at as many points as he thinks necessary, to a
> depth of about an eighth or a sixth of an inch each. A small
> basin is now held under the mouth of the speculum to catch
> the blood, and its flow is assisted by the injection of warm
> water.[77]

Like Fenwick, other members of the profession not only
continued to depend on bloodletting; some also introduced

rather novel approaches. In Germany, for example, physicians occasionally prescribed bleeding for psychological reasons; and in London, Christian Simpson and G. Harley claimed great success with *visceral phlebotomy*. In this latter operation, Harley extracted blood directly from the liver while Simpson penetrated into the lungs. "The day is not far distant," Harley wrote in 1893, "when the old-fashioned . . . mode of withdrawing blood cutaneously, will be totally abolished in all cases of inflammation and congestion of internal organs." Instead he claimed various successes with piercing the enlarged liver with a catheter and tapping it for blood. He said: "I feel perfectly safe in thrusting an eight-inch long trocar up to its very hilt. This was done with the hope that during its penetration it might wound one or more bloodvessels of sufficient calibre to yield a free stream of blood."[78]

Experiments carried out by Isaac Levene in the late 1890s to determine if bloodletting had any beneficial effect upon disease seemed to demonstrate conclusively that the resurgence of opinion favoring the lancet had been based on unsound scholastic reasoning. In experiments on rabbits, Levene observed that animals injected with a specific amount of diptheria toxin died within forty-eight hours. Having established a basis for comparison, he began bleeding animals that were inoculated with the toxin to test their response. In every case bleeding shortened the life of the animal. The same was true for animals inoculated with pneumococcus cultures and ricin. Then too, animals that were bled died sooner than those that were left alone. From these experiments, Levene concluded that bloodletting, "if it was of any effect at all, was deleterious."[79] As late as 1916, however, an assistant professor of clinical medicine at Jefferson Medical College in Philadelphia noted that the lost art of bleeding had been rediscovered and was again being used as a successful therapeutic agent. "It is indeed unfortunate," he wrote, "that a procedure so valuable as venesection should have been considered a fad and was for a time almost completely abandoned by the majority of the members of the medical profession."[80]

Throughout the centuries the lancet stood unrivalled amid the welter of therapeutic regimes and exalted drugs. It remained the underpinning of constitutional pathology—

the crowning achievement of medical rationalism—which rarely disappointed those seeking to justify their actions on grounds other than experience. Having existed before and beyond all precedent, it provided an air of authority for those facing the harsh realities of the sickroom. However, as the paradigm of nineteenth-century medical science shifted to accommodate the weight of germ theory and the innovations in pathological research, the lancet proved to be more of a burden than a passport to health and happiness. While critics cast dark shadows and talked of vanquishing the practice altogether and older practitioners became touring trumpeters to its continued use, the majority of doctors acknowledged the controversy and pleaded for compromise. On the whole the persistent reliance of the medical profession on the lancet, even while accommodating new medical discoveries and practices, reflected what G. K. Chesterton once regarded as the great Victorian compromise, the ability to accept change without allowing it to interfere with conventional beliefs.

3

*The Aging Materia Medica**

THE FALSE AND PRESUMPTUOUS EXAGGERATIONS of the materia
medica in the nineteenth century were no small obstacle to
the development of a truly sound medical approach. Public
credulity, combined with the temptation of some physicians
to indulge in their own deification, fostered habits that only
served to place medicine on an unsound if not pretentious
basis. "Much of the positive medication of the present day,"
William Hooker, M.D., commented in 1850, "will probably be
proved by the tests of a rigid observation to be aimless, but by
no means harmless."[1] Nowhere was the combination of public credulity and medical pretense more clearly evident than
in the materia medica, which felt the full impact of medicine's coming of age. Gone were the excessively complex
drugs, such as mithridate and Venice treacle with their fifty
and sixty-five ingredients respectively.[2] True, polypharmacy
continued into the early nineteenth century among a dying
generation of adherents, but typical drug usage turned toward heroic draughts of opium, quinine, calomel, antimony,
arsenic, and assorted other drugs.

The dogged determination of both European and American doctors to employ doses of cure reinforced the feeling of
a people whose national habits had already taken on a pecu-

---

*Portions of this chapter were previously published as "The History of
Tartar Emetic in the Nineteenth Century Materia Medica," *Bulletin of the
History of Medicine*, XLIV (1975), 235–57; "Samson of the Materia Medica:
Medical Theory and the Use and Abuse of Calomel in Nineteenth Century
America," *Pharmacy in History*, XIII (1971), 27–34 and 67–76; "Therapeu-
tic Mule: The Use of Arsenic in the Nineteenth Century Materia Medica,"
Pharmacy in History, XVII (1975), 87–100.

liarly monolithic strain. Oliver Wendell Holmes caught the essence of this phenomenon in American medicine when he wrote: "How could a people which has a revolution once in four years, which has contributed the Bowie-knife and the revolver, which has chewed the juice out of all the superlatives in the language in Fourth of July orations, and so used up its epithets in the rhetoric of abuse that it takes two great quarto dictionaries to supply the demand; which insists in sending out yachts and horses and boys to out-sail, out-run, out-fight, and checkmate all the rest of creation; how could such a people be content with any but 'heroic' practice? What wonder that the Stars and Stripes wave over doses of ninety grains of sulphate of quinine, and that the American eagle screams with delight to see three drachms of calomel given at a single mouthful?"[3] The young republic, as Holmes could attest, had created a solipsistic vision of its own worth and had every intention of spreading that vision among the ranks of even the most unregenerate. American doctors were no longer content with the simple righteousness of their pathological theories but insisted upon extending drug applicability to an almost endless list of patients and diseases; and they preached a philosophy that spoke to the rationality of their ideas and the universality of their therapeutic regime.

Triumphal Chariot: Antimony

Few metals in the materia medica of the nineteenth century acted so energetically upon the human system as antimony. It performed its function so violently that physicians regarded it as an active poison with a therapeutic use that required the most careful discrimination. Although employed as an eye paint by the ancients under the name *stibium* or *stimmi* and later as an astringent to the eyes and a caustic in cancer and hemorrhoids, it did not come into popular use until the seventeenth century, when chemiatrist Johann Thöld, using the pseudonym of a mythical fifteenth century Benedictine monk of Erfurt, Basil Valentine, wrote the earliest known treatise on the medical use of antimony. The pseudo-Valentine supposedly derived the name *antimony* (*anti-moine, anti-monk,* or *monks' bain*) from the fact that it had proved fatal to several monks to whom it had been given as medication. Thöld claimed to have used the metal in nearly all of his medicinal preparations; and in his *Currus triumphalis antimonii* (1604), he urged practitioners to prescribe antimony for syphilis, melancholy, chest pains, the plague, and at the onset of fevers. As a result of Thöld's treatise, a host of antimony compounds were employed during the seventeenth and eighteenth centuries, although, because of frequent accidents, the therapeutic use of antimonials suffered alternate periods of fame and controversy. The Faculty of Medicine in Paris, for example, forbade its use in the materia medica from 1566 to 1666, calling it a virulent poison. Guy Patin (1601–72), the dean of the Paris faculty, one of the more famous phlebotomists, and an opponent of the school of iatrochemistry, strongly opposed its use; even after doctors successfully treated Louis XIV for typhoid fever in 1657 with an antimonial mixture known as *Poudre de Chartres*, Patin vehemently denied its curative effects.[4]

Despite notable hostility physicians prescribed the Kermes Mineral (precipitated sulphide of antimony), first introduced by Johann Glauber in 1651, as a diaphoretic, alterative, and emetic, in epilepsy and hectic fevers. The popular James's Powder (*Pulvis Jacobi Verus*), made from one part oxide of antimony and two parts phosphate of lime, was first employed in 1747 as a sedative and diaphoretic in febrile diseases, and remained a basic remedy throughout the nineteenth century. Because of its tastelessness, doctors prescribed the fever powder for children when quinine was difficult to administer. Thus, as an antiperiodic and antipyretic in intermittent fevers of children, the antimonial was administered almost as regularly as quinine. Eighteenth century therapeutist John Fothergill (1712–80) recommended a combination of calcined antimony, aloes, scammony, and colocynth, which subsequently became known as Fothergill's Pills. Plummer's Pills, introduced in the 1730s by a professor of chemistry at Edinburgh, contained calomel, sulphurated antimony, guaiacum, and treacle and was prescribed for cutaneous eruptions, secondary syphilis, gout, apoplexy, and diseases commonly classified as plethoric, in which doctors employed antimony as a diaphoretic and emetic to equalize and quiet the circulation. Along with these preparations, doctors used sulphurated antimony and flowers of antimony (oxide of antimony) as a diaphoretic and alterative in scrofula, rheumatism, and cutaneous diseases, antimony iodide as an alterative, and antimony trichloride, better known as butter of antimony, as an external caustic.[5]

Among the antimonials, tartar emetic (antimony and potassium tartrate) stood unrivalled in the eighteenth and nineteenth centuries as a diaphoretic and emetic. Although said to have been discovered by the Dutch chemist Adrian de Mynsich in 1631, the drug may have been identical with an earlier mixture known in the 1620s as the Earl of Warwick's Powder. Formerly introduced into the pharmacopoeia of the London Royal Society of Physicians under the name *Tartarus Emeticus* in 1721, its preparations varied in strength and purity—the London, Edinburgh, and Dublin Colleges of Medicine each claiming a superior form of preparation.[6] According to the dose given and the interval between doses, tartar emetic acted as an emetic (often called "pukes"), diaphoretic, expectorant, sedative, cathartic, and irritant. Believing that the mechanical or shock effect brought on by perspiration, nausea, and vomiting would check fevers and other inflammatory diseases if treated at the outset, humoralists relied on tartar emetic with a faith bestowed on few other drugs. They used powerful vomiting to interrupt the morbid chain of symptoms by removing or preventing the local congestions that constituted the disease. In this manner, humoralists unloaded the slowly circulating blood in the hepatic vessels and *vena porta*.[7] Physicians varied the dosage to meet the needs of the moment—small doses were given for diaphoretic or expectorant effects, particularly for catarrhal affections, while larger doses were administered to quickly affect the system and induce vomiting in serious cases of croup or severe inflammation of the lungs. Although doctors usually administered the drug in pill form or as a powder mixed in syrup, molasses, or thick gruel, they also prescribed an antimonial wine[8] and later, as the theory of its modus operandi changed, as antimonial ointment[9] and antimonial plaster.[10] Tartar emetic also became the main ingredient in such noted patent medicines as Analeptic Pills, Ayer's Cherry Pectoral, Jayne's Expectorant, Piso's Cure for Consumption, Wistar's Balsam of Wild Cherry, Ransom's Hive Syrup, and Tobia's Derby Condition Powder.[11]

Edward Jenner (1749–1823), the founder of preventive inoculation, recommended tartar emetic as a suppurative and counterirritant in place of excessive bleeding, scarification, or blistering agents for mania, chorea, epilepsy, hysteria, and deep-seated pains and inflammations of the chest. Believing in true Boerhaavian fashion that the diverted blood and humors would redistribute at a spot away from the disease, Jenner applied tartar emetic in inflammatory diathesis following moderate bleeding. The application of the ointment, Jenner suggested, was far superior to normal blistering agents such as cantharides, croton oil, mustard, boiling water, or liquid ammonia, since it seldom caused gangrene and always gave relief when it produced an eruption. But tartar emetic accomplished much more. Physicians had at their command an agent that would "at the same time *vesicate* and produce diseased action on the *skin itself by deeply deranging its structure* beneath the surface." This was why it acted so differently from cantharides and other irritants. By mixing a drachm of tartar emetic with an ounce of hog's lard, for example, doctors could produce papular eruptions on the seats of pain or below, and, in the course of absorption, draw the inflammatory disease to the surface. The antimonial ointment transferred the disease from those parts necessary to life to the skin, where it could be more easily treated with external remedies.[12]

In the 1820s and 1830s physicians in both Europe and America who were influenced by William Cullen's (1712–90) contributions to therapeutics, particularly his criticism of medical restraint in the use of opiates, calomel, antimony, emetics, and purgatives, turned to heroic doses of antimony, asserting that the novel treatment produced neither vomiting nor sweating "but merely a peculiar state of the system which appears to be incompatible with the existence of inflammatory action." When physicians created this so-called state of tolerance, in which the patient could support large quantities of the drug without nausea, they discovered that antimony possessed "the remarkable property of subduing inflammatory action in the internal organs of the body."[13]

While this remedial approach was used as early as the 1750s by Marryatt of Bristol, its more general acceptance grew out of medical practices of French and Italian physicians at the beginning of the nineteenth century, especially

Giovanni Rasori (1766–1837) and René Théophile Laënnec (1781–1826).[14] Known as the founder of the contrastimulant school, Rasori had modified the earlier Brunonian theory (name given to the ideas of John Brown) of sthenic and asthenic diseases by suggesting that diseases were states of either stimulus or contrastimulus diathesis. Rasori believed that proper diagnosis of disease could only be ascertained by observing the effects of bloodletting. If the patient tolerated large losses of blood, he diagnosed a stimulant diathesis and corrected the system with sedatives, opium, antimony, and more bleeding. If, on the other hand, the patient's condition worsened from the venesection, he diagnosed a contrastimulant diathesis and prescribed heroic doses of gamboge, aconite, ipecac, or nux vomica. Rasori first employed tartar emetic in 1799 in the treatment of epidemic fever victims in Genoa, where he prescribed large doses "with a view to an *effect on the system* and on the *disease*, entirely *independent of any evacuation whatever*" (Rasori's italics). Rasori gave his patients from twelve to thirty grains of antimony after one or more bleedings, and in several cases, upwards of sixty grains in twenty-four hours, depending on the morbid state of the disease. He wrote, "The fitness of the living organism to support large doses of the salt without producing vomiting, or any other symptom of powerful action on the intestinal tube, belongs only to the *morbid state, is limited to this, and lasts only so long as this.*"[15]

Advocates of the contrastimulant school attributed the condition of tolerance to the peculiar morbid state or inflammatory condition of the system which allowed the body "*to support with impunity* . . . the different doses of the medicine.*"[16] As soon as the condition of tolerance made its effect on the constitution, the nauseous action of the drug stopped and the contrastimulant properties took charge. When tolerance took place, St. Louis physician L. C. Boislinière remarked in 1856, patients could readily take forty or fifty grains of tartar emetic daily without purging, vomiting, or perspiring. At this level of tolerance, the drug exerted its elective or specific action on the mucous membrane of the lungs and was afterwards carried away by the kidneys.[17] But when tolerance was not established, patients risked their lives with continued treatment of heroic doses. Physicians were warned when applying the Rasorian treatment not to repeat doses if the preceding dose had caused ill effects.[18]

Occasionally, when physicians used the antimonial as a contrastimulant, they found that the chest and abdomen broke out in pustular eruptions that spread to the arms, legs, and genital region.[19] These eruptions were usually interpreted as a sign of cure. Boisliniere, for example, argued that antimony cured pneumonia by producing "a toxic substitutive action" on the lung membrane which occasionally manifested itself on the skin through pustular eruptions. Antimony's effects on the mucous membrane of the lungs extended to the skin "by virtue of that continuity of tissues and reciprocity of functions"; the pustular eruption became proof that the medicine was working its effects on the lungs.[20]

The Frenchman François J. V. Broussais (1772–1838), who claimed that all disease was merely the result of inflammation of a gastro-enteritic origin—a change in the effects of heat on the humors that engendered disease through localized irritation—objected to the Brunonian theory of sthenic and asthenic states and especially to Brown's contention that most diseases were asthenic and required a heroic regime of stimulants. Believing that most illnesses were sthenic, demanding sedation, Broussais vehemently opposed the ingestion of most of the articles of the pharmacopoeia, preferring instead to rely upon bleeding and leeches. But while physicians identifying with the Broussaisian school extended their antipathy to the point of almost rejecting antimony from the pharmacopoeia, preferring instead to employ copious bloodlettings and large numbers of leeches, most doctors could not bring themselves to do so. They admitted that antimony had been employed indiscriminately, a situation which occasionally aggravated the disease or subverted the diseased action to the point of establishing a new one. They also criticized the fashionable procedure of beginning the treatment of chronic ailments with antimony to remove the "foul stomach" and then following with the Brunonians' favorite agents, laudanum and whiskey. Yet, despite these abuses, doctors continued to prescribe antimony as a necessary agent in controlling inflammatory fevers. The drug not only subdued "preternatural action" through its effects, but also evacuated irritating substances from the system and effected a "derivation of action from some other part, by the impression which it made upon the mucous membranes."[21]

Exemplary of this approach was that of James Kitchen, M.D., who, writing in the *North American Medical and Surgical Journal* of Philadelphia in 1828, rejected the Broussaisian antipathy for the drug. Although once a student and admirer of Broussais in France, he began to question the extremes of antiphlogistic regime and the monistic theory of gastro-enteritis. Shortly afterwards he learned from Laënnec's extensive pathological observations of autopsy examinations that there was no justifiable evidence for irritation of the mucous surface.[22] Later, while in residence in Paris under Laënnec's tutorship, Kitchen administered contrastimulant doses of tartar emetic in various chest diseases, without the least nausea or vomiting, by first bleedng the patient twenty ounces and then immediately administering antimony in increasing doses until the drug took effect, acting "more like an opiate than an emetic."[23]

In one of the more sophisticated studies on tartar emetic written in the early decades of the nineteenth century, physician William Balfour of Edinburgh found himself involved in the Asclepiadean controversy resulting from the successes of Rush in America and Rasori in Italy. Along with most nineteenth century practitioners, Balfour recognized the nauseant properties of tartar emetic, but hoped that its sedative or febrifuge powers in acute inflammatory diseases would become more generally accepted.[24] He agreed with the contrastimulant school of Rasori that it was possible to subdue febrile action, soothe irritation, and preserve the equilibrium of the circulation without inducing nausea and vomiting in the system. Along with Kitchen and Laënnec, he was also skeptical of the Broussaisian practice of heroic bloodletting. Why, he asked, should doctors abstract sixty, one hundred, or even two hundred ounces of blood from pneumonia victims when tartar emetic might easily lower arterial action and resolve the congestion with little danger to the patient?[25] Balfour predicted that when physicians learned the full powers of antimony, they would use it in place of bloodletting and thereby save patients who could not withstand the depleting process.[26] Physicians who relied on the lancet alone to equalize the nervous power of the system carried the patient to the point of collapse, when tartar emetic could subdue the inflammatory action and soothe irritation without producing nausea, debility, or "any sensible effect whatever on the skin."[27] Using the drug over a period of months, practitioners could also promote the excretions in a "powerful degree" without injuring the digestion.[28]

With this in mind Balfour recommended tartar emetic for persons predisposed to consumption. Could it not be concluded, he wrote, "that a medicine possessed of such power, is capable of expelling from phthisical constitutions, that acrimony which facilitates consumption?" Though catarrh was generally a mild disease in people of sound constitution, it frequently, through recurrence or neglect of health, produced phthisis or pneumonic inflammation and even occasioned hemoptysis (bleeding from the lungs) and the formation of tubercles in the lungs.[29] "If, therefore, catarrh consists in an afflux of fluids to the mucous membrane of the nose, fauces, and bronchiae, accompanied with inflammatory action of these parts—if this afflux and this action are occasioned by diminished perspiration, and increased by fresh accessions of cold repelling the fluids from the surface—if Emetic Tartar is powerful in equalizing the circulation, in determining to the surface, and in subduing inflammatory irritation; then it must also be considered a powerful preventive of phthisis from catarrh."[30]

Similarly, Balfour recommended the antimonial as a substitute for bloodletting in apoplexy, gout, quinsy, idiopathic fever, inflammation of the mammae, chronic hepatitis, nephritis, and asthma. He also encouraged its use as a nauseant in cases of insanity where debility was due to the "increased tension and fulness of the vessels of the brain." There the antimonial put an end to oppression of the brain by restoring the functions and equilibrium of the nervous power. "Yawning, and stretching, and sneezing," he wrote, "are evidently efforts of nature to preserve the balance of the circulation; and the forcible concussion given to the whole body by the action of vomiting must contribute powerfully to the same end." He likewise speculated that had vaccination not been discovered, tartar emetic would have proven a powerful moderating influence in the ravages of smallpox by lessening the violence of the eruptive fever. In addition, he suggested that Europeans traveling in tropical climates would find it expedient to carry tartar emetic with them to alleviate the dangers of tropical fevers.[31] His advice was taken, for a physician in Jamaica in the early decades of the twentieth century referred to tartar emetic as a "sheet anchor" in problems of tropical mania; he administered small doses of the medicine as an antiphlogistic and sedative to subdue the excited imagination of his mania patients. Small doses, combined with henbane and digitalis, not only calmed the pulse but also warded off the paroxysms of convulsive excitement.[32]

Physicians in both Britain and the United States added yet another feature to the drug when they used it as a substitute for ergot in obstetrics. Evory Kennedy of the Lying-In Hospital in Dublin prescribed tartar emetic in cases where patients suffered "grinding pains" due to the premature propelling of the child against the cervix before it was sufficiently dilated. While most accoucheurs preferred bleeding and warm baths in these instances, Kennedy recommended nauseating doses of tartar emetic to relax the pelvic muscles. He also used the drug in "irritable" or violent labor where the mother kept changing posture, and a combination of tartar emetic and copious bleeding for puerperal convulsions.[33] Were it only for its success in puerperal mania, Kennedy wrote, tartar emetic would be esteemed the most valuable article in the materia medica. "The moment a patient was observed to exhibit any incoherence after delivery, attended, as it usually is, with rapid pulse and wild expression of the eye," he wrote, "she was placed under its nauseating influence, and retained so for twenty-four or thirty-six hours, or longer if necessary." In almost every case the disease yielded, "the real ills produced by the medicine taking the place of the imaginary ones previously occupying her attention." He also prescribed tartar emetic for obstructed and inflamed mammae. The rationale for this latter treatment was based on the principle that nauseating doses of tartar emetic relieved the ducts and tubes of the breasts "by facilitating the transit and escape of the milk when secreted" without causing too rapid "a determination to the breasts."[34]

One of the more difficult problems arising from the application of tartar emetic was determining where the medical and therapeutic use of the drug ended and criminal intent began. Numerous court cases involved antimonial poisoning, but presenting a case in medico-legal language was almost impossible, given the lack of sophistication of nineteenth-century toxicology and conflicting therapeutic theories. Some physicians argued that the presence of antimony in the dead body proved nothing, since it may have been the result of the lawful administration over many previous years. Others contended that finding the metal in the liver, heart, or kidneys did not prove ingestion during life but only absorption from the stomach after death. If, on the other hand, antimony was found in the contents of the stomach and bowels, doctors argued that it did not prove ingestion immediately before death, simply "that the mucous membrane of the stomach and bowels was an eliminating surface to the liver and kidneys." The presence of antimony in any of these organs suggested only that antimony had been taken at some time antecedent to death—a time period that would justify its medical as opposed to criminal use. As an example, it was common for women to purchase tartarized antimony under the name of "quietness powders," which they secreted in food to cure their husbands' drinking habits. The fact that antimony had been discovered in the tissues and that none had been prescribed or that the nature of the victim's illness was such as to have prohibited its use proved negligible in such instances.[35] As a result of these complications, criminal trials involving antimonial poisoning found jurist, toxicologist, physician, and lawyer in one of the more difficult medico-legal problems of the day. Legal disagreements often degenerated into pettiness, name-calling, and serious questions of professionalism and served to warn the medical community of its responsibility in preparing thorough and irrefutable testimony in future medico-legal trials.[36]

Mastodon in Harness: Calomel

Like antimony, calomel (mercurous chloride) ranked foremost in the materia medica, yet the history of its application remained clouded in divisive conflicts over correct pathology and therapeutics.[37] The earliest advocates of calomel labored

in the area of first principles, deriving their therapeutics
from certain a priori beliefs concerning the body's functions:
both their pathology and therapeutics grew from a logical
derivation of those first principles. These so-called rationalists interpreted disease as the result of "venous congestion," a
state of the whole body, which they removed principally
through a combination of bloodletting and "bilious evacuation." The acceptance of constitutional pathology led many
practitioners to the almost exclusive use of calomel as the
"best bilious purgative" and, in general, they prescribed the
drug until the patient's tongue turned brown or until he began to salivate.[38] Armed with calomel, the lancet, and a few
other purgatives and believing that disease was a condition
the philosophy of which they had mastered, doctors considered themselves prepared to treat successfully almost every
case that presented itself.[39]

Much of the speculative pathology that lay behind the
rationalists' use of calomel resulted from the influence of
William Cullen and the Edinburgh School, which taught that
first principles—not observation into the processes and functions of life—were the mainstay of successful therapeutics.
In keeping with the Enlightenment's cosmic view of things,
Cullen and his disciples insisted that medicine was an exact
and predictable science measurably and logically deduced
from basic principles. Theories derived from anatomical
study of body parts and functions were "vain speculations,"
and those professing such ideas were "more ignorant than
many an uneducated nurse in a hospital."[40] Benjamin Rush
(1746–1813) of Philadelphia, once a disciple of Cullen and
the Edinburgh School (1768), provided the leadership for
much of America's monistic pathology and therapeutics. According to Rush, illness resulted from an underlying state of
the body; patient health depended upon a remedial application that overcame the state and returned the body to a
healthy balance. But, as medical historian R. H. Shryock remarked, Rush "had no confidence in Mother Nature, and insisted that she be driven from the sick room as one would a
stray dog or cat." Though Rush's theory of disease underwent various modifications in the nineteenth century, his
high regard for purgatives and antiphlogistics remained the
backbone of American medical practice; doctors tended to

oversimplify pathology, with the result that they administered oversimplified cures.[41]

But there were other doctors influenced by Gaspard Laurent Bayle (1774–1816), Auguste-François Chomel (1788–1858), Jean Nicolas Corvisart (1755–1821), and Pierre Charles Alexandre Louis (1787–1872) of the Paris clinical school, who criticized the systems formulated by their predecessors and looked instead to empirical evidence derived from observation, symptoms, forensic pathology or generalizations based on a statistical or numerical method. American doctors like Elisha Bartlett (1804–55), William Wood Gerhard (1809–72), and James Jackson, Jr. (1810–34), who were pupils of Louis and other French clinicians, blamed the Edinburgh School for the popularity of the system approach in America, claiming that their medical opinions confused and even contradicted structural pathology and nosography. Bartlett, professor of theory and practice of medicine at the University of Maryland, chastised his medical colleagues for their armchair pathology and their rationale for heroic doses of purgatives. As he wrote in his *Essay on the Philosophy of Medical Science* (1844), medical therapeutics required a foundation built upon solid hospital experience rather than procedures deduced from a priori principles. Since causation still lay beyond the reach of existing knowledge, therapeutics required a proper understanding of the morbid condition of the body and of the substances used in arresting and controlling that condition. Medical pathology, as he liked to remind his colleagues, was exclusively an empirical art with the emphasis placed on observation rather than philosophical deduction.[42] Those system theorists—men like Rush, Samuel Thomson, John Brown, Samuel Hahnemann, Rasori, and Broussais—had claimed "unadulterated and arrogant dogmatism" for what was essentially a priori reasoning based upon pure speculation.[43]

Bartlett lamented the lack of medical books used in America from countries other than England. He likewise criticized American medical students who restricted their training abroad to either Scotland or England and avoided the hospital medicine available on the continent.[44] It was the French clinical school, he emphasized, which had made the greatest advances in the analysis of morbid phenomena. The physician

Louis, whose name came to represent the Paris school, had rejected a priori reasoning and speculation for observations developed from numerical analysis. According to Bartlett, Louis represented the "true protestant school of medicine," since he repudiated the blind authority of tradition and, alone among the multitude of dogmatic regulars, romantic homeopaths, and flighty eclectics, sustained his pathology from observations derived from experience.[45]

Among his own generation of American physicians, Bartlett took special exception to the medicine practiced by John Esten Cooke (1783–1853), professor of medical theory at Transylvania University and later at Louisville Medical Institute. Cooke, like the systematist Rush, recognized but one fever, one disease, which caused an accumulation of blood in the venous system. Accordingly, disease affected the liver and those areas of the body "more distensible than others and less protected by valves."[46] Along with the other system pathologists, his therapeutic regime consisted of "removing the sanguineous engorgement of the liver" through the use of cathartics, such as calomel, aloes, and rhubarb, and by bleeding.[47] In his *Treatise of Pathology and Therapeutics* (1828), Cooke gave one of the best documentations of heroic treatment of a patient with calomel. From March to April of 1824, he treated a man with heroic doses of calomel, rhubarb, aloes, and jalap; and then, because the patient's condition grew worse, Cooke moved him to his own home, where in the course of the next ten weeks he supplied the patient with 249 grains of calomel, along with rhubarb and aloes. When the man continued to deteriorate, suffering from thirst and internal burning, Cooke supplied him with an even greater dose for fourteen days—410 grains of calomel, 270 grains of rhubarb, and 20 grains of jalap and scammony. Then from the tenth of August to the end of September, the patient consumed 836 more grains of calomel, 983 grains of scammony, 840 grains of rhubarb, 630 grains of jalap, and 560 grains of aloes. When the unfortunate man died, Cooke summarily placed the cause of death on "an improper diet, and the use of brandy." In another situation, however, Cooke treated a cholera victim with a pound of calomel in one day; and, except for softening of the gums, loss of teeth, and disfigurement, the patient survived as testament to the drug.[48]

The majority of physicians in nineteenth century America found themselves seeking positions somewhere between the heroic extremes of Cooke and the clinical stance of Bartlett, a situation which helps explain the mixture of opinions, often contradictory, that pervaded the era. Physicians seemed anxious to borrow from both the Edinburgh and Paris schools if only to justify the innumerable situations where they applied calomel and the patient's condition improved. The importance ascribed to calomel was consistent with the medical spirit of the day. Inevitably the profession used the drug, and nearly every disease seemed to fall within the parameters of its therapeutic charms. Ignoring the presence of mounting criticism, the typical practitioner administered calomel with almost scholastic devotion. Nineteenth-century physicians were headstrong defenders of their opinions and like their patients, who demanded a thorough conviction, were liable to extraordinary delusions. Their exemplary reasoning was typical of the *post hoc, propter hoc* (a patient gets well after taking a medicine, and therefore in consequence of it) rationale of the times. It also justified the derisive poetry of skeptics.

> Take some calomel
>   The more you take the better
> Mix it with a drop
>   Or two of cistern water.
>
> Feed some to your dog
>   It will make him vomit,
> And, may be, see stars
>   And perhaps a comet.
>
> One in each half hour,
>   Take a rousing portion;
> Say, a tumbler-full
>   If it suits your notion.
>
> Should you chance to die,
>   As you're almost sure to,
> You may safely swear,
>   That it did not hurt you.[49]

Part of the confusion surrounding the use of calomel grew out of the failure of nineteenth-century physicians to determine the exact modus operandi of the drug. Whether it acted by absorption or through the medium of the nervous system, or both, remained a puzzle. There were those, for example, who ascribed to the theory that the metal acted by direct stimulation of the hepatic cells; others claimed it irritated the mucous membrane of the duodenum and caused, by reflex action, a contraction of the gallbladder and hepatic ducts. What proved bothersome to the system theorists was how the drug could be absorbed so that the metallic globules could reach all the glandular tissues and the whole extent of the mucous membrane. In the end they concluded that the stomach acids converted calomel into a bichloride that then entered the bloodsteam. English physician John Hunter theorized that two poisons could not exist in the body at the same time; so in cases of syphilis he administered the strong mercurial medicine to expel the syphilitic poison from the system.[50] But others thought that as syphilis acted upon certain elements of the blood and broke them down, mercury seized upon the syphilitic agents, disintegrating and expelling them from the system. When the humoralist David Hosack, M.D., of New York attempted to revive the system approach in the 1820s with such designations as "morbific lentors" and "acrimony" in the blood, he precipitated much of the controversy over the modus operandi of calomel. While the Rushites or "solidists" argued that calomel did not enter the blood, Hosack and his defenders attempted to show that it did just that. Several investigations were undertaken to study the percentage of calomel which remained in the system after purging, the implication being that the percentage unaccounted for had circulated through the system via the blood; and, hence, calomel acted as a system cure rather than a functional cure. But there were many who argued that calomel acted as both. The confusion and outright doubts held by doctors regarding the modus operandi of calomel, however, had little immediate effect on the drug's usage. Doctors continued to prescribe it as a cholagogue, antisyphilitic, antiphlogistic, diuretic, antiseptic, tonic, and depressant.[51]

Throughout most of the eighteenth and early nineteenth centuries, physicians tended to be superficially cautious in their use of mercury, administering small amounts at a time, frequently over long periods. But early efforts by French and

Italian physicians at determining the modus operandi of the drug quickly led to the realization that calomel (like tartar emetic) acted as a sedative when administered in single heroic doses; indeed, knowledge of the phenomenon encouraged physicians to seek an even wider range of application. In small amounts calomel acted as a stimulant, stopping violent "hepatic derangements" by promoting biliary secretion; it also checked "chronic diseases of the cutaneous surface." But in the regime prescribed by Rasori and the contrastimulant school, large doses of calomel created a sedative effect, which not only stopped vomiting, but also moderated "debilitating catharsis in some of the most alarming and fatal forms of disease."[52]

In 1852 physician J. Annesley of India presented one of the earliest documentations of the effects of calomel in large and small doses. It became common practice, he wrote, for army physicians on the subcontinent to apply the medication in small amounts for an indefinite period, until the mouth became sore, with patients considered effectively doctored only when they salivated or when the mouth turned brown or showed evidence of a mercurous odor.[53] As a believer in contrastimulant therapeutics, Annesley observed that large doses of calomel created a sedative action on the system, causing less irritation and injury to the body functions. Ironically Annesley and a whole generation of more pathologically oriented doctors were responsible for the drug's most pernicious effects. "Small doses of calomel," Annesley wrote, "will purge, and keep up a considerable degree of irritation in the stomach and bowels, when twenty grains will not."[54] To test the validity of this thesis, Annesley performed experiments on dogs and found that a single excessive dose of calomel diminished vascular activity rather than excited it, while scruple doses of calomel caused almost immediate irritability of the stomach and produced vomiting. Further study on the effects of calomel led him to conclude that calomel did not act upon the vascular system or the liver as so many physicians had formerly believed, but rather that the medicine acted both chemically and mechanically upon the secretions, loosening the matter and "rendering it more fluid" while at the same time opening a passage for discharge.[55]

But there remained no real consensus on the proper use of calomel. So mixed were its applications that it was variously listed as a sialagogue by William Cullen, Nathaniel Chapman, and John Eberle; as a stimulant by A. T. Thompson and Vavasseur; as a sedative by Bertele and Horn; and as a tonic, revulsive, and hyposthenic by Murray, Begin, and Giacomini.[56] Besides the confusion regarding the drug's actual effect on the system, doctors also disagreed on just what constituted a large or small dose. One doctor writing in the *Transylvania Journal of Medicine* in 1837 objected to giving patients large doses of calomel and thought that a normal dose might amount to twenty-five or thirty grains.[57] Yet, in 1842, the editor of the *Western and Southern Medical Recorder* designated a large amount to be twenty or more grains, and a small dose from one to five grains. On the other hand, Martyn Paine's *Institutes of Medicine* (1860) recommended an initial 120-grain dose of calomel for Asiatic cholera, followed by sixty grains every hour.[58] Whatever the dosage, physicians agreed that calomel carried herculean powers; in fact, they were veritable Ciceros as they waxed eloquent in their praise of the metal.

In conclusion, then, with these facts before us, and the powerful and effective energies of our mal-treated remedy freely acknowledged, shall we, because in careless and injudicious hands, or in idiosyncratic temperaments it may have, occasionally overleaped the prescribed bounds of its therapeutic action, and done violence to the human constitution,—consent to cower to the out-cry of blind prejudice, or ignorant and interested empiricism, and, before the eyes of the living myriads whom it has rescued from the jaws of the grave, deliberately pronounce the blistering curse of Science upon its head, and consign it to the reproach of maledictions of posterity? No, never!—Sooner let the fate of the lacerated and engulfed multitudes, who have fallen under the explosive power of uncontrolled Steam, and found their winding sheet in the ocean wave, authorize the utter expulsion of this great agent from the civilized world, when ten thousand burning axles are rolling under its impulse and bearing with the speed of the winds, and exchanges of intelligence and commerce to rising and expectant nations. And yet who is prepared for such a national sacrifice?—None. The voice of Civilization is the voice of Reason, and the world obeys;—hear it—Study more profoundly your science—strengthen your cylinders,—

modify your machinery, and increase your circumspection, but still retain THE MASTODON IN HARNESS, to do the work of an AGE in a YEAR.[59]

Physicians in the newly opened lands of the South and West commonly avowed that calomel was their most important medicine. For one thing, "the peculiar condition of the atmosphere and climate [generated] an extraordinary susceptibility to biliary diseases."[60] A doctor from Jefferson County, Georgia, arguing that the environment had a particularly evil effect upon the system, advised "herculean doses" of forty to eighty-five grains of calomel, to be repeated every four hours, to cure hepatic derangements. He suggested this in the belief that calomel was one of the finest antiseptics, not only purging the system, but cleansing it thoroughly, and removing the deleterious remnants of disease.[61] Daniel Drake (1785–1852), one of the noted physicians west of the Alleghenies and author of *Diseases of the Interior Valley of North America* (1850–54), recalled a Louisiana doctor who boasted of having prescribed enough calomel to load a steamboat.[62] According to Charles R. Curtis, M.D., writing in the *Western Medico-Chirurgical Journal* for 1852, calomel had become a necessity for the western farmer because of his heavy diet of animal food and the scarcity of fruits and vegetables.[63] Indeed, the West's peculiar environment and dietary problems were "so thoroughly imbued in the public mind," another western physician wrote, "that a man would hardly dare to visit our beautiful country without first providing himself with a double supply of some celebrated Anti-Bilious Pills."[64]

Because children were known to survive higher febrile temperatures than adults, it became common practice among doctors in the early nineteenth century to prescribe calomel for children in doses larger than those given to adults. Physician Moore Hoyt of New York remarked in 1826 that children with a "high grade of arterial action" could consume twenty or more grains of calomel with perfect safety. He warned, however, that it was only "a certain grade of arterial action above the standard of adult health, in which calomel is exhibited with safety and advantage in large doses." Despite his qualifying remarks, doctors appeared all too willing to prescribe calomel in heroic and often fatal amounts. Parents, too, were infatuated with the metal and fed their children Storey's Worm Cakes, Cling's Worm Lozenges, or similarly destructive patent and proprietary medicines, which contained hazardous quantities of calomel mixed with jalap and scammony. In many of these instances, the mercury treatment produced salivation, followed by ulceration of the mouth, sloughing of the gums, and necrosis of the alveolar process of the lower jaw. While children sometimes recovered from the violence of the mercurial poisoning, many victims were unable to separate their jaws and were obliged to spend the remainder of their lives sucking food through apertures left by the loss of bone.[65]

In 1853, in the *Transactions* of the College of Physicians of Philadelphia, Samuel Jackson, M.D. (1787–1872), who held the chair of physiology for twenty-eight years at the University of Pennsylvania, caused immediate excitement in medical circles by condemning the salivation of children or the use of any amount of mercury that would affect the breath and gums in the slightest. He recalled one instance in his own medical practice where he had prescribed five grains of calomel to a three-year old who had suffered from an inflammation of the lungs. He administered the drug twice a day as an expectorant; and while the cough and inflammation abated, the child's breath became "intolerably offensive" and on observation he found that the lower teeth and gums had fallen off. In another case where he had prescribed several ten-grain doses of calomel over a period of several days to a child suffering from "epidemic remittent fever," the teeth had fallen out and gums had become gangrenous. Before the gangrene had been halted, a large piece of the maxilla bone had to be removed. On the basis of his own unfortunate experiences, he urged doctors to heed the advice of Benjamin Rush, who had steadfastly refused to salivate children under six years of age.[66]

The controversy surrounding the use of calomel reached new heights when, on May 4, 1863, Surgeon-General William A. Hammond surprised the medical world by directing that calomel "be struck from the [Army] Supply Table and that no further requisitions for this medicine be approved by Medical Directors." Hammond's edict stemmed from evidence that calomel had become "an abuse, the melancholy effects of which, as officially reported, have exhibited themselves not only in innumerable cases of profuse salivation, but in the not infrequent occurrence of mercurial gangrene."[67] As could be expected, the decision of the surgeongeneral caused an immediate furor among army surgeons in particular and the medical profession in general. A letter published in the *Chicago Tribune* called upon "the benevolent for a donation of rags to absorb the abominable flux from the salivation of the soldiery at Cairo."[68] But the Cincinnati Medical Association condemned the decision as unproved and libelous, and it continued to praise the remedial effects of the mineral. The following June, the American Medical Association appointed a committee to review Hammond's decision. On the basis of its deliberations, the committee concluded that Hammond's order was "unwise and unnecessary"; moreover, it requested that the surgeon-general modify his order because "the charge of wholesale malpractice [was] unjust to the army surgeons."[69] Other critics of Hammond's Circular No. 6 accused him of affiliating with the Thomsonians, eclectics, and homeopaths of the day, making a "senseless concession to 'anti-Mineral' knaves and fools."[70]

The Baltimore Medical Association took up the question of Hammond's decision at its meeting in January of 1867. One member of the association commented that the whole idea of mercurous chloride as a treatment for general inflammation grew initially from the discovery that calomel, used both internally and by fumigation, had cured syphilitic iritis. Subsequently physicians "thought because it was good in one inflammatory disease that it was good in all, and from this dates its introduction into general practice, and its abuse." But in no disease, with the exception of syphilis, was there any evidence that calomel had done any good. Notwithstanding this criticism, others at the Baltimore meeting were just as adamant about the drug's utility in pneumonia. One advocate related how he treated all pneumonia patients with "depletion" doses of mercury, since "salivation was salvation in pneumonia." Calomel, he said, acted upon the inflammation by reducing the strong pulse and the overactive heart. The same held true in cases of dysentery, where he insisted that patients be "depleted" with mercury before body repair could begin. He recalled having successfully administered to soldiers who suffered from dysentery and pneumonia at Fort Marshall and elsewhere. He did admit, however, that army physicians had no business treating gunshot wounds with calomel or administering mercury to emaciated and battle-weary soldiers who were unable to endure the harshness of the mercury treatment.[71]

Still others at the Baltimore meeting were astonished at the continued defense of calomel. The Civil War, one critic argued, "had satisfied the profession in regard to the use of calomel." As an army surgeon, he had found that calomel had not benefited pneumonia patients and that in those cases where it was employed most had died. Similarly, another physician thought Hammond's decision to ban the use of mercury had come at an auspicious moment. In the western war theater, army physicians had administered unusually large doses of calomel, resulting in profuse salivation, ulceration, and necrosis of the jaw. "When wounded men were subjected to the use of calomel," he wrote, "they did not get well as soon as those that were not. I noticed this in an Ohio regiment; the convalescence was protracted two or three weeks. The abuse became notorious."[72]

During the postwar decades, southern doctors gave little heed to Hammond's warnings and proceeded to dose patients with heaping spoonfuls of the metal, arguing that the prejudices aroused by botanics, eclectics, and homeopaths had unjustly condemned the "claims of the old giant."[73] As late as 1884, R. J. H. Hatchett, M.D., of Virginia was calling calomel the "Samson of the Materia Medica"; and though he admitted its destructive powers when improperly given, he remained impressed with its therapeutic effects, particularly for those patients who required a sedative. As soon as the drug reached the mucous membrane of the stomach, he wrote, there was an instantaneous sedative impression conveyed through the nervous system. During his residence in the swamplands of the Mississippi Delta, he discovered that calomel acted promptly on nearly all cases of convulsions, fevers, and spasms common to that climate. As a substitute for the lancet, cupping, and leeching, Hatchett found calomel to be a superior depleting measure in all acute attacks of fever and inflammation. But he warned against overuse of the preparation as an antiphlogistic. "The inflammation is a fire that is consuming the vitals," he wrote, "and calomel is the water with which we may moderate and control the fire, and with which, if carried too far, we may extinguish it, even to the last vital spark; for after calomel has subdued the morbid excitement, if persisted in, it will continue its warfare on the remaining excitement, that which is necessary to life and health."[74]

Calomel continued as the stock-in-trade of the laity as well as the physician in the southern states. One South Carolina doctor reported in 1891 that calomel was surely the most frequently used household remedy for everything from toothaches to ingrown toenails. He recounted individuals so accustomed to its usage that they seemed to have acquired "the calomel habit," though few cases of chronic mercurial poisoning resulted from this indiscriminate use. Persons who rarely went to physicians for treatment, generally blaming the liver for all their complaints, trusted calomel above all else. In effect, the language of the earlier humoral pathologists had "passed into the popular tongue" to the extent that people complained that their livers were "locked up," "torpid," or simply would not "act." As Elisha Bartlett, M.D., had remarked some forty years earlier:

> Almost every ailment to which the body is subject—functional or organic—trifling or grave—chronic or acute—each of these ailments can be removed in only one way,—by the restoration of the biliary secretion,—by inducing the liver "*to act*"; and this can be accomplished with certainty, only by one infallible remedy—calomel. This substance is proclaimed to be, not only the most efficacious and important article in the materia medica, but, also, one of the safest and most inoffensive. It is constantly administered—on all occasions—in all diseases—and in all their stages. It has, literally, in some instances, been made an article of daily food—sprinkled upon buttered bread, and mixed with it before baking! I suppose it is no exaggeration to say that there is more calomel consumed in the valley of the Mississippi and its tributaries, than in all the world beside.[75]

The system pathologists remained a vocal part of medical opinion late into the nineteenth century. In the *Cincinnati Lancet-Clinic* for 1899, for example, physician C. J. Funck

wrote that calomel remained the most important drug in removing poisons from the body. While nature allowed that in
some illnesses certain parts of the body might remain in
health, for the most part organs of the body acted in unison.
Accordingly, it was necessary only "for the physician to grasp
the tendencies and forces in the body, and through them, by
the help of more favorable circumstances, artificially produced, to bring to pass the possible neutralization of lesions."
Clearly the physician's task was to unload the body's humors
of their hepatic, pancreatic, intestinal, renal, salivary, and cutaneous secretions. Funck urged doctors to return to the
glandular (eliminative) medicines that had been popular in
the early part of the century. He objected to the investigations of Hughes Bennett's Edinburgh Committee and the
later experiments, in the 1880s and 1890s, of Roehrig, Vig-
nal, and William Rutherford, who had shown that calomel did
not act uniformly on the various glands. Their conclusions
were invalid, he reasoned, because they applied calomel to
healthy animals rather than to diseased ones. Similarly he objected to the prevailing condemnation of salivation. He wrote,
"Incalculable harm has been doubtless wrought by these false
arguments and have brought this medicine, a veritable king
and giant among remedies . . . almost into disrepute."[76]

The Therapeutic Mule: Arsenic

Arsenic was yet another drug that served the medical profession from the empirical age through the heroic period of
medicine and into the critical and experimental era ·of
therapeutics. Its progressive ascent from the alchemist's laboratory to the apothecary's cabinet reflected a history of observations and hypotheses that culminated in the early years
of the twentieth century in the development of synthetic
preparations that were far less toxic than their inorganic
time-honored ancestors. But the art of employing arsenic, as
so many physicians learned after trial and error, consisted of
controlling the pharmacological action of the mineral to
make it serve therapeutic aims.

The sulphides of arsenic were well-known medicants
among the physicians of ancient times. Hippocrates administered orpiment (As_2S_3) and realgar (As_2S_2) as escharotics

and as remedies for ulcers, while Dioscorides referred to orpiment in the first century as a valuable depilatory. In the eighth century, Schabir roasted realgar to obtain white arsenic (As_2O_3) and gave to it the name it still bears. Centuries later Jean de Gorris (1503–77) recommended arsenic as a sudorific, Angelus Salva and Donzellus used it as a specific (amulet) against the plague, and Lentilius (1684) and Friceius (1710) employed it in the treatment of malaria. Yellow sulphuret of arsenic formed one of the principal ingredients in Lanfranc's collyrium, which physicians prescribed for nearly two centuries as a remedy for ulcers. Frère Comé's paste, composed of red sulphuret of mercury, arsenious acid, the ashes of burnt shoesole, and dragon's blood, was also applied in the external treatment of ulcers and cancer. Orpiment became known as Rousselot's arsenical powder and was one of the major ingredients in Hellmund's ointment for cancer. Monsieur Le Febure of Paris recommended arsenic as a radical cure for cancer and administered it in much the same fashion as corrosive sublimate was used for venereal disease—external application and fumigation.[77]

Throughout the centuries, physicians prescribed arsenic both externally and internally. While pure metallic arsenic had no therapeutic use, doctors employed the arsenides and salts as alteratives, antiseptics, antispasmodics, antiperiodics, caustics, cholagogues, depilatories, hematinics, sedatives, and tonics.[78] Some sixty different preparations were tried therapeutically in the history of its use, and probably twenty or more were still in circulation by the end of the nineteenth century, including Aiken's Tonic Pills, Andrew's Tonic, Arsenauro, Gross's Neuralgia Pills, Chloro-Phosphide of Arsenic, and Sulphur Compound Lozenges. The potash solution of arsenious acid remained the most popular arsenic-based drug, while preparations such as De Valagin's mineral solution (arsenious acid in dilute hydrochloric acid) and Donovan's solution (iodide of arsenic and mercury) were frequent substitutes. Also popular were iron, quinine, sodium, and strychnine arsenates and the later cacodylates of sodium and mercury used in the treatment of pellagra, malaria, and sleeping sickness.[79]

Although the sulphurets of arsenic had been used for external and internal treatment, not until doctors boiled arsenious acid with an alkali to make it more soluble in water, did arsenic therapeutics change perceptibly from external to internal administration. As a result the popular Jacob's, Brera's and Hein's solutions were introduced into medical use. When Thomas Fowler, M.D., physician to the General Infirmary of the County of Stafford, suggested potassium arsenite for the treatment of intermittent fever in 1786, his solution soon superseded all others. Until then the "Tasteless Ague Drops," "Asiatic Drops," and "Asiatic Pills" (arsenic and black pepper) were popular antiperiodic remedies. In his *Medical Reports on the Effects of Arsenic in the Cure of Agues, Remittent Fevers and Periodic Headaches* (1786), the Edinburgh-educated physician related how he became interested in the "Tasteless Ague Drops" that were prescribed in the Stafford hospitals in the 1780s. Having examined the drops with the help of the infirmary's apothecary, he then tried to imitate the preparation. Soon Fowler recommended his "Solutio Mineralis," which later bore the name Fowler's Solution, as a substitute for the ague drops and costly Peruvian bark. In 1809 the solution became recognized in the London pharmacopoeia.[80]

In a series of well-received articles prepared for the *Edinburgh Medical and Surgical Journal* in 1809 and 1810, surgeon G. N. Hill blamed the past difficulty with the use of arsenic on the sanguine wishes of practitioners "to attack violent diseases by very enormous doses of medicine, thinking to mow down, as it were, all opposition to their wishes, by a *coup de main*." The mineral solution of arsenic, however, did "not admit of loose and inattentive application." Physicians who used the drug had the responsibility for administering it in the most exacting manner and in doses small enough to cure, and careful of every precaution.[81] But while physicians like Hill administered no more than a few drops of Fowler's Solution, partisans of heroic therapeutics believed that arsenic could be given in much larger doses without ill effect. One heroic advocate was D. Theodore Coxe, M.D., of Philadelphia who prescribed fifty to one hundred fifty drops of solution daily for weeks on end.[82] "It will not do to rest contented with such timid doses as might be worthy of a homeopathic quack," another doctor observed. "It must be exhibited in increasing doses and persevered in until the toxic effects show themselves, in sickness, a sense of fainting, formication in the toes and fingers, dryness of the fauces, and white tongue."[83]

Two of the more vocal supporters for the use of arsenic in the early nineteenth century were Thomas Hunt, M.D., and James Begbie, M.D., whose articles in *Lancet, Edinburgh Medical Journal,* and *Transactions* of the Provincial Medical and Surgical Association helped to support Fowler's introduction of the mineral into the pharmacopoeia. While agreeing that some doctors had been reckless in their heroic application, the two physicians felt that sound therapeutical reasons remained for its proper application as a tonic, antiperiodic, febrifuge, and as a powerful alterative. In the hands of the experienced physician, arsenic became a drug whose abandonment was as senseless as rejecting the steam engine because of its superior power. "Let us use the medicine," Hunt argued, "but use it discreetly. Let us not repudiate it; but let us beware of its overdose."[84] The most evident signs of the healing powers of arsenic were increased heat and dryness of the skin, quickened pulse, itchiness of the eyelids, conjunctivitis, and perhaps even swollen and tender gums, salivation, nausea, vomiting, nervous depression, faintness, and tremor. Physicians also looked for a change in skin coloring to a "dirt-brown, unwashed appearance." When these signs manifested themselves in the patient, the observant physician knew that arsenic was in "full operation over the disease."[85]

In addition to skin diseases, neuralgia, malarious disorders, and syphilis, Hunt and Begbie recommended arsenic for lumbago, dyspepsia, hypochondriasis, carcinoma, scrofula, and epilepsy. During the 1830s and 1840s, physicians working in the Ohio and Mississippi Valleys announced that arsenic had also relieved problems of menorrhagia, leucorrhea, and dysmenorrhea.[86] Soon afterward doctors were prescribing arsenic for threatened abortion, postdelivery hemorrhage, spermatorrhea, and functional impotency.[87] And although the exact modus operandi remained a puzzle, physicians also advocated arsenic for advanced stages of rheumatism, but warned against its use in the milder stages. John Jenkinson, M.D., of England wrote, "We must be content to know the fact and sit down with a conviction of our inability to solve the enigma."[88]

In mid-century, the medical world was surprised to learn that peasants living in the areas of Lower Austria and Styria were not only habitually eating arsenic, but were actually thriving on it. It was said that itinerant peddlers procured the mineral from the chimneys of lead and copper smelting furnaces and sold it under the name *hidri*, a corruption of the word *hütten-rauch*, meaning smelt-house smoke. According to Dr. Von Tschudi, whose original discussion of the habit became popularized in James F. W. Johnston's *The Chemistry of Common Life* (1855), Styrian peasant women consumed from one-half to five or six grains of arsenic daily to obtain a "fresh healthy aspect," which, defined in peasant language, meant a certain degree of obesity. The habit, particularly popular among young women, tended to favor them with a blooming rosy-cheeked complexion and a "strikingly healthy exterior," which on the whole was quite agreeable to the male population.[89] Johnston wrote that the peasant girl saw in arsenic-eating a "love-maker," a "harbinger of happiness," which through its effect upon her weight and complexion, soothed her "ardent longings" and bestowed "contentment and peace" upon her character. "Stirred by an unconsciously growing attachment," he added, "confiding scarcely to herself her secret feelings, and taking counsel of her inherited wisdom only—really adds, by the use of *hidri*, to the natural graces of her filling and rounding form, paints with brighter hues her blushing cheeks and tempting lips, and imparts a new and winning lustre to her sparkling eye." Beauty that lay dormant under oppressive peasant life flourished with the use of arsenic and brought to her feet young men who sang her praises and became suppliants for her charms.[90]

Peasant men, on the other hand, consumed arsenic for its tonic effects, which according to them, improved the appetite, invigorated digestion, gave them a strong sexual desire, excited muscular and nervous functions, and even facilitated respiration. After placing a crumb of arsenic in their mouths and allowing it to dissolve, they were soon able to ascend mountains "which previously they could only climb with great difficulty in breathing." The reason for this phenomenon, according to Johnston, lay in the power of the arsenic to arrest the metamorphosis of tissues, lessening the waste of the body and diminishing the quantity of carbonic acid discharged from the lungs. This meant that inhalation demanded less oxygen and allowed for "greater ease in breathing under all circumstances." Moreover, food, which otherwise would have been used to supply carbonic acid to be given off by the lungs, was deposited in the cellular tissues beneath the skin. What worked for men also worked for horses. Arsenic mixed into stable feed enabled peasants to obtain a greater amount of labor from those animals used to perform heavy work. On the other hand, those horses that did not toil as much tended (like the peasant women) to improve in appearance and gain weight. In Vienna and other parts of Europe, grooms and coachmen fed small amounts of arsenic to their carriage horses to produce a fuller look, a glossier coat, and a foaming mouth.[91]

There were those, too, who ate arsenic in order to build up an immunity to its poisonous effects. Charles Boner, M.D., writing in *Chambers's Journal* in 1856, related how Napoleon had himself become an arsenic-eater from fear of being poisoned. "Now, whether true or not that Napoleon did take arsenic—though his known inclination to stoutness, later in life, might seem to lend additional probability to the story—it is sufficient," Boner remarked, "that such report was *current* to show that arsenic-eating not only existed, *but was generally known to exist*." But arsenic eating often became a necessity after continued use. Like the Indian opium-eater, the Polynesian betel-chewer, or the Peruvian coca-chewer, the arsenic-eater found it difficult to abstain once the system became accustomed to the habit. Those who omitted their daily dose showed symptoms of illness that closely resembled arsenical poisoning, and the only means of relieving the symptoms consisted of returning to the practice.[92]

There were a number of reported arsenic-eaters in the late nineteenth century. The superintendent of the arsenic factory near Salzburg was actually advised by M. Boüsch, professor of chemistry and mineralogy at Eislenben, to consume small amounts of arsenic in order to prevent poisoning from factory fumes. "I advise you, nay, it is absolutely necessary," Boüsch remarked, "that besides strictly abstaining from spiritous liquors, you should learn to take arsenic; but do not forget when you have attained the age of fifty years, gradu-

ally to decrease the dose till, from the dose of which you have
been accustomed, you return to that which you began or
even less." Taking the professor's remarks at face value, the
superintendent began by eating three grains of arsenic daily
and gradually increased his dosage until by the age of forty-
five, he was consuming twenty-three grains of pure white arsenic daily![93] Similarly, in a paper read before the Medical Society of Quebec and subsequently published in the *Boston
Medical and Surgical Journal* in 1866, F. A. H. LaRue, M.D.,
professor of legal medicine and toxicology at Laval University, discussed the case of a man who for years consumed
eight grains of arsenious acid to prevent consumption. According to LaRue, the man began using arsenic for fear of
dying of the same dread illness as his parents; in addition to
eating arsenic, he also smoked a grain or two mixed with tobacco in his pipe.[94] This practice, it appears, was not unusual.
Chinese were known to smoke arsenic in combination with
tobacco so that "their lungs acted like smith's bellows; and
they were as red as cherubs."[95] There was also an English
physician who believed that arsenic diffused in the air mer-
ited further investigation, since in those areas near the smelting of copper, the vaporized arsenic had provided an immunity from fevers.[96]

News of arsenic-eating spread quickly through Victorian
culture. Tschudi's remarks were published in the major English journals and were also discussed in over thirty-two
French, German, Italian, and Swiss newspapers and ma-
gazines. Following the example set by the Styrian arsenic-
eaters, Victorians began to "doctor" themselves with arsenic
for everything from venereal disease to tapeworms. Arsenic
in its various forms became so popular a tonic that eminent
Victorians like Robert Browning, Thomas Huxley, Herbert
Spencer, Thomas Carlyle, and even Charles Darwin may well
have been its victims. Each of them suffered for years from
what they diagnosed as chronic dyspepsia. This Victorian
malady, which physicians sometimes identified as neurasthenia, may well have resulted from the toxic effects of
Fowler's Solution. Women drank the solution for their complexions, employed it as a cosmetic wash, and even purchased white arsenic as a hair-powder.[97] Doctors Daniel G.
Brinton and George H. Napheys, in their *Laws of Health in*

Relation to the Human Form (1870), condoned moderate arsenic-eating (*pour rajeunissante*) by women to obtain a healthy
appearance without the use of cosmetics but hoped that they
might eventually substitute flowers of sulphur in milk or
wash solutions of cucumber juice or horseradish root, which
were far less troublesome.[98]

While the claims of the Styrian arsenic-eaters were subjected to occasional criticism, physicians generally approved
of the practice and praised the virtues of minute doses of the
acid on the human organism. Writing in the *Provincial Medical Journal* in 1893, physician C. F. Brown suggested that doctors consider administering arsenic to healthy persons during epidemics so they might remain immune to disease. He
mentioned case histories of individuals who had taken arsenic during epidemics of scarlet fever, influenza, and diphtheria, and had remained unaffected. Drawing upon the experiences and claims of the Styrian peasants, he suggested
that moderate doses might be efficacious in building up an
immunity in the system. He also encouraged surgeons to
prepare their patients a few days before operations with
small doses of arsenic, believing it would render them immune to postoperative complications.[99]

The arsenic-eating habits of the Styrian peasants provided
a new rationale for doctors who substituted pure arsenic acid
for quinine in periodic fevers. According to A. P. Merrill,
M.D., of Memphis, arsenic was a nerve tonic as well as an
antiperiodic; and in its action upon the blood vessels and
the bronchial tubes, it induced an "expansion, by which the
circulation is facilitated, and congestion, hypertrophy, and
hemorrhage were relieved." Reflecting on the habits of the
Styrian peasants who consumed arsenic to increase lung capacity, Merrill suggested that the effects upon the tubular vessels induced similar phenomena "to all structures of that kind
in the body and caused an increase of animal heat and of muscular power and endurance, enabling men to encounter fatigue, withstand the tenuity of the air and cold on lofty mountains, and accomplish in every way an increase of physical
exertion." In its ability to invigorate circulation and respiration without precipitating undue excitability, arsenic became a
remedial agent in scrofulous and tuberculous persons, guarding the system from pulmonary diseases that so frequently

led to consumption. Rejecting earlier fears of arsenic-eating
as a catalyst in consumption, Merrill recommended arsenical
medication as "the main reliance of persons in any way pre-
disposed to consumption." When taken in full dose, arsenic
diminished febrile disturbances, prevented nocturnal sweats,
lessened general excitement, and retarded development of
the tubercules by arresting their evolution and "softening
the old [tubercules], rendering them abortive and latent, and
not allowing them to pass beyond crudity." [100]

Arsenic earned the nickname therapeutic mule of the materia medica not only because of its dependability but also
because of the stubborn persistence with which it acted, together with the capricious nature of its toxic powers. One
doctor wrote in 1912 that arsenic was his therapeutic mule
because it performed "the hardest kind of work under the
most adverse conditions, with the least amount of exertion." [101] Along with mercury and antimony, arsenic became
one of the mainstays of drug therapeutics in the nineteenth
century and only reluctantly yielded to new drug formulas of
the twentieth century. Yet, as late as 1906, *Abbott's Alkaloidal
Digest* list of 198 diseases contained 51 that called for the use
of arsenic. In 1909 Ehrlich's experiments with arsenic led to
the widespread use of Salvarsan (arsphenamine), often called
606, which, until its replacement by penicillin, remained the
treatment for syphilis for nearly forty years. Taken internally
in either liquid or solid form, injected hypodermically, in-
haled as a vapor, administered intravenously, applied externally, and in rare occasions given in enema form, arsenic
proved to be one of the most popular drugs of the materia
medica. [102]

Retrospect

Considering the biforated nature of medical education in
nineteenth century America, it was not surprising that doctors continued to reinforce the weaknesses rather than
strengths of the profession. As in previous centuries, physicians relied too heavily upon the virtues of the materia medica and not enough upon the recuperative powers of nature.
Armed with cups, lancet, and leech and provided with calomel, tartar emetic, arsenic, and an assortment of other

drugs, doctors proceeded to bleed, blister, puke, purge, and salivate patients until they either died from the combined disease and treatment or persevered long enough to recover from both. Recuperation from these heroic regimes was long and arduous, with some patients never recovering fully. Doctors seldom questioned the reliability of older remedies, and fewer still were willing to experiment except by increasing dosage or extending the range of the drug's applicability. If patient mortality was high, it was no worse than most doctors experienced and no less than the public expected.

In viewing the first half of the nineteenth century, it is clear that the materia medica bore the stamp of the system builders, who were famous for their generalizations and for a nosology that reduced nearly all diseases to liver complaints, gastroenteritis, biliousness, nervous debility, psora, or the vapors. They mistook the internal logic of their theories for universal truth and not only insisted that all obey the principles deduced from their axioms, but closed their minds to ideas and facts that fell outside their neat intellectual worlds. Indeed, they labored in building intricate systems out of rough observations and a few chance results; and their risk of error was enormous when, as often happened, the specific instances of cure were more imagined than observed. In most instances the medical theories of the system-builders reflected and sometimes even exaggerated the dominant characteristics of the culture. The extent to which drug therapy became an ogre by mid-century simply mirrored the gusto of American society. European observers like Tocqueville and James Bryce no doubt would have commended Oliver Wendell Holmes for his perceptive view of heroic therapeutics and America for its heroic self-portrait.

4

Transcendental Medicine

As in the political arena, where intellectual ferment frequently interrupted the machinery of government with groundswells of revolutionary reform, so the spirit of medical dissatisfaction with etiology, pathology, and treatment of disease eventually caused patients to translate their practitioners' doubts into a more general loss of confidence. The newer tendencies in heroic therapeutics, the massive use of mercury, tartar emetic, arsenic, and opium and its derivatives, and the proliferation of mechanical contrivances, elixirs, patent and proprietary drugs had brought medicine to the frontiers of medical nihilism. The tendency for brinkmanship therapeutics resulted in the spawning of countless system-builders, each seeking to replace traditional medicine with a newer mode of treatment. Mesmerism, Thomsonianism, mind-cure, faith-cure, baunscheidtism, Christian Science, electropathy, hydropathy, vitopathy, and chemopathy had all but abandoned the older specifics for promises of quick and harmless cures. These medical heresies rivaled the religious sects, political parties, movements, and fads that emerged, along with the common man, in the early decades of the nineteenth century. Unfortunately, few of the systems did more than compound the errors of the past. As medical science searched for better methods and procedures, the public wandered amid an endless list of *pathies*, the claims of which rivaled the eschatological dreams of the era's religious and political leaders. The spirit of heresy was rampant and worshipers eagerly gathered before the newer medical shrines in search of cures.

Mesmer and the Art of Magnetism

Many of the sectarian healers of the late eighteenth and nineteenth centuries owed their popularity to the influence of Friedrich Anton Mesmer (1734–1815) of Mersburg in Swabia, whose theories on animal magnetism captivated the attention of Europe and America during the closing decades of the eighteenth century. A student of Gerard Van Swieten and De Haen at the University of Vienna, Mesmer demonstrated an early interest in astrology, and for his doctor's degree in 1766 wrote a thesis entitled *De Planetarium Influxu* in which he theorized that the sun, moon, and fixed stars, in accordance with the principle of attraction, exercised a direct influence over the earth, its sea, and atmosphere, as well as on the nervous systems of living things. Through the effects of animal magnetism, which he considered analogous to but independent of mineral magnetism, human life had become as susceptible to the forces of gravitation as the tides, as proven by the influence that gravitation held over the monthly flux of women and the remissions occurring in diseases.

The sources for Mesmer's ideas included Paracelsus, who claimed it was possible to transplant diseases into the earth, and the exorcist treatment of the Swabian priest Johann Joseph Gassner, who gained a huge following in the Austrian Tyrol through a combination of exorcism, suggestion, and drugs. Mesmer also owed much to the "etheriall sperm" of the English Rosicrucian Robert Fludd, Sebastian Wirdig's *New Medicine of the Spirit* (1673), William Maxwell's *De Medicina Magnetica* (1679), the mercury and earth magnet of Father Kirchner, and the reputed cures of Father Maximillen Hell, a Jesuit priest and astronomer in Vienna who began treating disease in the 1770s with the use of magnetic plates of steel. In 1774 Father Hell explained his technique to Mesmer, who in turn experimented with the magnetic plates. When Mesmer concluded that animal magnetism was a radically different force from simple mineral magnetism, he broke with the Jesuit astronomer and ceased using magnets in the treatment of disease. Instead, Mesmer claimed that he could produce the same therapeutic effect by passing his hands downward toward the patient's feet. Despite his replacement of mineral magnetism with this innovative technique, magnetic theory continued to play a dominant role in Mesmer's treatment. Between 1773 and 1778 Mesmer traveled through Switzerland, Swabia, and Bavaria, sending accounts of his successful cures to the leading scientific societies of the day. Although his accounts received little attention in medical circles, Mesmer took up residence in Paris, where he soon won favor with Marie Antoinette, Comte d'Artois (the future Charles X), LaFayette, and other fashionable people of the court; and he proceeded to treat patients with magnetism in the belief that the humors were readily affected by the action of the "magnetic vapour." His novel treatment received great notoriety after the conversion of Charles d'Eslon, physician to the king's brother and doctor regent of the Faculty of Paris, who later established a successful practice of his own patterned after Mesmer's principles of animal magnetism.[1]

Combining the scientific notions of magnetism with his own theories regarding animal magnetism, Mesmer constructed a huge oak tub or *baquet* filled with bottles of magnetized water, powdered glass, and iron filings to give the appearance of a gigantic galvanic cell and provide the condenser and conductor effects of animal magnetism. In group treatment that more resembled a séance than a medical examination, patients assembled around the *baquet*, each holding a rod (*baquette*) that projected from the lid of the tub to the diseased area. In addition, Mesmer passed a cord around the bodies of the patients, who sometimes held hands to form yet another magnetic field. To increase the magnetic influence, Mesmer provided his consulting room with soft music, the scent of perfume, and dim lights. Then at the proper moment, he entered dressed in lilac colored silk, carrying a magic wand, which he passed over each patient, suggesting that magnetic currents emanating from himself and the *baquet* were healing the disease. On occasion Mesmer held his group exercises outdoors, where, with the aid of various magnetized trees or fountains, he continued to achieve remarkable cures.[2]

Like the Greeks, Mesmer believed that disease developed to the point of crisis; and since women composed a majority of his patients, he encouraged crisis through the employment of male assistants (*valets toucheurs*), who positioned themselves in close physical contact with the woman's knees enclosed between their own. They then proceeded to place "subtle pressures upon the breasts with the finger tips" and applied their hands over the ovaries and "in the neighborhood of the most sensitive parts of the body." The general excitability of the female patient, as analyzed by the French commission appointed in 1784 to study Mesmer's claims, caused her to throw caution to the wind as she entered the crisis stage. As one woman became agitated, others soon went through jerking, hiccoughing, crying, laughing, and hysterical movements. The commission, whose membership included the astronomer Bailly, the chemist Lavoisier, the naturalist Jussieu, Dr. Guillotin, and Benjamin Franklin among its investigative members, concluded that Mesmer's activities, along with the services provided by his assistants, could not "be otherwise than dangerous for morals," since the convulsions experienced by women disarmed their modesty and natural virtue. This was particularly true when Mesmer provided a special room (*salle des crises*) for their crises.[3] Since Mesmer chose only the most handsome young men for the delicate task of inciting a crisis, abuses not only occurred, but, according to the commission, "many of the women who went to Mesmer did not go to be magnetized!" As one popular song suggested:

> Que le charlatan
>   Mesmer,
> Avec un au autre frater
> Guérisse mainte
>   femelle;
> Qu'il en tourne la
>   cervelle,
> En les tâtant ne sais où,
>   C'est fou,
>   Très fou,
> Et je n'y crois pas
>   tu tout;
> Mais je pense qu'il
>   magnétise
> Par la sottise.[4]

Mesmer's ideas quickly spread abroad through the efforts of men like Abbé de Faria, Bergasse, Joseph Deleuze, Richard Chenevix, George Winter, James Braid of Manchester, and John Elliotson, professor of medicine at University College Hospital in London, who experimented with hypnotism as an anesthetic in surgery. In 1838 Mesmer's system likewise traveled to the United States with the French lecturer Charles Poyen (who received encouragement from John Greenleaf Whittier of New England), and with the subsequent notoriety of American advocates, such as President Francis Wayland of Brown University, Silas Wright, Professor J. Stanley Grimes, La Roy Sunderland (pathetism), Charles Morley, Robert H. Collyer (psychography), Dodds, Buchanan, and Roswell Park (pantology). Despite this support one critical observer noted that the leading American practitioners of mesmerism "were men . . . of less general culture and possessing inferior qualifications for scientific investigation, so that the movement was marked by greater extravagance, and seems to have obtained less scientific recognition in America than in Europe."[5] Mesmerism in America was most often portrayed under the aegis of "electro-biology," where, for example, the patients of John Reid and John R. Wroe were hypnotized by staring at a disk and then made to carry out the suggestions of the operator.[6] In time the advocates of mesmerism merged into the larger mainstream of romantics, magnetic clairvoyants, transcendental mystics, hypnotists, and the outpouring of spiritualists that ran the gamut from Andrew Jackson Davis, the so-called seer of Poughkeepsie, who claimed that both Galen and Swedenborg had appeared to him, to the Kentucky peddlers of Bibles and nostrums like Oil of Smoke, and the mysterious rappings of the Fox sisters.[7]

Samuel Hahnemann and His "Shaking Doctors"

Far less extreme than the magnetic vapors of Mesmer but still outside the mainstream of medical orthodoxy stood the spiritual and vitalistic theory of Georg Ernst Stahl (1660–1734) of the University of Halle in Germany, court physician to the King of Prussia. Stahl's "animism," with principles borrowed from Paracelsus (1493–1514) and the "sensitive-soul" concept of the Belgian mystic Jean Baptiste van Helmont

(1577–1644), suggested that a rational soul governed the economy of man and was the protective power of the body and the actual healer of its diseases. Stahl observed that the soul possessed an inherent power to protect itself from external dangers that threatened health; it had the capacity to initiate certain bodily motions that would heal the constitution in disease. Although writers like Hippocrates, van Helmont, and Cullen had attributed such powers to what they variously called φύols, *archeus*, *vis conservatrix*, or *vis medicatrix naturae*, Stahl elevated his "anima" to the principal remedial element in the treatment of disease. In practice this meant that doctors should employ medicines only insofar as they aided nature. The followers of Stahl's system naturally objected to potent drugs, such as opium and bark, and rarely resorted to bleeding, vomiting, or the more powerful purging agents. Critics, on the other hand, accused Stahl and his followers of curing by expectation, employing only the most inert medicines, and trusting the powers of nature to be superior to treatment from their own hands.[8]

In the nineteenth century, the homeopathic system of medicine devised by Samuel Hahnemann (1755–1843) became one of the more successful descendants of Stahlian animism. The years of Hahnemann's intellectual development paralleled some of the most shattering events of the eighteenth and early nineteenth centuries. Revolution and the overthrow of age-old institutions and authorities occurred during the period Hahnemann was making his own break from traditional medicine. He graduated from medical school during the period of the American Revolution; and he lived through the agonies of the French Revolution, the overthrow of the Bourbon monarchy, and the military glories of Napoleon. His homeopathic system was the product of a turbulent era, full of speculation and high hopes, maturing prior to the great advances in pathological anatomy and chemistry that thoroughly revolutionized medical science. His system of homeopathy, as one doctor remarked in 1869, marked "the last remnant of the Dark Ages of medicine which has come down to modern times."[9] Hahnemann's aposticism was not without precedent, as ideas of earlier medical men had often matured during times of political and social turmoil. Paracelsus, for example, presented his major contributions at the time when Europe was awakening to the discovery of America and the impact of Luther's reformation of Christendom.

Homeopathy also came at an auspicious moment in medical science—a time when medical men were beginning to question several longstanding procedures, such as bleeding, cupping, heroic dosage, and salivation. Perhaps it was not so much what Hahnemann said or claimed to represent as the time frame in which he challenged existing therapeutics that made the history of homeopathy so important and its influence so pervasive. Significant in its faddish popularity among the upper classes, it also represented the last of the major medical systems to flourish before the onrush of extensive advances in germ theory, treatment of infection, pathology, and pharmaco-therapeutics. Although homeopathy emerged from the backwash of eighteenth century revolutionary speculation, it matured into a sophisticated medical system, half scientific, half spiritualistic, and decidedly high brow and upper class—a sort of metaphysical retreat for those tender consciences fleeing the brittleness of Victorian values. For many American and European intellectuals, homeopathy reflected an illusory escape from an otherwise materialistic century.

Samuel Christian Friedrich Hahnemann, the author of the homeopathic system, grew up at Meissen in Upper Saxony. He studied medicine first at the University of Leipzig and then at the University of Erlangen, where he supported himself by translating English and French works of medicine into his native language. Somewhat a ne'er-do-well during the first part of his medical career, Hahnemann perhaps established a record for having practiced in twenty-four different places by the time he was forty-eight years old—a situation that also reflected the depressed state of the medical profession in the latter part of the eighteenth and early nineteenth centuries. Because of a chronic lack of patients, a problem aggravated by residence in remote villages, he continued translating books, contributing to various scientific journals, and devoting his spare moments to chemistry, botany, and other interests. His translations included Stedtmann's *Physiological Essays and Observations* (1777), Nugent on *Hydrophobia* (1777), Ball's *Modern Practice of Physic* (1777), Cullen's *Treatise on the Materia Medica* (1790), Donald Monro's *Medical and Pharmaceutical Chemistry* (1791), John Grigg's *Advice to the Female Sex in Pregnancy* (1791), and Haller's *Materia Medica* (1806). His own writings during this period included essays on arsenic, washing soda, plumbago, glauber salts, tests for impure wine, the use of anthracite coal in baker's ovens, and the prevention of salivation.

In his translation of Cullen's *Treatise on the Materia Medica* in 1790, Hahnemann inaugurated an investigation that eventually culminated in the formulation of his own medical system. Dissatisfied with Cullen's discussion of the antipyretic virtues of Peruvian bark, he began a series of experiments on himself, discovering in the process that on taking the bark while in good health, he was attacked by what he interpreted as the symptoms of intermittent fever. Surprised at the similarity between the intermittent fever brought on by the bark and the intermittent fever of malaria, he concluded that the drug possessed the power of causing in healthy persons the same symptoms it cured in the sick. He became convinced that the paroxysm was actually caused by the bark and from this circumstance suspected that the curative properties of the bark depended upon this singular peculiarity. Subsequent experiments with belladonna produced a sore throat much like that evidenced in scarlet fever; sulphur caused an itch or eruption very similar to that for which it had so long been prescribed; and mercury produced symptoms that resembled syphilis. When he established a similar peculiarity with other medicinal agents, he divined that he had unraveled one of the great mysteries of medical science—a discovery as remarkable as Newton's law of gravitation. "It was the dawn of that bright light which now shines in the treatment of disease," he wrote, "for it led me to establish and demonstrate the law that disease can only be cured by remedies which produce symptoms in the healthy body similar to those of the disease to be relieved."[10]

Hahnemann thus concluded that the curative basis of medicines in the materia medica stemmed from their power to induce in healthy persons symptoms analogous to the diseases for which they were administered. He considered those medicines which best produced these symptoms to be the most efficacious in the pharmacopoeia. This meant that doctors should employ purgative medicines in cases of diarrhea, emetic remedies for vomiting, and opium and astringents for costiveness. Hahnemann, who claimed that no other physician except Albrecht von Haller had emphasized the importance of drug experimentation on healthy subjects, eventually built from his own experiments the foundations of his epic work *Organon of Homeopathic Medicine* (1810). Hahnemann named the book after Bacon's *Organon* to support his claim that the homeopathic system had been based on experiment and inductive reasoning. As far as he was concerned, medical science had at long last emerged from twenty-five centuries of Hippocratic confusion.[11]

In the same year in which Hahnemann published his *Organon*, he returned to the University of Leipzig as a public medical lecturer on the principles of his system. It was there, too, that he publicly attacked orthodox medicine, vilifying it for vulgar practices and crude therapeutic procedures. Hahnemann's first principle of therapeutics became *similia similibus curantur*, or like cures like, and the followers of this system distinguished their school with the term *homeopathy* (from the Greek word *homoion, similar,* and meaning analogous suffering or the use of remedies that produce effects like the disease) and designated their opponents as allopaths (from the Greek word *alloion, different,* meaning the use of remedies whose effects differed from but were not directly opposite to the disease) or antipaths (meaning the application of remedies that produced effects opposite to the disease). Hahnemann regarded most physicians who came before him as so much "learned lumber" and unblushingly recommended his own system as the only certain method of curing disease. His pretensions and those of his followers led homeopaths to follow a strict sectarian path, defying developments in anatomy and pathology and considering themselves the exclusive professors of medical truth. "The day of the true knowledge of remedies, and a true system of therapeutics will dawn," Hahnemann wrote, "when physicians shall abandon the systems and opinions which have heretofore swayed the minds of the profession."[12] Before long the maxim *similia similibus curantur* became the watchword of the new school. "I am persuaded," Hahnemann observed in his *Organon*, "that diseases yield to remedies which produce analogous affection (*similia similibus*)—burns are cured by keeping the parts affected before the fire—frostbite by applying snow or cold water—inflammations and contusions by spirituous lotions." [13]

Actually, Hahnemann did not originate the principle *similia similibus curantur*. Hippocrates, the father of physic, had called notice to it two thousand years earlier; and the Danish philosopher and physician Stahl had pointed it out nearly a century before Hahnemann. There were, in fact, numerous writers, both in and out of medicine, who had commented on the principle.

> Some diseases can be treated best by contraries and some by similars. Hippocrates, 460–370 B.C.

> Diseases are cured by remedies which affect the organism similarly to the disease. Theophrastus, 370–286 B.C.

> A hot disease has never been cured by cold remedy, nor a cold disease by a hot remedy. Like attacks its like and never its contrary. Paracelsus, 1493–1541.

> Like cures like but contraries do not. Basil Valentine, circa 1602.

> I am persuaded that diseases are subdued by agents which produce a similar affection. Stahl, 1660–1734. [14]

What incurred the wrath of the regulars was not so much Hahnemann's first principle as the heretical assertions that quickly followed, including his belief that diseases resulted from neither mechanical nor chemical changes of the body but from spiritual, dynamic disturbances of life. He once remarked, "Disease will not, out of deference to our stupidity, cease to be dynamic aberrations, which our spiritual existence undergoes in its mode of feeling and acting—that is to say IMMATERIAL changes in the state of health." [15] In a condition of good health, the spiritual force that animated the material body ruled supreme. However, in sickness, "this spiritlike, self-acting vital force, omnipresent in the organism, was alone primarily deranged by dynamic influence of some morbific agency inimical to life." In making this distinction, Hahnemann steered his homeopathic system away from orthodox medicine. For him disease had no anatomical basis; functional disturbances of the body resulted from a pertur-

bation of the body's spiritual force rather than from a molecular, chemical, or structural derangement. In other words,
a universal harmony (*a summum bonum*) ruled over the physical world, with disease resulting from a dysfunction in the
harmony between man and nature. Disease existed by virtue
of the dynamic alterations of vital force between matter and
spirit, and the morbid symptoms felt by the patient constituted the only form of disease.[16]

The role of the homeopath lay in finding the dynamic,
specific medicinal agent to influence the vital force and destroy the disease. "Drugs become curative remedies capable
of obliterating disease," Hahnemann once remarked, "only
through their power of creating certain disturbances and
symptoms; that is, by producing a certain artificial diseased
condition, they cancel and exterminate the symptoms already present, that is, the natural diseased condition which it
is intended to cure." Borrowing from John Hunter's idea
that two similar diseases could not exist in the body because
the stronger would eventually expel the weaker, Hahnemann
concluded that drug-induced diseases made a more powerful impression on the body than spontaneous diseases. A
drug given to the ailing patient expelled the disease, and
then its own effect—which was limited in duration, since it
was artificially produced—slowly subsided.[17]

Once Hahnemann determined which medicines were most
efficacious in curing, he began to experiment with proper
dosage. At first, he employed full doses of medicine according to the common practice among regulars in the profession. He found, however, that medicines normally prescribed
(provided they were administered according to the law of
similars) were usually successful in removing disease but
were unnecessarily harsh on the patient's constitution, often
to the point of aggravating the symptoms. Having determined that disease was nonmaterial, he proceeded to deny
the relevance of existing drug therapy by insisting that crude
or "vulgar" drugs could not free the vital force brought on by
morbid disturbances except through the "spirit-like alterative powers of appropriate remedies." By gradually diminishing the dosage, he attempted to ascertain at what point the
medicine still retained its power over disease.[18]

In experimenting with dosage, Hahnemann discovered

that he could reduce the reliable amount of drug to a minis-
cule amount; accomplishing this, he began to suspect that the
manner in which he prepared his medicines had added to
the medicinal potency of the properties. From Baron Stoerck
of Vienna he borrowed the procedure of triturating his medicines with sugar of milk (*saccharum lactis*)—of mixing or rubbing the crude drug into the medium (sugar of milk) in
which it was administered. From these elements Hahnemann
erected the doctrine of potentization or dynamization, which
stated that as medicines underwent attenuation they were
increased in power by the very process of being rubbed or
shaken; a dynamic or spiritual power was transferred into
the crude drug during the preparation of the dilution.
Hahnemann compared the friction of the medicine with its
medium with that of striking flint or rubbing dry sticks together to create fire. He explained:

> It appears that it was reserved for me, to discover this prop-
> erty, the influence of which is such that by virtue of it, sub-
> stances which are never known to possess medicinal proper-
> ties, acquire a surprising energy. Thus, gold, silver, and wood
> charcoal, are without action upon man in their ordinary state.
> The most delicate person could take several grains of gold or
> silver foil, or charcoal, without the least medicinal effect.
> From the constant rubbing for an hour of one grain with one
> hundred grains of powdered sugar of milk, there results a
> preparation already possessed of considerable medicinal vir-
> tue. But, take a grain of that preparation, rub it for another
> hour, with a hundred grains of sugar of milk, and continue
> the same process until each grain of the last preparation shall
> contain only the quadrillionth part of a grain of gold, you will
> then possess a preparation in which the medicinal virtue of
> the gold will be so developed, that it will be sufficient to put
> one grain of it into a phile, and to cause a melancholy person
> whose disgust of life has brought him to the verge of suicide,
> to breathe it for a few seconds, when in one hour, the
> wretched being will be relieved from the wicked demon, and
> restored to a relish of life![19]

Some have suggested that Hahnemann borrowed the idea
of potentization from the third chapter of Cervantes' *Don
Quixote*: "In the plains and deserts no aid was near, unless
they had some sage enchantress for their friend—who would
give them immediate assistance by conveying, in a cloud

through the air, some damsel or dwarf with a phial of water, possessed of some virtue that upon tasting a single drop of it, would instantly become as sound as if they had received no injury." Others traced the source to the Prince of Orange, who at the seige of Breda in 1625 reputedly revived his sick and exhausted soldiers by passing among them several phials of chamomile, wormwood, and camphor, claiming them to be potent medicines whose single drop would restore health. The influence of Anton Mesmer must not be ignored either, since Hahnemann believed that the shaking process produced a spiritualization or electrization of the medicine in which the particles underwent a radical change from a crude form into a dynamic curative force. Hahnemann probably borrowed this principle from Mesmer's reputed ability to communicate extraordinary power to inert substances such as trees, chairs, tables, and iron rods. Hahnemann had, in fact, endorsed mesmerism; he wrote in his *Organon* that "none but madmen can entertain doubt of its curative powers." He observed that the homeopathic system for curing disease could profit from the assistance of a mesmerizer, particularly when a homeopathic dose produced a state of excessive irritability over the patient. "Under such circumstances," he commented, "the hand of the mesmerizer gently sliding down and frequently touching the part affected, produces a uniform distribution of the vital power through the system and rest, sleep, and health are restored." [20]

Until Hahnemann moved in the direction of his infinitesimal doses, much of his theory brought praise—albeit grudgingly—from the regulars. He had favored less heroic procedures in medicine, encouraged experiments with drugs on healthy persons, endeavored to cure disease with single remedies and uncomplicated prescriptions, and demanded a high standard of purity in the preparation of medicines. But for Hahnemann the doctrine of infinitesimals signaled an equally significant change in medical therapeutics, one that would challenge such traditional medical procedures as cupping, leeching, blistering, counterirritation, liniments, fomentations, poultices, and ointments. Now doctors could replace the most violent emetics with a thirteenth dilution of pulsatilla, or cure an overloaded stomach in two hours with a single whiff of a globule of sugar impregnated with the thirty-

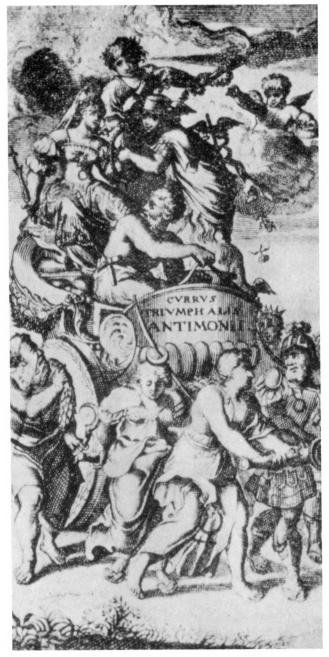

Basil Valentine, *Triumphal Chariot of Antimony*, frontispiece.
Courtesy of Indiana University.

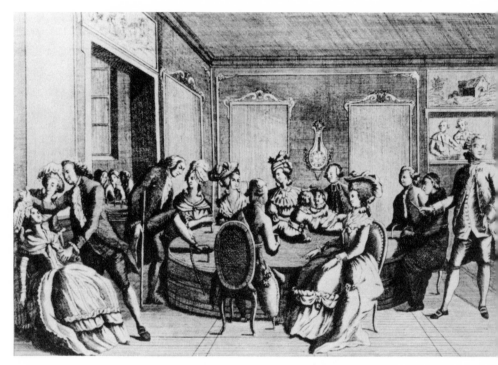

Mesmer (right), wand in hand, moves around the baquet surrounded by persons from various walks of life. Conspicuous are the military with decorations (front center), the religious with habit and skullcap (right), and the lawyer with distinctive collar (rear center). Courtesy of Historical Pictures Service, Inc., Chicago.

ninth dilution of pulsatilla and energized by a simple mesmeric touching.[21] In an age when the doctrines of John Brown, Benjamin Rush, and F. J. V. Broussais were terrorizing patients with heroic purgings, bleedings, and opiates, homeopathic practitioners were successfully treating patients "not because of deeds of commission, but by deeds of omission."[22]

Hahnemann usually carried his attenuations to the thirtieth power; but others like Franz Hartmann of Germany and Korsakoff of St. Petersburg diluted their medicines as many as fifteen hundred times without, they claimed, a diminution of energy. As one critic explained it, "the sulphur existing in one humming bird's egg is more than enough to impregnate millions of hogsheads to the fortieth dilution, and not only abundantly sufficient to supply all the homeopaths in this world, but in all worlds, if they are filled with homeopaths."[23] Another skeptic suggested a parallel. "Take one pound of flour, and by rubbing it in a mortar, you gain enough nutriment to feed twenty men. Carry your grinding still further, and you can perform a greater miracle than our blessed Saviour did when he fed the . . . multitude with the few loaves and fishes."[24]

Along with sulphur, which Hahnemann prescribed as the principal cure-all of homeopathic medicine, his six-volume *Materia Medica Pura* (1826–28) listed an arsenal of more than two hundred additional drugs, including flint, clay, chalk, and common table salt. When properly potentized, salt became a "powerful and heroical medicament, which can only be administered to patients with the greatest caution."[25] In addition to the more common drugs, such as conium, belladonna, red pepper, pulsatilla, bryonia, and aconite, the homeopathic pharmacopoeia also contributed cockroach (*blatta Americana*) and skunk fluid (*mephitis*), along with West Indian spider (*tarantula cubensis*) and bed bugs (*cimex*) for ulcers. Dr. Samuel Swan, who sold homeopathic remedies in New York, advertised a witch's brew of pharmaceutical curiosities in his *Catalogue of Morbific Products, Nosodes, and Other Remedies in High Potencies* (1886), including pus from rectal and septic abscesses, pus from caries of os calsis, "vomito—blood from yellow fever patient while moribund," gravel from lungs (*calcaria pulmonum*), secreted salt from a "gentleman's scalp," chimney soot (*fuligo communis*), moonlight, sunlight, constipation of newborn infant (*colostrom*), tears of a young girl in great fear and suffering (*lachryma filia*), body lice (*pediculus corporis*) from Boston, and menstrual blood from a woman who had warts (*verucca menstruo*).[26]

Unlike the regulars in medicine who employed the word *symptoms* to refer only to those affections which accompanied disease, homeopaths applied the term to medicines as they affected both healthy and diseased individuals. The ingestion by healthy persons of an attenuation of sulphur, for example, produced some two thousand symptoms or "provings," aconite over five hundred, arsenic with sulphur over one thousand, pulsatilla about eleven hundred, oyster shell (*calcarea*) over one thousand, and plumbago nearly six hundred. Numerous drugs in Hahnemann's *Materia Medica Pura* caused peculiar symptoms or provings in the reproductive functions. Aconite, for example, produced an "itching of the prepuce, with increase of sexual functions," angustura incited "voluptuous itching at the tip of the glands, which forces one to rub," nitrate of silver produced an "effusion of semen almost every night," arnica montana brought on "violent sexual desire and continued erections," camphor caused an "increase of sexual desire," and ambra grisea in a dose of a millionth of a grain caused "violent itching of the pudendum, which has to be rubbed." This seeming emphasis upon the sexual nature of the body induced one critic to suggest that the partisans of "this moonshine and mosquito system of medical practice are a very libidinous set of fellows."[27]

Despite these eccentricities, the provings of homeopathy spelled out a clear therapeutic approach to disease. Responsibility lay in ascertaining the symptoms that accompanied a patient's illness and then finding the proper medicine from among the drugs that produced a similar set of pathogenetic symptoms or provings. In effect, the homeopath became a cataloguer of symptoms who compared notes made in the sickroom with the list of provings in the *Materia Medica Pura*. Each major sensation was subdivided into a multitude of more specific forms. Homeopaths divided pain into simple, obtuse, compressing, bending, jamming, pinching, twisting, gnawing, scratching, and jerking. According to Gottlieb H. G. Jahr, one of the major oracles in homeopathic practice, there was a specific for each symptom: one for blueness of the nose, along with one for blueness of the lips or face; one for clammy perspiration of the cheeks, longing to get out of bed, wishing to cry, and ringing in the ears; and even one for fear of death. When the symptoms of the disease matched the symptoms created by the medicine on the healthy constitution, the homeopath knew he had found the true specific. Popular homeopathic textbooks, including Boenninghausen's *Therapeutic Pocket-Book*, Jahr's *Symptomen-Codex*, Hahnemann's *Materia Medica Pura*, and countless *Repertories* contained multitudinous lists of symptoms that aided the physician in selecting the proper remedies. As a result of this emphasis on symptoms, homeopaths were accused of discarding anatomy, physiology, and pathology as the worn-out baggage of an earlier medical era.[28]

Soon after Hahnemann announced his claims to the world, various governments ordered experiments to judge the veracity of the system. In 1829 the King of Naples appointed a commission to test homeopathic remedies under strict rules of supervision. After a trial period, the commission concluded that homeopathy had no effect in treating disease and that in some cases its use had actually prevented the employment of remedies capable of curing. In tests conducted in Berlin, doctors discovered that the effects of sugar of milk were virtually the same as when triturated with medicine. A medical council established to make recommendations on the basis of these experiments concluded that patients in both instances were cured *vis medicatrix naturae*; and, following the council's advice, the German government prohibited homeopathic practice. The Russian government forbade the system after the failure of tests in several military hospitals. Homeopathy was likewise banned after experimental studies in Vienna and Rome proved it unefficacious. In 1834 a German homeopath petitioned the Egyptian government to test the system in the Hospital of Cairo, claiming that its relative cheapness would greatly benefit the government and people. After an unsuccessful experiment designed to demonstrate the effectiveness of the attenuations, the Egyptian Council of Health decided that those cures which did occur "were due simply to the hygienic and dietetic treatment adopted and not at all to the infinitesimal doses."

Distinguished French homeopath Guerard attributed the

failure of experiments at the Hôtel Dieu de Lyon in 1832 to the "deleterious miasma" that pervaded the hospital. The very remedies that worked so well in his own private practice, he argued, were ineffective "owing to the emanations from the bodies of persons collected together, which neutralized the infinitesimal doses." A similar experiment conducted in the Hôpital de la Pitié of Paris under the supervision of Gabriel Andral also proved ineffective, and hospital administrators had to direct that the patients be treated with regular medicines. When the Homeopathic Society of Paris petitioned for the establishment of a hospital and dispensary in 1835, the Academy of Medicine conducted yet another test. On the basis of its negative results, the Academy argued that to grant the petition would only encourage every other form of quackery, including mesmerism and animal magnetism, to petition for hospitals of their own. On the advice of the Academy, the Minister of Public Instruction refused the petition.[29]

Orthodox American medicine preferred to regard Hahnemann's system as a by-product of Germany's political and social turbulence. Alexander N. Dougherty, M.D., wrote in 1848, "A country where thought on political subjects can have no vent, because of the surveillance of the censorship, and because of an organized all-pervading system of espionage, almost demanding the secrets of men's hearts, is just fitted to foster metaphysical vagaries of the wildest order, rivaling in their fantastic gambols the poetic flights of Grecian and Roman mythology." He viewed homeopathy as one avenue of escape from Germany's authoritarian society. Just as the soul had become the active principle for the body in the metaphysical philosophies of Kant, Hegel, and Fichte, so also in Hahnemann's *Materia Medica Pura* "the matter of medicine merely encloses a spiritual essence; and as the soul must be freed from its gross corporeity to exhibit its full perfections, so the matter of medicines must be divided infinitesimally to allow their spiritual essence to work best on the human spirit."[30]

Dougherty's remarks were perceptive but inconclusive, since homeopathy had actually made its greatest converts in France and later in America. Even Hahnemann recognized the potential response to his system outside Germany. "Let homeopathy but reach Paris," he wrote, "and it is saved." In making this remark, the author of the homeopathic system merely confirmed what Prince Metternich had reputedly said to the phrenologist Franz Joseph Gall: "Go to Paris; if you can only get Parisians to laugh at your bumps, you will not fail of reputation." Perhaps Dougherty's analysis was little more than a visceral reaction to the growing numbers of German immigrants who sought political asylum in America after the turmoil of the 1848 revolutions in Europe, bringing with them ideas of homeopathic medicine. But homeopathy had already made successful inroads among the German families that had migrated from Saxony to Northampton County in Pennsylvania. As early as 1825, Swedenborgian homeopath Hans Burch Gram (1786–1840), an American of Danish extraction, set up practice in New York. Samuel Gregg, one of the founders of the American Institute of Homeopathy, practiced in Massachusetts in the late 1830s. Other early converts included John F. Gray and Abraham D. Wilson in 1829, A. Gerald Hull in 1830, and William Channing (cousin of William Ellery Channing) in 1832. Channing, an adherent of the physiological system of Broussais, converted to homeopathy in mid-life as a result of successfully employing camphor, veratrum, and cuprum as prescribed by Hahnemann for cholera. With his conversion came a number of other American physicians, along with political and religious liberals, including first Unitarians and then zealots of Transcendentalism. Noted American believers in homeopathy included William Wadsworth Longfellow, William Lloyd Garrison, Nathaniel Hawthorne, Julia Ward Howe, Louisa May Alcott, Daniel Webster, William Seward, and John D. Rockefeller. While Gram and the New York homeopaths administered the equivalent of first and second centesimal dilutions, the New England homeopaths promptly accepted the potentizing theory of Hahnemann and observed the founder's faith in high triturations. This latter group, which imbibed heavily in the flightly transports of American romanticism, found Hahnemann a welcome bedfellow to their native philosophical delights.[31]

In 1835 Swiss immigrant Henry Detwiller, who converted to homeopathy in the late 1820s, and Constantine Herring (1800–1880), who is often called the father of American homeopathy, established at Allentown, Pennsylvania, the Nordamerikanische Akademie der Homeopathischen Heikunst to instruct students in the German language. The academy closed its doors in 1841; and in 1848 Herring and an associate, William Wesselhoeft, obtained a charter for the Homeopathic Medical College.[32] The first periodical devoted to homeopathy published in the United States appeared in 1835 under the title *The American Journal of Homeopathia*. It was soon followed by the *Homeopathic Examiner* (1840–47), *Miscellanies on Homeopathy* (1838–39), *The Homeopathic Pioneer* (1845–46), and *The South Western Homeopathic Journal and Review* (1847–50). By the 1840s converts to homeopathy increased with the publication of Jahr's *Manual*; and men like A. Haynel of Baltimore, G. M. Taft of New Orleans, James B. Gilbert of Savannah, Robert Rosman and P. P. Wells of Brooklyn began proselytizing Hahnemann's system throughout the young republic. Dr. Storm Rosa, who held a position in the Cincinnati Eclectic Institute, became the first homeopathic teacher in the West, and in 1850 the Cleveland Homeopathic College opened its doors. Perhaps a sense of theoretical security amid massive changes in medical therapeutics and of metaphysical simplicity amid the growth of scientific skepticism brought a continual stream of converts to seek solace in Hahnemann's monistic therapeutics.[33]

Another reason for Hahnemann's popularity stemmed from the troubled spirit of the American romantics during the decades preceding the Civil War. The burgeoning prosperity of the new nation, the travails of industrialism, the awakened response to new individualism, and the uneasy religious conscience, a relic of the Puritan past, left their mark upon a generation of intellectuals seeking new sources of truth and righteousness. While some sought the solace of nirvana through the rapturous mysticism of Swedenborg or communed with Nature through the transparent eyeball of Emerson, still others, who were more antinomian in character, set out to reshape society through perfectionist organizations that varied as widely as the solipsisms that motivated their thought. Not too surprisingly, the anti-institutional bias of these transcendental voyagers fell equally hard upon traditional medicine, although the onus they displayed stemmed less from a seasoned critique of orthodox therapeutic practices than it did from a passionate distrust of anything bearing the stamp of tradition. As protagonists for an awakened consciousness that blossomed amid the harshness of the factory system, the evils of slavery, and the temptations of demon rum, those same romantics, not inconsistently, became vague kinsmen of Hahnemann's medical theories.

Orthodox Reaction

Regulars relished every opportunity to accuse Hahnemann of being an arrogant medical vaporer, whose real "sheet anchor" was a compound of water and time and whose system was no more than a well-disguised plan to carry out the expectant treatment for disease. One form of popular criticism included the well-published poem entitled "Homeopathy."

> Take a little rum,
>   The less you take the better;
> Mix it with the lakes
>   Of Werner and of Wetter.
>
> Dip a spoonful out—
>   Mind you don't get groggy.
> Pour it in the lake
>   Winnipisiogee.
>
> Stir the mixture well,
>   Lest it prove inferior;
> Then put half a drop
>   Into Lake Superior.[34]

Doctors were fond of comparing Hahnemann's theories with those of the metaphysical idealist Bishop George Berkeley (1685–1753), who had once advocated tar water as a specific for nearly all the ills of man. But as Oliver Wendell Holmes caustically remarked, Berkeley "was an illustrious man, but he held two very odd opinions; that tar water was everything and that the material universe was nothing." And when the bishop took ill suddenly, Holmes added, "there was not time enough to stir up a quart of his panacea."[35] According to one New England physician, homeopath was just another name for those physicians who had degenerated into "listless waiters upon providence." The homeopath was "a sort of medical Micawber, waiting for something to turn up:

and this more than oriental fatalism does not always disappoint, for something does turn up, and it is generally the toes of the patient." Fortunately for the country, he concluded, "these transcendental speculators mostly infest the large cities."[36]

The belief in the recuperative powers of nature was certainly not a novel idea for the nineteenth century. Many of the earliest medical theorists had recognized the importance of the body's own life forces. As Celsus once wrote: *"Natura repugnate, nihil proficit medicina."* ("If nature does not cooperate, the medicine is useless.") According to orthodox critics, however, homeopaths had made the doctrine all and the medicine nothing. Admittedly homeopaths did not deny the reparative powers of medicine, but their infinitesimal doses encouraged others to draw that conclusion. Critics of Hahnemann suggested that in those cases where homeopathic treatment had proved successful, imagination had probably been a major factor. "Mental stimulus of hope is one of the best of medicines," a practitioner remarked in the 1830s, "and if it can be exhibited in a globule of Homeopathic sugar, the latter will effect wonders."

Remembering the reputed cures of Mesmer's *baquet* and of the patented "magnetic tractors" of the Connecticut charlatan Elisha Perkins in 1798, doctors were reluctant to fall prey to yet another sectarian. Opponents of Hahnemann concluded that the cures attributable to homeopathy were nothing more than the product of suggestion and imagination, the very sources to which Benjamin Franklin and his colleagues in the French Royal Commission had attributed the cures of Mesmer's animal magnetism. "While, then, we acknowledge the powerful influence of the mind upon disease, and the value of securing the confidence of our patients, and the importance of sustaining their hopes," a doctor observed in 1838, "let us be careful that we do not confound effects purely mental, with the inherent properties of medicine."[37] The evil of homeopathy, L. A. Dugas, M.D., of Georgia explained, came not just from its unwholesome effect upon the imagination of the doctor, but from its efforts "to enthrall the patient . . . in the misty mazes of [the doctor's] absurdities, by having him also to believe in the remedial potency of inert doses." Although most practitioners at some time in their career employed a placebo for the imagined ills of a complaining hypochondriac, it was another matter for physicians to interpret the inert substance as an actual remedial agent. Perhaps, Dugas remarked, doctors should try to enlighten patients more to the truths of medical science. He confessed, however, that of all the forms of charlatanism, he preferred homeopathy, since it dealt with harmless medicines rather than with serious mischief.[38]

Edward Waldo Emerson, physician and son of the transcendentalist, urged practitioners to hold a middle course between the extremes of expectant medicine and heroic therapeutics. Like his father, the son gave ample license to the yearnings of the age, but stood apart from any formal commitment to sectarian claims. Since medicine was not an exact science like mathematics, the gaps in medical knowledge made "all the more room for growth, for genius" to enlarge the scope and methods of physicians. With clear observation, responsible experimentation, and proper scientific usage, physicians could grow in both knowledge and humanity. A good doctor must be able to apply what was tried and safe, yet be willing to challenge the past with a healthy skepticism that was solidly based in new observation and scientific knowledge. "We must take large views, stand apart, like the artist, and follow his rule," Emerson wrote, and "look three times at the figure of the ideal physician to once at our poor copy of him."[39]

Homeopaths strongly resented being identified as heretics by the medical orthodoxy but grudgingly credited the regulars with consistency. In 1870 homeopath A. D. Lippe wrote, the regulars "admit only such persons to membership in their various medical societies as are fully qualified practitioners, and who adhere to what they, as a body, take the liberty to consider legitimate practice; and they will summarily expel any member from their societies who violates their rules or code of ethics." Unfortunately, he observed, homeopaths were not as consistent. For a system that proclaimed superiority over allopathy, it not only tolerated excessive freedom of medical opinion to the point of subverting the principles of its founder, but it also freely admitted persons into its medical colleges merely because they claimed to be homeopaths. Across America, Lippe pointed out, self-proclaimed homeopaths were practicing a sort of "mongrel allopathy" by following Hahnemann's advice in compounding their own prescriptions but then administering drugs in traditionally heroic dosages. Growing numbers of men and women who identified themselves as homeopathic physicians were consistently ignoring the laws of homeopathic therapeutics. Lippe hoped that homeopathic physicians would imitate the strictness of the regulars when it came to self-government by expelling those who refused to practice the rules taught and promulgated by Hahnemann.[40]

Winds of Change

With the exception of its New England disciples, American homeopahy never slavishly imitated Hahnemann's complete system. Despite the mental affinity that attracted many to his doctrines, converts were willing to work out compromises between the conflicting tendencies of matter and spirit. As early as the 1840s, American homeopaths began improvising on the doctrines of their founder. While they continued to admit the efficacy of Hahnemann's attenuations, they interpreted the dynamization principle as analogous to infection by miasma. Accordingly, "the active principle of the drug being set free by the destruction of the matter, it communicates itself to the vehicle [the miasma of syphilis, sycosis, or psora] and becomes infected and as active as the drug itself."[41] More changes followed, and the rise in popularity of the new system resulted in the creation of the American Institute of Homeopathy in 1844, the Homeopathic Medical College in Philadelphia in 1848, and the unsuccessful but vigorous attempt in 1857 to set aside one-half of New York's Bellevue Hospital for the practice of homeopathy. The New York Medical College and Hospital for Women, chartered in 1863, was not only a homeopathic clinic, but also the first woman's medical college in America. During the Civil War, Senator James W. Grimes of Iowa introduced a bill that would have opened the medical department of the army to homeopathic appointments and placed a select number of hospitals in the District of Columbia under homeopathic supervision. Although Lincoln signed the bill into law, homeopaths obtained only a negligible number of commissions as surgeons in the army—usually under the aegis of orthodoxy—and the government refused to permit any hospitals to come under their control.[42]

By the 1870s the majority of American homeopaths neither confined their therapeutics to the single principle of similars, nor relied wholly upon infinitesimal doses or potentization; in fact, many were unabashedly treating disease with dram doses. Although they loudly condemned remedies like bleeding, cupping, and blistering, some homeopaths willingly employed these very methods in their medical practice. One prosperous St. Louis homeopath, for example, made frequent use of Victor Theodore Junod's enormous cupping boots, which were applied to the entire lower half of the body to artifically establish a powerful derivation of blood.[43] Despite Hahnemann's reluctance to employ anything but homeopathic medicines, his American disciples turned to electric shocks, cold water douches, water baths, bloodletting, leeches, metallic chains, and hypnotism. Gynecologists who practiced homeopathy relied on an assortment of mechanical devices, surgery, dress and diet changes, and adopted methods of cure strikingly similar to those employed by the regulars.[44] After facing repeated criticism from regulars concerning infinitesimal dosage, the relationship of homeopathy to animal magnetism, psychotherapy, and the dynamization of its drugs, homeopaths began to give ground by refusing to accept literally and unconditionally the doctrines of Hahnemann. As German homeopath Heischel observed, the *Organon* had to be read "*cum grano salis.*"[45] The internal changes in their therapeutic principles were so extensive that the New York *Homeopathic Medical Times* noted in the 1880s that the system had divided itself between the high and low potency parties, each advocating theories considered subversive by the other.[46] The extent of these changes became evident in 1877, when the president of the British Homeopathic Society urged a union of allopathy and homeopathy on the ground that the views of Hahnemann were "extravagant and incorrect," and infinitesimal doses were practically abandoned by the school.[47] According to A. B. Palmer, in the *North American Review* in 1882, "there is not a tenet, as presented by the founder of the system, which has not been rejected by members who are regarded as of high authority in the homeopathic fraternity."[48]

The realization that Hahnemann's provings and symptomatology were far less scientific than the knowledge of microscopic and chemical changes in tissues and organs brought homeopaths even closer to the position of the regulars. "In making drug-provings," a homeopath remarked in 1874, "we should not be satisfied with the manifestations of mere subjective or general functional symptoms, but in accordance with the scientific knowledge of our day also include in the field of our observations the finer pathological, physiological, anatomical, and chemical manifestations." [49] Perhaps the most revealing statement came from an editorial in the *Homeopathic News* of 1892. "We venture to assert," the author stated, "that had not our school drifted away from the practice of forty years ago, it would have been dead and buried long since."

> We have drifted away from the practice of giving a pellet of the two-hundredth or higher, and waiting thirty or sixty days for its curative effects; from the prescribing of a high dilution by smelling the dry pellets, those same pellets "grafted" by shaking a thousand pure pellets with one medicated by the ten thousandth.
>
> We have drifted away from a belief in provings made by taking a single dose of the one-thousandth, thirtieth, or third even, and then recording all the symptoms felt by the prover— natural symptoms, colds, diarrhoea, etc., for the next sixty days!
>
> We have drifted away from the carrying of a pocket repertory to the bedside of the patient, and recording the symptoms in columns, and a weary search in said repertory until a mechanical similimum was found.
>
> We have drifted away from the narration of miraculous cures with the highest attenuations, which were not cures at all, but a spontaneous finale of a self-limited disease.
>
> We have drifted from the days when our practitioners would sit by the bedside of a woman dying of uterine hemorrhage, hunting in the repertory for the "indicated remedy," while the vital fluid was ebbing away, without recourse to the tampon or ergot. [50]

One major reason for the retreat from the doctrines of Hahnemann was the glaring lack of textbooks written by homeopathic doctors. The fact that homeopathic colleges of medicine relied heavily on old-school authorities became a serious indictment of the internal developments in homeopathy after the death of its founder. The inability of the system to keep pace with the developments of orthodox medicine forced its medical schools to fall back on the standard texts of the regulars despite the fact that orthodox texts presented medicine in a manner opposed to their own. Ironically, the reliance on standard medical texts meant a gradual tightening of the homeopaths' own standards and, more important, a growing consistency in overall medical practice. By the 1880s and 1890s, the requirements for graduation from the Hahnemann Medical College of Philadelphia were remarkably similar to most orthodox medical schools of the day. The three-year program included courses on anatomy, physiology, chemistry, surgery, therapeutics, pharmacy, and toxicology. The books used for its courses—Wood's *Therapeutics*; Taylor on poisons; Mann on prescription writing; Stillé and Maisch's *Dispensatory*; the *U.S. Pharmacopoeia*; Gross's *Surgery*; Draper, Ganot, Fownes, and Attfield in practical chemistry; Gray, Wilson, and Leidy on anatomy; Dalton, Foster, and Green on pathology; Tyson's *Urinary Analysis*; Agnew's *Surgery*; Playfair's *Obstetrics*; Duhring on *Diseases of the Skin*; and Reese's *Medical Jurisprudence*—were identical with those used in the schools of the regulars. Not surprisingly, many homeopaths, upon graduation, declined to connect themselves publicly with the doctrines of Hahnemann and refused even to use the name homeopath in their own identification.[51]

By the later decades of the nineteenth century, reform homeopathy had achieved sufficient respectability to suggest the need for compromise between the two schools. Sensing this the State of New York passed a law recognizing homeopathy and directing state commissioners to examine license applications in both homeopathy and allopathy. Scarcely eighteen years after Oliver Wendell Holmes denounced homeopathy as "dilute moonshine" and predicted the quick extinction of the heresy, the City Council of Boston gave a banquet for the members of the American Institute of Homeopathy. In fact, by the 1890s, Massachusetts homeopaths boasted of several Hahnemannian societies, a dispensary, a surgical hospital, the Westborough Insane Hospital, Boston

University School of Medicine, and five hospitals that offered both allopathic and homeopathic treatment. The New York Ophthalmic Hospital passed into the hands of homeopathy; and, even more significantly, the State of Michigan in 1875 directed its legislature to establish a homeopathic medical college at the University of Michigan. Signs of change also included an appropriation of $400,000 by the New York legislature for the establishment of a homeopathic insane asylum, a decision by the Common Council of St. Louis requiring professors of medicine to admit homeopathic medical students to hospital clinics, a New York court decision that fined a physician for accusing a homeopath of quackery, the increasing failure of allopaths to control the state licensing system for medical practice, and a statistical report by a life insurance company in the 1880s indicating that the homeopathic system was as effective in safeguarding human life as the allopathic system.[52]

Although homeopathy capitulated to the regulars' position by becoming less sectarian, the system achieved a surprising degree of success and recognition. For one thing, orthodox medicine adopted homeopathic drugs, such as *cocculus indicus* for paralysis, *pulsatilla nigricans* for uterine problems, *drosers rotundifolia* in whooping cough, *apis mellefica* in rheumatism, and the popular aconite and veratum. A regular remarked in 1882, "We cannot now, as we could twenty-five years or so ago, hurl at the homeopath . . . the epithet of quack, for he is now, as a rule, no longer an 'ignorant pretender'."[53] By the turn of the century, there were 143 homeopathic medical societies, 112 homeopathic hospitals, 59 dispensaries, 35 medical journals, and 14,000 practicing homeopaths (of whom 1,158 were women) who were graduates of some 20 homeopathic colleges.[54] In 1900 American homeopaths even dedicated a monument to Hahnemann in the nation's capital. Hahnemann had succeeded in giving impetus to the systematic study of physiological action of medicines, compelled men to question the heroic doctrines of the past, including the use of the lancet, blistering, and polypharmacy, and had given strong encouragement to the pharmaceutical preparation of fresh drugs. Finally, he had urged regulars to have more understanding and appreciation for *vis medicatrix naturae* by questioning whether medication alone could cure disease. From both the mesmerist and homeopath, the profession also learned something of the relationship of mind to cure. Medicine had traveled a great distance from venesection to the homeopath's use of aconite; from Alexander's Golden Antidote containing seventy-seven ingredients to the single remedies of Hahnemann; from the cruelties meted out to the insane to the nonrestraint system Hahnemann introduced in 1792; from salivation and blue mass to infinitesimal doses of mercury; from the use of blisters, setons, issues, caustics, and cauteries to the use of moist heat; and from the heroic consumption of purgatives to mild laxatives.[55]

By the closing decades of the century, homeopaths had retreated from their doctrines to the degree that they no longer based their practice on exclusive dogma to the exclusion of the accumulated experience of medical science and the aids furnished by anatomy, physiology, pathology, and organic histology. This position was reiterated in a resolution passed by the Homeopathic Medical Society of the County of New York in 1878 stating that the law of similars "does not debar us [homeopathic physicians] from recognizing and making use of the results of any experience, and we shall exercise and defend the inviolable right of every educated physician to make practical use of any established principle of medical science, or of any therapeutic facts founded on experiments and verified by experience, so far as in his individual judgment they shall tend to promote the welfare of those under his professional care." This admission, probably the most compromising of the homeopathic system, encouraged the American Medical Association to look more favorably upon those attempting to bridge the chasm between the two schools.[56]

Of course the purists within the homeopathic system steadfastly refused to accept an appeasement policy. At a meeting of the American Institute of Homeopathy in 1880, a splinter movement that struggled to prevent the further erosion of homeopathic ideas founded the International Hahnemannian Association, dedicated to the true principles of their founder. Fearing that true homeopathy would lose in any effort to bring the old and new school proponents into closer harmony, the movement adopted the following platform:

Whereas, We believe that *Organon of Homeopathic Medicine* as promulgated by Samuel Hahnemann to be the only reliable guide in therapeutics; and

Whereas, This clearly teaches that homeopathy consists in the law of similars, the totality of symptoms, the single remedy, the minimum dose of the dynamized drug, and these not singly, but collectively; and

Whereas, Numbers of professed homeopaths not only violate these tenets but largely repudiate them; and

Whereas, An effort has been made on the part of such physicians to unite the homeopathic with the allopathic school; therefore

Resolved, That the time has fully come when legitimate Hahnemannian homeopaths should publicly disavow all such innovations;

Resolved, That the mixture or alternating of two or more medicines is regarded as non-homeopathic;

Resolved, That in non-surgical cases we disapprove of medicated topical applications and mechanical appliances as being also non-homeopathic;

Resolved, That as the "best dose of medicines is ever the smallest," we can not recognize as being homeopathic such treatment as suppresses symptoms by the toxic action of the drug;

Resolved, That we have no sympathy in common with those physicians who would engraft on homeopathy the crude ideas and doses of allopathy or eclecticism, and we do not hold ourselves responsible for their fatal errors in theory and failures in practice;

Resolved, That as some self-styled homeopathists have taken occasion to traduce Hahnemann as a "fanatic," as "dishonest" and "visionary," and his teachings as "not being the standard of homeopathy of today," we regard all such as recreant to the best interests of homeopathy;

Resolved, That for the purpose of promoting these sentiments, and for our own mutual improvement, we organize ourselves into an International Association, and adopt a Constitution and By-Laws.

But for all of that, true homeopathy continued to exist in little more than name alone. In 1892 James B. Bell, president of the International Hahnemannian Association, admitted that there were probably fewer than 150 true Hahnemannians in the world and that the majority of those practiced medicine with the means and methods of the regulars. A few avowed adherents of the school persisted in espousing Hahnemann's sectarian creed; the majority of practicing homeopaths had compromised all the concepts of symptomatic treatment—the prohibition of local treatment for local diseases, of dynamization imparted to the crude drugs by the process of attenuation and shaking, the limitation of single remedies at a time, the doctrine of similars, and the provings and cures produced by the high potencies.[57]

The Healers

At the same time when doctors were seeking to rid medicine of its sectarianism, nineteenth-century society began manifesting an interest in psychotherapy that went far beyond the spiritual transports of even the most dogmatic homeopath. The turbulence of medical controversy in mid-century had precipitated an assortment of metaphysical and magnetic faith healers, phrenopathists, sun curists, medical clairvoyants, esoteric vibrationists, occultists, psychic scientists, advertisers of magnetic cups and positive and negative powders, viti-culturists, and venopathists. On the periphery of these radical sectarians were the Peculiar People, the Holiness Society of West Virginia, Fire-Baptized Holiness Associations, Pennsylvania hex charms, and colleges of fine forces—all claiming to cure what medical science seemed unable to achieve except through the rigorous path of pragmatic observation and experiment.[58]

In Christian tradition, faith healing had a Biblical basis—people had been cured of disease by a direct response from God to prayer. Divine healing was a phenomenon based not on demonstration but on faith; believers were therefore disposed to reject medical examination as having no material bearing on the process of cure. The same divine hand that offered salvation also healed; and, inasmuch as religion in the nineteenth century had gone far beyond the predestinarian Calvinism of the seventeenth century, certain sects predictably proclaimed that those who had faith must inevitably be cured of their diseases. Failures fell heavily upon the individual patient who remained uncured only for lack of the healing faith. Success depended in the last analysis on the individual seeking cure—"that any particular prayer not answered is evidence that the patient did not have sufficient faith." Faith healing involved the very process of salvation; and, as some seeking salvation were not saved, so too, some cure seekers were not cured.[59]

Faith healers defended themselves against accusations of spiritualism by claiming that the cures wrought among heathen nations, Voodoos, and Indian medicine men were either clever tricks, the effects of will power or, in some instances, were actually performed under the direction of the devil. But, for all their claims, there was little difference between Christian faith-healing practices and those of pagan spiritualists, clairvoyants, or magnetic healers. Skeptics contended that faith healing did not parallel the works of Christ or the apostles and that purely natural causation could explain the many claims attributed to faith cure. Furthermore, by their promise to work miracles, healers had relegated to themselves powers that even the greatest Christian reformers—Calvin, Knox, Luther, and even Augustine—denied ever having.[60]

In an effort to understand the nature of faith healing, the Society for Psychical Research in Philadelphia appointed a committee in 1885 to investigate the matter. The chairman of the committee, James Hendrie Lloyd, M.D., instructor of electro-therapeutics at the University of Pennsylvania, intended the investigation to examine not the subject of prayer but simply those individual cases of reputed faith cure. Despite personal requests to known healers, advertisements in the press, and various public announcements, the committee found it difficult to obtain case histories of healed persons. The few who did respond to the committee's request couched their remarks in a manner that made the results of the inquiry almost negligible. "Doubtless some healed ones would innocently submit to a medical examination," Captain Robert Kelso Carter wrote to the committee. "I would not, believing it to be dishonoring to my great Physician. I give my testimony—and I say Jesus cured me. I do not propose to submit to tests, to endorse God's notes of promise by the signature of men."[61] In October 1885 the committee presented a questionnaire to a convention of faith curites in Philadelphia who responded by tabling the request. One indignant faith curist remarked, "I should as soon expose the sanctity of my home life to the public eye, as the sacred work of God in human bodies . . . to scientific criticism." Another faith curist, a Reverend John E. Cookman, was equally incensed with the committee's request. He wrote scathingly, "A society for psychical research might have been formed in Jerusalem, Judea, Samaria, or Galilee, in the days of our Divine Lord, to investigate the causes of healing wrought by Him with as much pertinency as your present society."[62]

According to the medical profession, the danger of faith healers lay not in their reputed cures but in their refusal to countenance needed medical care for patients. Ignorant of pathology and physical diagnosis, and dogmatically insistent that intelligent medical therapeutics was wholly unnecessary to achieve cure, faith healers had contributed to the deaths of countless believers—a problem aggravated by the fact that the children of believers, as well as the general public, often became their innocent victims. Doctors faced the dilemma of parents who refused medical treatment for children with diphtheria or scarlet fever and who then compounded the tragedy by refusing to recognize quarantine laws. In 1889, when diphtheria broke out among several families of the New Evangelists of Brooklyn, parents refused medical treatment for their children and only permitted the services of two nurses to look after them. The nurses, who were themselves members of the New Evangelists, proceeded to spread the disease to children of other families in the church. After several unsuccessful attempts to spur the Board of Health into action, doctors were eventually empowered, with the aid of the attorney general, to take forcible possession of the children and place a quarantine over the houses involved. When the parents and nurses disobeyed the quarantine order, they were arrested on charges of endangering the public health.[63]

The claims of faith healers rippled from one end of the country to the other. Charles Cullis, once a homeopathic physician from Boston, transformed his triturations into "faith work" and extended his therapeutic powers from Virginia to California and even to missions in India. Another well-known healer and self-proclaimed Elijah, who produced cures from touching, was the Reverend John Alexander Dowie of Chicago, General Overseer of the Christian Catholic Church of Chicago and editor and publisher of *Leaves of Healing*, a weekly newspaper devoted to divine healing. Besides Dowie's newspaper, there were Charles and Myrtle Fillmore's magazine *Modern Thought*, the essays of H. Emile Cady, Julia Anderson Root's *The Healing Power of Mind* (1884), and Helen B. Merriam's *What Shall Make Us Whole, Or Thoughts in the Direction of Man's Spiritual and Physical Integrity* (1888). Among the more popular traveling healers were James Moore Hickson, who practiced in New York and Kansas City by the laying-on of hands; Canadian evangelist Aimee Semple McPherson, who was active in Texas and Denver; A. F. Hock of Los Angeles; and Francis Schlatter, who came to America from France in 1884 and began a two-year walk through the southwest. Claiming to be Christ and following the commands of "Father," Schlatter preached to thousands and sold blessed handkerchiefs to induce cure in the afflicted. Other divine healers included J. Barbera of New York, who anointed patients with oil; John Cudney of New Orleans, who practiced under the name of Brother Isaiah; and Reverend W. T. Reynolds of Pennsylvania. There was also a variety of "faith homes," which were allegedly supported by donations from women believers who had left their husbands and families for a life with God.[64]

Mind Cure and Christian Science

As early as 1857, efforts were underway to connect homeopathy with Christianity and to see Hahnemann as "the new evangelist" for a truly Christian medicine. One staunch advocate of homeopathy announced that Hahnemann's system was not merely science "but also for those who comprehend it, a sublime devotion, a form of religion, a divine rainbow of union, holding out to mankind the promise of speedy regeneration." Doctors who were shocked by the homeopathic doctrine of potentization were even more opposed to homeopathic religion and denounced it as a "blasphemous infidelity" concocted by "a few crazy transcendentalists."[65] Nevertheless, the homeopathic doctrine of infinitesimal dosage did bear fruit among philosophical idealists in America; and although the doctrine adopted the title of "Christian" or "mind-cure" medicine, it was more closely related to mesmerism than to the faith cures of Christian healers. Mental healing, transcendentalism, Grahamitism, and religious utopias, such as Oneida, existed on the fringe of religious liberalism—a teasing philosophical position for the educated—while faith cure remained an offshoot of the stark literalism of fundamentalist religion, appealing strongly to the lower levels of the social and economic order.

Equally significant in the development of mind-cure therapeutics was the multitude of cosmic theories that followed in the wake of Darwin's *Origin of Species* (1859). The writings of Christian evolutionists Henry Ward Beecher and Lyman Abbott, of theists John Fiske and Joseph LeConte, and the evolutionary cosmology of Henry Drummond's *Natural Law in the Spiritual World* (1883) and *Ascent of Man* (1894) were but a few examples of late nineteenth-century efforts to spurn modern materialism and seek a new reconciliation between science and religion. These intellectual liberals picked up the romantic threads of the earlier transcendentalists and, using Darwin as their touchstone, wove broad analogies between the principles of biology and the new ethical man. Their theistic philosophy portrayed a new Christianity, cleansed by the fires of evolution, with man rising above his close structural association with the brutes and human nature evolving beyond the restraints of matter. The cosmic theism of Fiske became a tool for accepting both the century's achievements in science and the enduring beliefs of religious-minded persons. Chief among God's creatures, man had outgrown the bestiality of the lower primates and was moving quickly into a psychic realization of God's eternal plan. Evil, a brute inheritance, was quantitatively proportional to man's stage in evolution. As man advanced through the scale of evolution and intelligence took precedence over bodily change, man learned to conform with the Christian ethic and in time would look back upon evil as a relic of his primitive past. Fiske wrote in *Studies in Religion* (1902), "From the general analogies furnished in the process of evolution, we are entitled to hope that, as it approaches its goal and man comes nearer to God, the fact of evil will lapse into a mere memory."[66] In the future, the evolution of man would be in the direction of his spiritual nature, with a gradual ascendancy of mind over matter. Emerson, Beecher, and, later, Abbott and Fiske marked the guideposts for a whole generation of cosmic thinkers in the late nineteenth century. Those more daring in their metaphysical beliefs jumped from the cautious ideas of Fiske and Abbott to suggest that pain, disease, and even death operated under the same laws of evolution. Just as the physiological and psychological processes of life occupied successive stages in man's evolutionary ascent, so also had the etiology, pathology, and treatment of disease likewise ascended from material to spiritual form.

Phineas Parkhurst Quimby (1802–66), a mental healer from Belfast, Maine, influenced the ideas of many subsequent mind-cure movements, including phrenopathy and Christian Science. He began as a disciple of Mesmer and the Frenchman Charles Poyen, whom he had heard lecture once in his state. Quimby avoided the rigid fundamentalism incumbent upon the promoters of divine healing and held aloof from the dogmatisms so characteristic of the later Christian Scientists. He experimented briefly with hypnotism and traveled through New England giving exhibitions of the technique. Gradually he began employing hypnotic techniques to diagnose disease, and from that point on devoted his time to the relationship between disease and the mental state of his patients. Quimby eventually dispensed with hypnotism altogether when he discovered that it was unnecessary in effecting cure, particularly since many regarded it as a form of witchcraft. Instead he initiated quiet conversations with patients, convincing them through mental suggestion that disease was simply an expression of fear and untruth that manifested itself in the improper functioning of the body. He believed disease originated through certain erroneous lines of thought that could be removed by the establishment of different modes of thinking. Only through correct thinking could nature build and retain a healthy body. Besides effective conversation and reasoning, Quimby sometimes employed massage and even rubbed the patient's head with water. Although denying that his hands possessed any inherent power or healing property, Quimby was willing to exploit the technique for those who lacked confidence in his words alone and who sought reassurance in some physical contact.[67]

Mary Baker Eddy (1821–1910), whose character one doctor described as "hysteria mixed with a bad temper," became a patient of Quimby in the 1860s and later shaped the foundations of her own Christian Science movement from a combination of Quimbyism, Christianity, homeopathy, phrenology, and the mesmeric notions of Charles Poyen.[68] There was an elusive quality in the mind-cure ideas of Mrs. Eddy that tended to separate her Christian Science movement from those that preceded it. Although her ideas were as openly pretentious as the claims of clairvoyants and the supporters of animal magnetism, she dressed them attractively in a spiritual attenuation that was more fastidious than the most distinguished mind cures and incidentally, more diluted than the most triturated homeopathic medicine. Christian Science had the classic parentage of Plato, a lingering flavor of New England's transcendentalism, the fervor of the Victorian's faith in science, and the Christian's fascination with metaphysics. Like so many other New Englanders who had imbibed too heavily in the pleasing constructions of romantic idealism, Mrs. Eddy was reluctant to follow the arduous path laid out by Darwin's theory of natural selection; she sought instead a more peaceful excursion into the eighteenth century's Chain of Being, which she spiritualized to her own liking. As one who was more at home with Louis Agassiz's Platonic typology, who had heard of the mysterious rappings of the Fox sisters in the 1840s, and had read Jahr's *New Manual of Homeopathic Practice* and Charles Poyen's *Progress of Animal Magnetism in New England* (1837), she could find little in Darwin's thesis to move her soul.

> Theorizing about man's development from mushrooms to monkeys and from monkeys into men amounts to nothing in the right direction and very much in the wrong. Materialism grades the human species as rising from matter upward. How then is the material species maintained, if man passes through what we call death and death is the Rubicon of spirituality? Spirit can form no real link in the supposed chain of material

being. But divine Science reveals the eternal chain of existence as uninterrupted and wholly spiritual; yet this can be realized only as the false sense of being disappears. If man was first a material being, he must have passed through all the forms of matter in order to become man. If the material body is man, he is a portion of matter, or dust. On the contrary, man is the image and likeness of spirit.[69]

In the etiology of ideas, Christian Science owed many of its mind-cure concepts to the principles of homeopathy. Hahnemann's ridicule of nineteenth century medical practices and his insistence on the immateriality of disease were crucial factors in the formation of Mrs. Eddy's later medical beliefs. The homeopath's success with infinitesimal dosages had convinced her that mortal belief rather than drugs governed the therapeutic success of the *Materia Medica Pura*—that the least amount of medicine employed in treating disease, the more successful the result. As the material drug disappeared in its higher attenuations, matter was thereby reduced in proportion to the infusion of mortal mind.[70] "Homeopathy mentalizes a drug with such repetition of thought-attenuations," she wrote, "that the drug becomes more like the human mind than the substratum of this so-called mind, which we call matter; and the drug's power of action is proportionately increased."[71] In her *Message to the Mother Church* (1901), Mrs. Eddy remarked that her favorite homeopathic dosages were those in which a grain of crude drug had been triturated at least a thousand times, since in these highest attenuations, "it must be mind that controls the effect" rather than the materialism of the drug.[72] To prepare homeopathic medicines required a combination of time and thought, and the higher attenuations were proof that the power of the drugs was in the thought, "for when the drug disappears . . . the power remains, and homeopathists admit the higher attenuations are the most powerful."[73]

While homeopathy had carried the art and science of healing beyond the dangers of "the old-time medicine of matter," Mrs. Eddy believed it still suffered from the excessive influence of matter. For this reason she felt Christian Science must carry therapeutics beyond matter, administering its remedy in the form of Mind, the true Christian medicine.[74] Her book *Science and Health* (1875), which became the pharmacopoeia for the Christian Scientist, taught that Mind was synonymous with Good or God and therefore was one with Life or the principle of existence. "Christian Science," she wrote, "exterminates the drug, and rests on Mind alone as the curative Principle, acknowledging that the divine Mind has all power." Only Christian Science operated true to its rule. "If you fail to succeed in any case," she argued, "it is because you have not demonstrated the life of Christ, Truth, more in your own life,—because you have not obeyed the rule and proved the Principles of divine Science."[75]

Throughout its early history, Christian Science sought to establish scientific mastery (both religious and curative) of the original teachings of Jesus and the monotheism of the Old Testament. Its followers believed that when Christ directed his disciples to preach the gospel to the world, he also instructed them to heal the sick. Christ based his method for healing not on drugs but on spiritual mind healing, which his disciples successfully used during the first three centuries of the Christian era. Like sin, disease was an abnormal condition curable "by a right application of the divine Principle of health and its laws." Sin and sickness were nothing more than delusions of the mortal mind—an improper apprehension of truth. The only effective agency in the cure of disease was the correct exercise of mind. If a sufferer was resolute enough, matter would yield to the spirit and the body would not become affected by disease. However, the decline of spirituality in the Christian world had resulted in the development of allopathy with its crude drugs and heroic therapeutics. Only slowly did medicine cast off its materialism by progressively moving first into the material attenuations of homeopathy and finally into the metaphysical therapeutics of Christian Science. In this sense Christian Science was neither a new religion nor a new healing process; rather, its healing work was "a revival of a lost element of the teachings and practice of Christ." The followers of Mary Baker Eddy intended to recapture the regenerative aspects of healing, which, through negligence and the temptations of materialism, had become "a lost art in the list of Christian privileges and duties."[76]

Christian Scientists believed that, as man removed the materialism that had hardened his reason and crippled his progress with false beliefs and made his way back to a more spiritual life of the mind ("the final unity between man and God"), he would abandon the sin, drugs, and sickness that had cluttered his path to righteousness. Just as man had sinned by giving material form to the deity, so also had he erred by transforming the materia medica into a Pandora's box of noxious drugs and mind-deadening vapors. "Idolatry sprang from the belief that God is a form, more than an infinite and divine Mind," Mrs. Eddy wrote. "Sin, sickness, and death originated in the belief that Spirit materialized into a body, infinity became finity or man, and eternal entered the temporal."[77] Only when man removed these material things from his faith would he move beyond the impediments of disease and death. The true self, "a wave in the eternal Divine ocean, a part of the All-pervading Spirit, the Universal Christ," was neither diseased nor sinful.[78] The true materia medica and the theology of Christ were one; and as man became more spiritual, his religion and medicine united in God to overcome the error of disease. Mind, which governed all the actions of the body, replaced the "fossils of material systems" that had blinded man's spiritual ascent. Only when man stopped trusting systems, whose principles were based on the laws of matter, would he attain the supremacy of the soul over sense, of mind over matter, of the risen Christ over the heathen gods of medicine.[79]

Properly speaking, Christian Science healers did not practice medicine, since they eschewed the use of drugs, surgery, and the techniques of past medical systems.[80] Instead they identified themselves as practicing a form of absolute idealism (that mind is divine, mind is all) as well as a genuine part of Christianity; and they demanded to be dealt with as a "religious act or system" rather than an offshoot of homeopathy, mesmerism, hypnotism, mind-cure, or other purely suggestive therapeutics. The true ascent from material medicine did not follow the path of animal or spiritual magnetism. "The currents of God flow through no such channels," Mrs. Eddy once wrote. Such systems only demonstrated the misuse of mind, by guiding the thoughts of others to serve the purposes of the human will and not the divine mind. The mesmerizer and hypnotist were disloyal to both God and man, by misleading the human mind along the channels of mortal needs and, while working to cure one disease, producing another.[81]

Eventually Mrs. Eddy accused the supporters of animal and spiritual magnetism of seeking to destroy her own movement with Malicious Animal Magnetism (M. A. M.). It was M. A. M., she claimed, which had originally made her an invalid, crossed her moods, thwarted her efforts, set people against her, and incited enemies to pervert the benefits of Christian Science. She blamed Richard Kennedy, who allegedly employed a combination of "Quimbyism" and "Eddyism" at the time of his expulsion from Christian Science, with using the "mental malpractice" of M. A. M. to bring a temporary lull in the Christian Science movement. Daniel Spofford, another heretic expelled for malpractice, was sued for causing "great suffering of body and mind and severe spinal pains and neuralgia and temporary suspension of mind" through the devious tactics of Malicious Animal Magnetism.[82]

Despite these eccentricities many liberal Christians welcomed the return of this metaphysical healing element to religious practice. What started out as a fin-de-siècle fad or drawing-room cult soon became a popular alternative to regular medicine and a metaphysical replacement for homeopathy among intellectuals who found the philosophy of Mrs. Eddy a soothing escape from the heroic claims of attenuated medicines, the pessimism of evolutionary naturalism, and the religious pablum of Henry Ward Beecher. Eventually the disciples of Mrs. Eddy gained support among upper-class businessmen, novelists, lawyers, clergy, and even a few doctors—like Judges Septimus J. Hanna, J. R. Clarkson, and William G. Ewing; medical practitioners J. Foster-Eddy, A. A. Suleer, and Julia Field-King; novelist Harold Frederick; clergymen H. G. Fiske, W. P. McKenzie, and George Tompkins; and businessman John V. Dittemore. By 1900 Christian Science had claimed the formation of nearly five hundred church organizations in Europe and America and the healing of almost two million cases of "hopeless disease." Its practitioners numbered some 3,156 in 1901, of whom 90 percent were women. And there was no end to their reputed cures. Mrs. Eddy claimed to have successfully "healed consumption in its last stages, the lungs being mostly consumed," cured "carious bones which could be dented with the finger," and even "healed in one visit a cancer that had so eaten the flesh of the neck as to expose the jugular vein so that it stood out like a cord."[83] Mark Twain, whose study of Mrs. Eddy had both a humorous and a serious side, relentlessly pursued her inability to write grammatically correct sentences (i.e., "Many pale cripples went into the Church leaning on their crutches who came out carrying them on their shoulders"). As Twain remarked, "None but a seasoned Christian Scientist can examine a literary animal of Mrs. Eddy's creation and tell which end of it the tail is on."[84]

Phrenopathy

The phrenopaths, whose founder was an ex-Methodist minister named Warren Felt Evans (1817–89), employed the teachings of Mesmer, Comte, Spencer, Swedenborg, and St. Paul to erect the foundations of a mental therapeutics that was strikingly similar to that of the Christian Scientists in both faith and practice. Evans borrowed from the positivist and synthetic philosophies of Auguste Comte and Herbert Spencer to support his belief in the unity of the various sciences, which, like the societies of man, were arranged according to their degree of complexity and dependency on others. From Swedenborg, Evans borrowed the idea that the body was only an external manifestation of mind or soul. Man was spirit and the body constituted "no essential part of his being and existence." The soul was the active, dynamic principle of the body and therefore the cause of all its muscular and physiological movements. By degrees this inner soul appropriated and directed the external nature of man and, when perfected, imitated the humanity of Jesus. "This," wrote Evans, "is the end of our creation, the appointed destiny of every created soul."[85] Since thought and existence were one and inseparable, "any change in our way of thinking must, by a necessary law, modify our existence." Thus disease, which was really only "an abnormal mode of existence," became "a wrong way of thinking, or a misbelief." Disease was a deflection of the mind from truth. In adopting from Swedenborg the "law of correspondence," which suggested that the outward manifestation of things (i.e., disease) was simply a representation of an internal spiritual disharmony, Evans maintained that cure consisted in restoring harmony to the mental state. By mixing Swedenborg and St. Paul, Evans formulated a method of cure that closely resembled the act of Christian conversion—a turning of the mind from a life of sense (untruth or disease) to one of spiritual thought and feeling. "When the psychical or natural man becomes the spiritual man, which transition from the lower to the higher degree of our being is called conversion," he wrote, "the change is described by Jesus as a passing from death into life. . . . So great a change as this ought to be nothing less than a transition from disease into health, both of mind and body." [86]

Like the Christian Scientists, Evans referred to Samuel Hahnemann as one of the pioneers in mind cure, since he had discovered that diseases were simply dynamic or spiritual disturbances that he had learned to combat with the spiritual essence of medicines. The magnetic influence of the homeopath's hand, along with the "imponderable essence of the drug," produced remarkable effects on disease. Infused with "sanative magnetic virtues" in the process of shaking, homeopathic attenuations changed from their material essence into one of spirituality. [87] Evans concluded that magnetism was the cohesive principle of life that pervaded the atmosphere in the form of mineral, animal, and mental forces and, under the proper circumstances, could be controlled by the "intelligent spirit of man." Homeopaths discovered that when they changed a neutral substance such as sugar of milk with magnetic forces it could absorb into the soul and cure disease. "I have experimented with these neutral substances for several years," Evans observed, "and when psychologically and magnetically medicated, they have proved themselves an efficient remedy." But homeopathy lacked the more subtle powers of phrenopathic mind cure. Those whose lives were "hid with Christ in God," he wrote, were able to take the power of magnetism one step further in the direction of spiritual science by discarding the homeopath's globules of sugar of milk and employing only the hands to transmit the forces of cure. "If a man is in vital union with God . . . the sphere of his presence will be full of a divine sanative contagion, that [through the mechanism of laying-on of hands] will infect the suffering, trusting patient with life, health and peace." [88]

Central to the phrenopathic method of cure was the law of

mental sympathy, which implied a state of "intercommunion of mind with mind" through thoughts, ideas, and feelings. By a process of "mental induction" (a phrase that bore the etiological earmarks of electrical theory), the mind acquired a diffusive power of reproducing its images, thoughts, etc., into the mental state of another. By transferring spiritual thoughts and feelings to the patient through the law of correspondence, a phrenopath was able to bring about cure; since disease had a fundamentally spiritual origin, it could be more efficaciously removed through phrenopathy than through homeopathy or the more primitive techniques of material medicine. The phrenopathic physician conceptualized a patient in thought and mentally affirmed perfect health in both spirit and body. If receptive to the physician's phrenopathic thought processes, the patient could receive this new supply of life energy, which then flowed through muscles, nerves, and veins, bringing strength and life to deficient parts. Although the healer usually transferred physical vitality through the medium of the hands, phrenopaths claimed they could also act at a distance. Since the spirit recognized no limitation in time, space, or materiality, the word of God spoken by the healer instantaneously reached its object. This later process became known as "absent treatment"—a practice used also by the Christian Scientists. Evans warned, however, that phrenopaths could not cure a diseased person by mental or verbal reasoning. Patients had the obligation to affirm—have faith—and not argue; they must allow the image of truth present in the mind of the healer to infuse their own diseased mind.[89]

For those who lacked the discipline required for phrenopathic mind cure, Evans supplemented his pseudo-Christian system with massage. Unlike the phrenopathic method, which first converted the patient and then brought him into harmony with the redeemed spirit, Evans's auxiliary magnetic-movement cure relied on a "nervo-tonic stimulation" (massage) to the muscular system and its effect on the reflex action of the cerebro-spinal system. An electric force, generated by friction of the physician's hands on the diseased part, vitalized the nervous forces of the patient, and the magnetic or psychic influence of the physician added to the stock of vital energy in the patient.[90]

Medical Response

For those physicians who had spent a lifetime in pursuit of a scientific medicine, the sectarian claims of faith and mind healers seemed scandalous. For the most part, the medical profession refused to recognize either their healing claims or their techniques as having any place in the armamentarium of therapeutic practice. In spite of this professional stance, however, doctors discovered that the power of mental stimulus or autosuggestion became increasingly important in the treatment of functional and neurotic diseases. In cases where mental anxiety and forebodings added to the sufferings of the patient, doctors found that their own presence had much more effect than drugs. In 1888 R. Lauder, M.D., asked, "Is not . . . the secret of all physicians' popularity that they inspire their patients with faith rather than that they are more skillful in the use of medicinal agents to cure disease, than others less successful?"[91] By encouraging a hopeful attitude, doctors furnished the right mental stimulus for enabling patients to turn a most serious illness toward recovery. Though not formerly recognized as such, there was always a space in every physician's repertoire for the exercise of psychic healing, particularly in those cases where the real disease was exaggerated, imaginary, or hysterical. It was also valuable in those situations where a bodily illness could benefit from a well-balanced mentality or when the mental attitude of the patient or his friends necessitated an encouraging outlook.[92]

In most cases doctors were reluctant to speak of this powerful ally known as autosuggestion, since over the centuries countless victims had been duped by humbugs and charlatans advertising miraculous cures through the use of prayer, laying-on of hands or hypnotic séances. Occasionally outspoken doctors would urge the regulars to speak openly of this mental factor and encourage its use with as much authority as they dispensed their drugs. Only then, they argued, would faith healers begin to lose their clientele. If the physician, with his power of diagnosis, his understanding of drugs, and his ability to employ autosuggestion, could not surpass the claims of the faith or mind healer, then—a physician remarked in 1898—he had no business being a doctor. "I see no good reason why we should allow the army of irregulars to carry away the best part of our business," he observed. If a patient acknowledges "that the miracle cure is no miracle, that we not only understand the miracle but the scientific reason for it, we have saved him, pocketbook and all."[93]

In an investigation carried out in 1898, Henry Goddard of Clark University concluded that there was nothing in the suggestive process of mental therapeutics that was incompatible with drug therapeutics and that, in fact, the two could actually reinforce each other in the general prophylaxis of disease. Although he found no basis in the contention that faith or mind cure had replaced the science of medicine, nevertheless there was sufficient evidence of the efficacy of mental therapeutics to establish that "the proper reform of mental attitude could relieve many a sufferer of ills that the ordinary physician cannot touch."[94] In effect, mental therapeutics provided a base on which the physician could build the science of medicine. According to Goddard, this meant that doctors had first to recognize the patient's psychic condition as equal in importance to the disease itself. This meant, too, that doctors had to be much more careful in what they said to patients, since many were genuinely affected by the knowledge doctors imparted to them concerning their disease. Unfortunately the lack of sufficient research by the medical profession into this area of study, its continued emphasis on drug therapy, and its refusal to officially appreciate the relationship between medicine and psychotherapy had caused the public to fall prey to the absurd claims of itinerant healers who fed on the imagination and the natural tendency of many diseases to be resolved without the need for medicine. The real tragedy came with the public's loss of faith in medicine and their willingness to seek help from less reputable sources.

Goddard believed that society should ignore the peculiar sectarianism evident among the forms of mental therapeutics. "What Christian Science has in common with Mental Science," he observed, "constitutes its sole claim to regard." As for mental science, it owed its value "to its effort to make practical and bring within the reach of all, the best idealism of heathen philosophy and the Christian religion." All mental therapeutics—whether called mesmerism, divine healing,

Christian Science, hypnotism, or mental science—was based on the common power of suggestion. "Suggestion is the bond of union between all the different methods," Goddard wrote, "and the law of suggestion is the fundamental truth underlying all of them, and that upon which each has built its own superstructure of ignorance, superstition, or fanaticism." The same could be said of the drummers of patent and proprietary medicines who appealed to the secret powers of their drugs; it could likewise be said of the quack doctor who preyed upon gullible clients with claims of special healing.[95]

As a result of his investigation into the various types of psychic healing, Goddard concluded that "the curative principle in every one of the forms is found in the influence of the mind of the patient on his body"; that the various forms of faith and mind cure have success as well as failure in the cure of disease; that "they all cure the same kind of diseases and the same diseases are incurable for them all"; that the percentage of success is about the same in all forms; and that there was a significant lateral movement of people from one form to another. "Some fail after trying all," Goddard explained. "Some fail to get cured by divine healing, but get restored by Christian Science, and vice versa." Faith was a valuable therapeutic agent, but the faith exercised by patients in their physician was the same in kind and degree as that employed by faith and mind healers, mesmerists, and Christian Scientists. The common denominator was the simple natural stimulus of autosuggestion.[96]

The Emmanuel Movement

The Emmanuel Movement undertaken in Boston in 1905 represented the extent to which medical men were willing to follow the suggestions put forth by Goddard. The Reverend Elwood Worcester, rector of the Emmanuel Church, and his associate Samuel McComb, with Isidor H. Coriat, M.D., and Joseph H. Pratt, M.D., of the Massachusetts General Hospital, administered a program of psychotherapy for the neuroses of the educated elite. They openly vowed to turn indulgent self-centeredness into a social gospel aimed at the problems of the tenement sections of the city's poor. This meant giving up the crutches of alcohol and drugs and treating the assortment of functional diseases of the mind with a social gospel of good works.[97]

McComb claimed that many of society's most productive leaders suffered from a nervous predisposition, the symptoms of which were evident in extreme self-consciousness, insomnia, melancholy, inability to work, alcoholism, spasms, and numerous disorders that fell under the category of neurasthenia. In neurasthenia, he wrote, the "nerve energy is depleted or exhausted, and the exhaustion gives rise to a sense of fatigue, to fleeting pains that come and go, to mental instability, and lack of moral poise." As a pre-Freudian, mind-cure urban agency, the Emmanuel Movement sought to achieve its goals through a harmony of brain, nerve, and religion by bringing the doctor, clergyman, and social worker into a coordinated work effort to alleviate disease, both real and imagined, that originated from "defects of character." Any person who sought the services of the Emmanuel Clinic was thoroughly examined by a physician and remained under medical care throughout the administration of psychic and moral remedies. Quite often the physician prescribed drugs, electricity, or baths to accompany other therapeutic measures prescribed by the minister or social worker.

Correct treatment called for the interdependence of mind and nervous system and the use of such tools as suggestion, education, and work. In the therapeutic sense, suggestion became a method of influencing the thought and feeling of the patient "through ideas which work . . . in that region of the mind which lies, as it were, below the threshhold of consciousness, and which . . . exercises a deep influence upon . . . mental, moral, and physiological life." The Emmanuel Clinic employed the spoken word, gesture, electrical and mechanical shock, or an inspiring personality to achieve this end. In some rare cases, suggestion was administered during hypnosis, but only by medical advice and under medical supervision. The most usual method was "waking suggestion," in which clinic personnel encouraged the patient to relax and then induced a state of mind favorable to the reception of suggestions.[98]

The clinic employed its second remedial technique, education, for those forms of nervousness that were deeply rooted.

McComb described this procedure as mental gymnastics. Just as suggestion was designed to influence the subconscious mind, education was to infuse in the conscious reason a conviction that the patient's disorder was curable. To achieve this the staff of the clinic tried to "exercise particular groups of thoughts and feelings until they dominated the mind and crushed out the influence of other thoughts and feelings that only rack and harass the nervous system." Accompanying the tool of reeducation was the process known simply as explanation, which meant that the patient should thoroughly understand the cause of his or her troubles. "The sufferer must be taught . . . not to plunge into the very conditions which throw him into despair, nor . . . to avoid them altogether." In this connection the clinic thought that many persons could benefit from moral and religious reeducation. Although society lived in an age overwhelmed by the inroads of materialism and skepticism, McComb believed Christian religion to be one of the best preventive medicines against the fear, worry, and disgust with life so prevalent among patients at the clinic. Faith gave the soul "safe anchorage amid the storms and stresses of experience." [99]

The final remedial tool in the armamentarium of the Emmanuel Movement was work. According to McComb most doctors were mistaken in their belief that overwork was the cause of most nervous disorders. Admitting that certain acute cases evidenced real physical fatigue that required prolonged rest, he nevertheless observed that most cases of nervous breakdown demonstrated only psychical fatigue brought on by worry, tension, insomnia, and certain emotions. "To give up work—the first instinct of man from whom nature exacts her penalty for some violation of her laws—is, as a rule, a mistake," he wrote. The skillful physician, minister, and social worker must discover what was wrong in the way a person worked and must then provide a more suitable alternative. For some this meant a reorientation of objectives; for others, especially middle- and upper-class women, whose interests were largely self-centered and who were without work and therefore without any conscious purpose in life, this meant finding a vocation that was altruistic in character. Worcester and his associates directed many of these women to charitable and philanthropic organizations where they could observe genuine tragedies of poverty and crime. In this manner nervous women were turned from their own personal sorrows, which "sank into a relatively insignificant place," and became absorbed in the plight of their fellow man, learning to love God and themselves through love of humanity.[100]

Worcester combined his concern for social problems with his psychological training in Germany under Gustav Theodor Fechner (1801–87) and Wilhelm Wundt (1832–1920), founder of the Institute for Experimental Psychology in Leipzig. Since his organization retained close relations with the medical profession, particularly with Philadelphia neurologist S. Weir Mitchell and Richard Cabot of Harvard Medical School, he was able to enjoy the confidence of many medical men. Only when the movement spread to cities like Chicago and San Francisco and fell under the influence of less competent persons did medical men finally withdraw their support. Historian Stow Persons observed that "perhaps the lasting contribution of the Emmanuel Movement was to furnish added inducement to the medical profession to enter the field of functional disorders, to recognize psychiatry as a legitimate branch of medicine, and to support research and practice in that important field."[101]

Retrospect

Although transcendental medicine bore the marks of an earlier medical age resplendent with fads and sectarian mischief, the antinomian tendencies which tempted these American sectarians to defy traditional medicine permitted few liberties that brought irrevocable harm to medical science. Their triumphs were won on those occasions when science left a fringe of inexplicable phenomena that was baffling even to those who were experts in the field. Given the temper of the historical moment and the assistance of an imprecise science, sectarians reveled in their momentary freedom. Like the pragmatic mold of American politics and morals, however, medical sectarians preferred flirting with excitement to real danger and the consequences of any imprudence. Throughout the nineteenth century, they acted as third party platforms by putting forth ideas espoused by a few fervent supporters, clamoring loudly in voices all out of proportion to their numbers, teasing and annoying the mainstream of medical thought. As in the century's political arena, where barnburners, locofocos, grangers, silverites, and populists were eventually absorbed or discredited by the two-party system, so also orthodox medical thinkers adopted the best of the sectarian ideas, thereby enriching American medicine with a boldness that carried into the twentieth century. By balancing propriety with the necessity for change, and sustained by the creative interests of an educated elite, the advocates of transcendental medicine enriched medical science during the long period of its apprenticeship.

5

Midwives in Britches

THE HISTORY OF MIDWIFERY parallels the history of mankind and antedates any record of medicine as an applied science. Among the Hebrews, Greeks, and Romans and, later, the Portuguese, Spaniards, and Italians, the term applied to the person attending confinement was feminine. From the Latin word *obstetrix* and *cummater*, which had no masculine, to the Italian *commere*, to the Spanish and Portuguese *commadre*, and the Anglo-Saxon *midwife* (*mid-wif*, with woman), no language prior to the seventeenth century referred to a male assistant during woman's confinement. The writings of Hippocrates and others in classical times reveal that male physicians and surgeons left obstetric work to the midwife and assisted only in abnormal cases, when they removed an impacted or dead fetus. In spite of the midwife's control over natural delivery, however, male midwives eventually became a reality for normal as well as difficult labor, and the history of that development marks one of the more protracted controversies in the annals of medicine. Beginning first with the dissemination of obstetrical knowledge and then progressing into actual practice, obstetrics fell gradually into the hands of male physicians and surgeons.[1]

Early History

For centuries Soranus of Ephesus (ca. 2d century A.D.) remained the chief source of European treatises on obstetrics and gynecology. His writings, along with those of Renaissance doctors who utilized the printing press for the instruction of fellow physicians and surgeons, brought greater stature to the male practitioner by offering a scientific alternative to obstetric folklore. No books on midwifery existed in English until 1540, when Richard Jonas translated Eucharius Röslin's *Rosengarten der Swangern Frawen und Hebammen* (1513), itself a reworking of the writings of Soranus and the manuscripts of Mochion, Aetius, Albertus Magnus, and Savonarola, Jonas's *The Byrthe of Mankynde*, otherwise named *The Woman's Boke*, helped to reassert the teachings of Soranus in a medium accessible to midwives and served likewise to reintroduce podalic version and the obstetric chair. When reissued by Thomas Raynalde, *The Byrthe of Mankynde* became one of the popular books on obstetrics in the sixteenth century and went through a dozen or more editions. The book also precipitated the appearance of complementary texts, such as Jacob Reuff's *Ein schön lustig Trostbüchle* in 1554, which became the basis for examination of midwives in Zurich. Other pertinent texts included *Practica Major* (1547) by Johannis Michaelis of Savonarola; *Medici Regii de Morbus* (1547) by Martin Akakia of Paris; *De Morbis Mulierum* (1591) by Geronimo Mercuriale; *De Generatione* (1555) by Maistre Nicolle du Hault; *De Affectibus Uterinus* (1557) by Giovanni Battista della Monta; and *De Conceptu et Generatione Hominis* (1580) by Louis de Mercado. Noted seventeenth century obstetrical books include *The Woman's Doctor* (1652) by Nicolaus Fontanus of Amsterdam; *The Directory for Midwives* (1651) by Nicholas Culpeper; *De Generatione Animalium* (1651) by William Harvey; and James Woolveridge's *Speculum Matricis, or the Expert Midwives' Handmaid*, published in 1671.[2]

Jean Astruc (1684–1766), author of *L'art d'accoucher réduit a ses principes* (1766) and medical consultant to Louis XV, dated the acceptance of the male midwife from the night of December 27, 1663, when Louis XIV allegedly summoned Jules Clément, a student of the eminent surgeon James La Fèvre, to attend his mistress, the Duchess de la Vallière. The event was shrouded in secrecy, with Clément chosen because the king feared the idle tongue of women, midwives in particular. The duchess received Clément in a mask to remain anonymous; and, to protect the honor of his mistress, the king observed the male midwife's conduct from behind curtains. In 1670 Clément attended at the birth of the Duc de Maine; in 1682 he delivered Louis de Bourbon, for which he received the title of "accoucheur." Soon afterward, according to Astruc, the employment of *sages-femmes en culottes* became fashionable, first among the *dames du grand monde* and then among the bourgeoisie.[3] However, there is ample evidence to suggest that midwifery had been more common than Astruc originally believed. As early as 1617 the midwife Louise Bourgeois (1563–1636), in her *Observations Diverses de la sterilité, perté de fruict, foecondité, accouchements*, lamented the growing favor given to the use of accoucheurs. Louise, who was sage-femme to Marie de Medici, wife of Henry IV, used her position to decry the male usurpation of the ancient rights of midwives.[4] In her book she frequently criticized the popularity of Maistre Honoré, an accoucheur and great favorite among ladies of the court. She was also much annoyed with the success of Maistre Jacques Guillemeau (1550–1613), whose *L'Heureux Accouchement des femmes* (1609) had earned him a lucrative employment as male midwife to fashionable ladies.[5]

Despite the prejudices of Louise Bourgeois and of those in the ranks of the medical profession itself, obstetrics occupied the increasing attention of physicians. Before long the fashionable use of male midwives for normal delivery spread from France to the rest of Europe. The London surgeon Peter Chamberlen the elder (1550–1631), a Huguenot refugee practicing in the early seventeenth century, became the first notable male midwife in English history. His son, Peter the younger, graduated as a doctor of medicine from Padua, and in 1628 became a fellow of the College of Physicians. His knowledge of midwifery, handed down from his father, secured for him an extensive practice in the London area. Another Peter Chamberlen, son of Peter the younger, attended the wife of Charles I of England in 1682. Sir William Hamilton in his *History of Medicine, Surgery, and Anatomy* (1831) attributed the preference for male midwives to the introduction of obstetrical forceps by the Chamberlen family. To be sure, physicians had employed forceps prior to the Chamberlens but only to destroy or remove the dead fetus rather than to facilitate delivery. Jean Palfyn (1650–1730) of Ghent later modified the forceps by contriving a *tier-tête* or head drawer. William Smellie (1697–1763) added flanges to the grooves and set down rules for its use, and Benjamin Pugh introduced the "pelvic curve" in 1754. Those who employed

forceps became known as instrumentarians, and the history
of obstetrics from the first third of the eighteenth century
onward became one of continued strife between midwives
and the usurping male physician.[6]

Along with the introduction of forceps, the establishment
of lying-in hospitals between 1749 and 1765 and the creation
of chairs of midwifery in medical schools contributed to the
acceleration of forces that caused the midwife to lose her accustomed place at the parturient's bedside. The University of
Edinburgh initiated the first professorship in obstetrics in
1726, with other universities quickly following suit.[7] Those
American doctors who obtained prominence as male midwives included John Moultrie of Charleston, who started his
practice in 1733; William Shippen of Philadelphia, who gave
lectures to women as well as to medical students in the 1760s;
Samuel Bard of New York, who received his medical degree
from Edinburgh and published *A Compendium of the Theory
and Practice of Midwifery* (1807); John V. B. Tenent of New
York, who lectured on the practice of midwifery at King's
College in 1767; and James Lloyd, a student of both William
Smellie and William Hunter, who practiced obstetrics in
Boston in the 1750s. Many of these early American male mid-
wives were students of London teachers, such as Sir Richard
Manningham, John Leake, William Osborn, Thomas Den-
man, and, of course, Hunter and Smellie.

Some forty years after the first English lying-in hospital
opened, Americans opened the New York Lying-in Hospital (1791) and the lying-in wards of the Pennsylvania Hospital (1803) and Boston (1832). Harvard College established a
professorship of midwifery as early as 1815 with the appointment of Walter Channing.[8] William Potts Dewees, whose
popular *Systems of Midwifery* (1824) went through twelve editions, provided American physicians with the obstetric experience of both British and French physicians, laying the
foundation for scientific midwifery in the United States.
J. Blundell's *Lectures on the Principles and Practices of Midwifery* became available to American medical students in the
1830s, followed by C. D. Meigs, *The Philadelphia Practice of Midwifery* (1838); R. Lee, *Lectures on the Theory and Practice of Midwifery* (1844); F. Churchill, *On the Theory and Practice of Midwifery* (1843); D. H. Tucker, *Elements of the Principles and Practice of*

Midwifery (1848); and R. Gooch, *A Practical Compendium of Midwifery* (1832). Books for more popular consumption included Alfred Folger, *A Domestic Medical Work: The Family Physician* (1845); Richard Foreman, *An Indian Guide to Health* (1849); and J. T. Schonwald, *The Child: A Treatise of the Diseases of Children according to the Laws of Nature* (1851). Hugh Lenox Hodge's *Diseases Peculiar to Women* (1860) and *Principles and Practice of Midwifery* (1864) became foremost works on gynecology and obstetrics in the nineteenth century. Prominent teachers of obstetrics in the Middle West included Henry Miller of Kentucky and William H. Byford, professor of obstetrics and diseases of women and children at the Chicago Medical College, who published his *Treatise on the Theory and Practice of Obstetrics* in 1870.[9]

The surgeon as an assistant in childbirth, employed initially in instances of difficult labor, gradually achieved respectability as a preference grew among women for those with knowledge that went beyond a midwife's learning from oral tradition and haphazard experience. Since men had long been teachers of obstetrics, it was only a matter of time before women began placing greater faith in physicians and surgeons than in midwives. "What more natural than that intelligent women should prefer the teacher to the inept pupil; should place their lives in skilled hands, than in those that were unlettered?" In 1876 physician and medical historian William Goodell argued that inevitably "the male physician, who was hurriedly sent for in cases of emergency, or was kept waiting in the ante-chamber for such an emergency, should, despite tradition, prejudice and religion—should, in spite of himself, for it was deemed dishonorable for him to practice midwifery—ultimately usurp the place of the midwife by the bedside of the woman in travail." From their surgical experience, dissections, and study of the human body, physicians found themselves ideally suited to improve upon the obstetric art.[10]

"Finger-Smiths"

Those physicians who employed forceps and followed in the footsteps of Smellie faced abuse from midwives and doctors who railed against their efforts to bring obstetrics to the level of a medical specialty. One eighteenth century midwife, Elizabeth Nihell, was notorious for her attacks on Smellie's "delicate fists" and branded his forceps as "agents of death."[11] In her *Treatise on the Art of Midwifery, Setting Forth Various Abuses Therein, Especially as to the Practice with Instruments* (1760), she described the disciples of Smellie as "self-constituted men midwives made out of broken barbers, tailors, or even pork butchers; for I know myself one of the last trade who, after passing half of his life in stuffing sausages, is turned an intrepid physician and man midwife."[12] Nineteenth century critics of Smellie included Sir Henry Halford, the president of the Royal Society of Physicians, who in a letter to Sir Robert Peel remarked that the practice of midwifery was "an act foreign to the habits of gentlemen of enlarged academic education."[13]

Purity jeremiads considered the male midwife a dangerous catalyst whose indecent "touching" provoked woman's constitutional instability and undermined the intricate web of etiquette that defined the parameters of middle-class respectability. John Blunt, M.D., pseudonym of S. W. Fores, a Picadilly bookseller, in his *Man-Midwifery Dissected* (1793), expressed moral outrage at the practice of vaginal examinations performed by male midwives as part of the delivery procedure. According to Blunt these "touching" examinations were an affront to the very decency of women and served only to rend the moral fabric of society.[14] "The practice of man-midwifery is among the noxious weeds which the rank luxuriance of civilization has produced," George Morant added, in his *Hints to Husbands: A Revelation to the Man-Midwife's Mysteries* (1857). He continued:

> What shock so terrible to a man who, rejoicing in the delightful sentiment of a wife's purity, discovers that all he held dearest and most sacred, all which he would shield from profanation with the last drop of his life's blood, has been invaded by the presence, and violated by the actual contact of the man-midwife? The doctor may be a sober, discreet, oily man, of staid appearance, and a very pattern of propriety; or he may be a vulgar, low-bred person in his leisure consorting with those of similar bent; or he may be a tippling, jovial fellow, who at some roystering party is always called on for "a good song," sure to have as its theme wine, love, and women—for

accoucheurs are mortals like other men; or he may be some
tyro in "the art," just let loose from his course of walking the
hospitals, strong in syphilitic cases, and with all the recollections of a young surgeon's life fresh upon him: nevertheless,
whatever he be, *the very inmost secrets of your wife's person* are
known to him, the veil of modesty has been rudely torn aside,
and the sanctity of marriage exists but in the name.[15]

The rules of medical etiquette placed severe limitations on
examinations of women. Both Samuel Bard, in his *Compendium of the Theory and Practice of Midwifery* (1807), and William
Dewees, in his *Compendious System of Midwifery* (1824), urged
the most stringent precautions when touching examinations
proved necessary. Dewees recommended that a third party,
preferably a nurse or a female friend of the patient, communicate information of any delicate sort to the female patient.
Moreover, he cautioned, "before you proceed to the examination, let your patient be placed with the most scrupulous
regard to delicacy, as the slightest exposure is never necessary." The examination was to be carried out in a darkened
room by manual touch, with the physician relying on previous instruction in anatomy and information gathered from
pictures to supplement the tactile examination. And when
delivery took place, the physician performed the task with
the mother properly covered.[16]

Despite these precautions, public reaction to the touching
examinations of the so-called "finger-smiths" was high-
lighted by the libel trial in 1850 of Horatio N. Loomis, M.D.,
whose article in the *Buffalo Courier* had criticized James P.
White, M.D., for demonstrative midwifery—examination of
a living subject during instruction in midwifery. Loomis accused White, a professor of obstetrics at Buffalo Medical College, of outrage against the rights of the parturient woman
by allowing a group of twenty medical students to observe
their preceptor's handling of a clinical case of natural labor.
Notwithstanding the fact that European lying-in hospitals
had long employed demonstrative midwifery as a teaching
aid, many American doctors took exception to exposing the
patient to view, even in cutting the cord, supporting the per-
ineum, or making vaginal examinations. Bryant Burwell, a
physician and surgeon for thirty-five years, regarded the
teaching of obstetrics by demonstration as "neither necessary

nor proper." He insisted that instructors of midwifery teach with pictures, mannequins made of buckskin that exhibited the fetus and female organs, and by hearing and touch; under no circumstances should a physician make a visual examination of the woman's pelvic organs. Even with the jury's verdict of not guilty, the venom generated by the "prudish 'Miss Nancies' of Buffalo" against demonstrative midwifery forced the medical profession to move more cautiously in sustaining the new teaching method.[17]

The American Midwife

In America, except for preternatural and tedious cases, midwifery remained almost exclusively in the hands of women until the middle of the eighteenth century. Throughout this period American midwifery differed little from that prevalent in Europe over the centuries. Midwives seldom read genuine obstetric texts, although many in both Europe and America had access to the "Aristotle" pamphlets that first appeared anonymously in England in the mid-seventeenth century and during the following two centuries went through countless editions and translations. These pamphlets, which drew upon the writings of Aristotle, ancient medical practices, the writings of Sylvius, the works of Ambrose Paré, and any number of Greek, Roman, and medieval myths, provided one of the few popular sources of obstetric knowledge. Variously titled *Aristotle's Master-Piece Completed,* the *Last Legacy,* and *Aristotle's Compleat and Experienc'd Midwife,* the manuals dealt with such subjects as puberty, coition, conception, development of the fetus, delivery, marking of unborn children, and sexual dysfunction. The pamphlets gave directions for midwives regarding normal as well as difficult labor; recipes for chicken, mutton broth, or poached fig in the event of tardy labor; advice on correct positioning of the parturient woman; and strict admonitions against the use of fingernails to burst the membrane. There were instructions on how to force the delivery and afterbirth with vomiting, fastening a ribbon to the leg of the child during breech delivery, advice to surgeons on the removal of a dead fetus, and the need to wrap the woman's belly in the skin of a freshly killed sheep after hard labor. There were few differences between Mrs. Jane Sharp's *Midwives Book* (1671), which advised such things as an eagle-stone "held near the privy parts" to draw forth the child "as the loadstone draws iron," and the countless suggestions put forward in the Aristotle pamphlets. Each provided an assortment of obstetric folklore mixed with common-sense advice. Although improvements in the obstetric art eventually removed the Aristotle pamphlets from the midwife's handbag, the pamphlets nevertheless served to apprentice countless women who were unable to benefit from the few existing teachers of obstetrics in Europe and America.[18]

Noted early American midwives included the widows Potter and Ruth Bradley and Goodwife Beecher of the New Haven colony, Mrs. Bridget Lee Fuller of the Massachusetts Bay Colony, Anne Hutchinson (1600–43), Trijn Jonas and her daughter Anneke in Manhattan during the 1630s, Ruth Barnaby (1664–1765), and Elizabeth Phillips (1685–1761) of Charlestown. The American Revolution, however, brought chaos to the education of midwives without, at the same time, replacing them with persons of competent obstetrical knowledge. In towns along the Atlantic seaboard, poorly trained physicians began to replace midwives except among the poorer classes who were unable to pay a doctor's higher fees. For those settlers spilling forth across the Appalachians, the state of medicine and midwifery deteriorated to the level of folklore or oral literature—albeit selective—among the frontier settlements.[19]

It was common practice for the American midwife to choose her successor from within her own family, training the woman with techniques handed down by word of mouth outside of men's hearing. A midwife's apprenticeship lasted several years. In typical situations the midwife delegated supportive tasks such as washing spoiled linens, ironing the cord dressings and then scorching the pieces in the oven, burning the dried cords, and burying the placenta. Soon she began helping the postpartum mother, performing household chores, bathing the newborn, dressing the cord, and reporting to the midwife on the mother's progress. In most instances an apprentice midwife did not observe a delivery until she had experienced labor herself. Indeed, most midwives had personal experience not only with birth but also with death. Eventually the midwife sent the apprentice ahead to stay with the parturient when delivery appeared imminent, and occasionally she delivered an early baby. Later she assumed responsibility for the midwife's night calls and gradually took more of the workload until she inherited full control when the midwife either retired or died.[20]

In a typical delivery procedure in the eighteenth and early nineteenth century, the midwife prepared the labor room by closing all windows and doors for fear that the woman might catch a chill. Like the physician, midwives regarded fresh air as a pernicious cause of childbed fever. The parturient remained dressed in ordinary day-clothes, since early labor consisted of walking about the room with one or two neighborhood women supporting her back when pains ensued. While this was occurring, the midwife prescribed hot tea and, in the frontier regions, whiskey and even a pipe. Obstetrical anesthesia was not used by midwives and faced the opposition of both doctors and theologians who believed that pains of childbirth were biblically as well as physiologically correct. Only when Queen Victoria resorted to the use of chloroform in the 1850s did obstetrical anesthesia obtain full respectability.[21]

When labor advanced to the point that the woman could no longer walk about, she went to a couch or chair, knelt on her knees or, in more typical cases, sat on a neighbor's knee (in some regions the wife sat on her husband's knees) while friends supported her back and legs, urging her to bear down. In difficult labor the midwife instructed the parturient to recline on a bed, which was moved before the fireplace for extra warmth. With the birth of the child, the midwife superintended the separation of the cord, while an attending woman or apprentice washed and dressed the child. The cord was cut and tied with two ligaments, and the placental end was fastened to the woman's thigh as a precaution against being drawn back into the womb. The mother then brought on the expulsion of the placenta through various exercises, forced vomiting, or the use of drugs, such as ergot or tartar emetic. In some cases of delayed placenta, feathers were burned under the mother's nose or snuff was blown into her nose to incite sneezing. On other occasions the parturient held salt in her hand to induce sweating and was encouraged to blow into a bottle. Finally, upon expulsion of the placenta, the midwife pushed a handkerchief or linen into the womb, where it remained for three days. In general, midwives were content to live with surroundings they met in the home rather than improve upon them by encouraging a more aseptic condition. They believed that the hemorrhage accompanying labor and the amniotic fluid were a form of filth that could be collected through similarly unsanitary techniques. Some midwives even avoided washing the woman after delivery. Indeed, mothers sometimes remained in a soiled bed for a week or more before sheets or clothing were changed.[22]

The midwife's instruments ranged from scissors, string, and lard to a vaginal speculum, axis-traction forceps, curettes, and a complete outfit for perineorrhaphy. For the most part, however, the lack of obstetrical instruments aided midwives, who, in their competition for patients, accused physicians of causing physical harm to mother and child with forceps and other instruments. No doubt, many women preferred to believe that midwives could induce natural birth without harmful instrumentation. Besides delivery, midwives tried to monopolize as much as possible the care of children and the preparation of young girls for menstruation. Their materia medica consisted of teas, "underfoot salve" (excrement of humans, cows, or hogs), sheep saffron (manure), and even a tincture of human placenta for chlorotic girls suffering from catamenial suppression. They prescribed a string of bear's teeth to make the child grow strong and cabbage hearts, bacon rinds, and beer for the baby's diet.[23]

Throughout the nineteenth century, American midwifery remained a form of collective behavior existing outside formal rules, which nevertheless matured within a long and sometimes close relationship with physicians. Most reputable midwives worked in conjunction with a doctor. In fact, they derived part of their prestige from their relationship with the local physician, who assisted in difficult deliveries and, as an authority figure, added immeasurably to their store of experiences. The earliest medical theories had given at least tacit approval to the midwife's techniques; and although the midwife perhaps employed these techniques longer than the bright new authorities on medicine, she probably was not much farther behind the times than many of the older practitioners in her district. From doctors she had first learned to keep patients bedded down in a dark room for a week or more, with bound abdomens, and strict diets. When drugs became available, she learned to prescribe calomel, spirits of hartshorn, opium, laudanum, paregoric, chloral, tincture of castor, and ergot; indeed, she was only too anxious to abandon older prescriptions and magic for the newer materia medica. Thus she replaced pepper tea and burnt feathers with ergot and substituted chloral for the ax under the bed or copper wires tied on the thighs. When in doubt she employed a combination of all the known magic, both ancient and modern. For the most part, midwives employed "a fund of outmoded medicine which they had acquired and were still largely putting into practice with the sanction of the older doctors." Ironically, doctors who attacked the midwife for her ignorant ways were simply striking at the last remnants of their own profession still practicing in that outmoded manner.[24]

Forcing Drops

The earliest use of ergot as an abortifacient and childbed remedy derived from fourteenth- and fifteenth-century midwives and empirics who first discovered its effects on cattle that ate spoiled grain and on pregnant peasant women who ate bread tainted with spurred rye. Before long doctors began distinguishing ergot (*mutterkorn* or *womb-grain* as it was called in German) with such soubriquets as *poudre obstetricale*, *forcing powders*, or more commonly, *forcing drops*. Following its interdiction by the French Parliament in 1774 as the result of misapplication, the drug went into brief eclipse until the publication in 1807 of a letter by John Stearns, M.D., of Saratoga County praising its parturient powers and encouraging its full employment. The Stearns letter, published in *Medical Repository*, a New York journal, designated ergot as a *pulvis parturiens*. Stearns had experimented with ergot several years before sending his letter and reputedly learned of the drug's effect from a German midwife. According to the letter, the action of the drug caused the uterus to contract upon any substance within its cavity. Stearns warned physicians to make certain before administering the drug that the orifice of the uterus was sufficiently relaxed and dilated. His directions were to never give ergot until true labor had commenced. Given prematurely or in too large a dose, "the violent uterine contractions which it would produce, would be in danger of rupturing the walls of the uterus; or of destroying the child." Notwithstanding the reservations voiced by Stearns, ergot quickly replaced borax, cinnamon, and turpentine as the most popular parturient agent.[25]

The employment of ergot reached dangerous proportions in the first half of the nineteenth century, partly because doctors used it as an expulsive agent when uterine contractions, however vigorous, seemed insufficient. In one sense its use corresponded with the quickened pace of medical practice; American doctors who fought disease with heroic doses from the materia medica were reluctant to sit passively by and await natural delivery. In other words, the use of ergot gratified the profession's desire to do something to facilitate nature. As men accustomed to a busy schedule, they were anxious to adopt a drug which would hasten delivery without endangering the life of the mother. One physician, reminiscing about his earlier student days, recalled a practitioner who had relied so heavily on ergot as a parturient drug that he "gave it freely and . . . had, during a long professional life, more instances of ruptured uteri, deadborn children, puerperal convulsions, and widowered husbands than any other physician I have ever known." Doctors who were tempted to accelerate nature's timetable by giving ergot before sufficient dilation of the cervix caused children to be literally destroyed by the violent contractions which thrust them against the undilated cervix.[26]

Despite initial enthusiasm for the drug, ergot was never universally welcomed by the medical profession. The editors of the *New England Journal of Medicine*, for example, agreed on the drug's parturient powers, but warned that the newborn child suffered greatly from its employment. In many cases where ergot had been used, children "did not respire for an unusual length of time after the birth, and in several cases . . . were irrecoverably dead." Subsequent studies by Doctors Holcombe and Ward of New Jersey concluded that unless born within forty minutes after ergot-induced contractions, the child would be stillborn. According to their analysis, more children had perished in a few years from the use of ergot than had died from the unwarranted use of the crochet hook during the preceding century.[27] John B. Beck, M.D., of New York deplored the fact that so many doctors employed the drug merely as a "time-saving agent." Believing, as a general rule, that nature was competent to insure safe delivery, he urged doctors to leave nature alone to accomplish its work. "Artificial and violent interference," he observed, "whether it be applied in the shape of instruments or by the use of ergot, cannot but be improper."[28] According to David Hosack, professor of theory and practice of physic at the University of the State of New York, the number of stillbirths had noticeably increased in his state since the introduction of ergot. While ergot had been called the *pulvis ad partum* because it hastened labor, Hosack suggested the more appropriate term of *pulvis ad mortem.*[29]

At a meeting of the London Medical Society in January 1833, members were conspicuously divided over the powers and efficacy of ergot. In 1837 a similar meeting of forty-eight medical men attached to Trinity College, Dublin, ended with only three defending its use. The Academy of Medicine of Paris likewise directed an investigation into the powers of ergot in 1850 and concluded that except in cases of miscarriage, in certain labors attended by hemorrhage, and occasionally at the conclusion of natural labor, the profession should avoid the use of ergot, since its contractions literally smothered the infant, shutting off blood and preventing oxygenation. In 1855 the prefect of the city of Paris sent a communication to the Academy of Medicine blaming the increased number of stillbirths on the unwarranted use of ergot. While investigating the claim, physician St. Claire Develle found that the rate of stillbirths in Paris had increased 6 percent over the twenty-five year period following the drug's general acceptance by the medical profession.[30]

Puerperal Fever and Ophthalmia Neonatorum

Over the centuries puerperal or childbed fever (postpartum infection) claimed the lives of both the primapara and the experienced mother. The medical profession judged puerperal fever to be of sporadic form, inflammatory in character, and involving a variety of tissues. In treating the condition, doctors commonly employed bleeding and opium, although some claimed results using a strong emetic, followed by heroic doses of carbonate of ammonia and quinine. Other remedies included warm poultices, foxglove, and castor oil. At the first sign of fever or pain that began in the uterus or ovaries and slowly spread through the entire abdomen, doctors employed local bleeding (twenty to twenty-four ounces), which they continued until the symptoms disappeared or the patient fainted, and then resumed after she recovered from syncope. Doctors believed that persistent bleeding would overcome the disease, provided they diagnosed the symptoms early enough. In most cases, however, both doctors and midwives mistook the pain for postdelivery aches and neglected prophylaxis until the infection became too advanced. Although too late for cure, doctors then plied their patients with opium to "soothe their passage to the grave."[31]

The medical profession continued to dispute the cause and prophylaxis of puerperal fever long after the Manchester surgeon and man-midwife Charles White (1728–1813) insisted on cleanliness in his *Management of Pregnancy and Lying-in Women*, published in 1772. Other warnings came in the form of a paper by Oliver W. Holmes, "On the Contagiousness of Puerperal Fever" (1843) and a book by John Stevens, M.D., *Man-Midwifery Exposed; Or the Danger and Immorality of Employing Men in Midwifery Proved; And the Remedy for the Evil Found* (1849). Stevens blamed doctors for the high incidence of puerperal fever and suggested as the cause their overly liberal attitude toward touching (vaginal examination).[32] Whether incited by reasons of prudery or otherwise, Stevens was surprisingly accurate in his assessment, since physicians were more apt to examine women before delivery than midwives and were, therefore, more prone to introduce infection. Although unaware of precise statistics, Viennese mothers were acutely conscious of the mortality differential between the department of obstetrics of the University (99.2 per thousand) and the School for Midwives (33.8 per thousand); and although the two departments were located in the same building, women formed long lines outside the Midwifery School, while the obstetrics department remained empty. According to medical historian Fielding Garrison, women begged in tears not to be taken into the obstetrical wards.[33] The Hungarian Ignaz Philipp Semmelweis (1818–65) provided clinical documentation of puerperal sepsis by demonstrating that infected materials brought into the labor room at the Allegemeines Krankenhaus in Vienna by medical students who had received obstetrical instruction on cadavers had been responsible for 11.4 percent of the puerperal mortality rate. Concluding that puerperal fever had become contagious through contact with infected materials, Semmelweis introduced a simple procedure of scrubbing with chloride of lime, which reduced the danger tenfold.[34]

Even after the achievements of Lister, Pasteur, and Koch in microbiology, physicians and midwives were slow to accept responsibility for puerperal fever. Despite efforts to introduce carbolic acid, bichloride of mercury, and the fingernail brush into obstetric practice, noted obstetricians and gynecologists like James Young Simpson, Lawson Tait, Hugh L. Hodge, and Matthews Duncan remained unconvinced of Listerian antisepsis and the germ theory of disease, preferring to place the blame on local suppression, crasis (humoral pathology), dissolution of the blood, or gastric-bilious conditions.[35] Hodge, professor of obstetrics at the University of Pennsylvania and author of *On the Non-Contagiousness of Puerperal Fever* (1852), rejected the idea "that you can ever convey, in any possible manner, a horrible virus, so destructive in its effects, and so mysterious in its operations as that attributed to puerperal fever." Likewise, Charles D. Meigs (1792–1869) of Philadelphia, professor of obstetrics at Jefferson Medical College and author of *The Science and Art of Obstetrics* (1849) and *On the Nature, Signs, and Treatment of Childbed Fevers* (1854), rejected the very thought of medical culpability in puerperal fever, referring to such suggestions as "jejeune dreaming of sophomore writers" and preferred to attribute puerperal fever "to accident or Providence of which I can form a conception, rather than to a contagion of which I cannot form any clear idea."[36] Indeed, both William P. Dewees, in *Treatise on the Diseases of Females* (1826), and Meigs, in *Philadelphia Practice of Midwives* (1838), taught the noncontagiousness of puerperal fever. In 1883, however, J. H. Garrigues demonstrated the efficacy of antiseptic techniques when he instituted massive changes in the New York Maternity Hospital on Blackwell's Island. By employing a 1:2000 solution of bichloride of mercury and heroic applications of soap and water to floors, beds, patients, and the hands of attendants, he reduced the hospital's high mortality rate to zero within three months.[37]

Even when it became clear that puerperal fever was blood poisoning or septicemia that most often resulted from negligence in personal cleanliness, doctors preferred to condemn the midwife rather than themselves. They were quick to characterize the midwife as "gin-guzzling . . . with her pockets full of forcing drops, her mouth full of snuff, her fingers full of dirt, and her brains full of arrogance and superstition."[38] Two noted portraits of midwives that served to stigmatize the profession in the nineteenth century were Dickens's gin-sodden, irresponsible Sara Gamp in *Martin Chuzzlewit* (1843) and Leigh Hunt's *The Monthly Nurse* (1846).

In attempting to explain the discrepancy between facts and accusations, P. W. Van Peyma, M.D., obstetrician to the Buffalo General Hospital and professor of obstetrics at the University of Buffalo, suggested that physicians were more inclined to report the infections that occurred in the practice of the midwives than in their own. Despite this reluctance, statistics available before 1860 of deaths from puerperal fever among Negroes and Caucasians indicated a higher mortality among the white women attended by physicians than among Negro women attended by midwives.[39] In 1909, in a borough of Manhattan, 71 percent of the deaths from puerperal sepsis occurred at the hands of physicians. Similar statistics available for 1910 indicated that physicians had attended 65 percent of puerperal cases, while midwives had attended the remainder. "The poorly trained physician," R. W. Lobenstine, M.D., remarked in 1911, "does far more harm than the midwife, as is abundantly shown by the various hospital records as well as by the records of the Board of Health."[40]

Doctors also insisted on blaming midwives for the high incidence of gonorrheal ophthalmia and its resulting blindness. They made frequent sport of midwives who treated sore eyes by rubbing them with the mother's placenta for two or three days or by using boric acid, mother's milk, lemon juice, lard, a solution of catnip tea and camphor, raw potatoes, scraped beef, and saliva.[41] But available statistics seemed only to confuse the issue. The Maryland State School for the Blind claimed that midwives delivered 79 percent of those babies whose blindness had resulted from opthalmia neonatorum.[42] It was not entirely clear, however, that responsibility rested solely with the midwife. Of 116 cases treated in 1909 at the Massachusetts Charitable Eye and Ear Infirmary, for example, 114 were known to have occurred in the practice of physicians. Similar statistics were available from the New York City Department of Health, the New York School of Philanthropy, and other agencies that advocated the use of silver nitrate as a prophylactic against the disease.[43] Of the 108 cases investigated by the New York Committee for the Prevention of Blindness in 1913, physicians accounted for 62, while midwives accounted for 43. The remaining 3 cases were emergency situations attended by neighbors. Overall, it appeared that the midwife, who looked to the physician for innovation in her practice, only reflected the chaos of the medical profession's own aseptic standards. The findings of S. W. Newmayer, M.D., of the Bureau of Health for the State of Pennsylvania, indicated that, notwithstanding the poor educational background of midwives, most were as competent to attend to the mother as the average physician.[44]

A private questionnaire sent by J. Whitridge Williams, M.D., of Johns Hopkins University to professors of obstetrics in some forty-three medical schools across the country indicated that the midwife was not as culpable for puerperal infection and ophthalmia neonatorum as doctors had led the public to believe. Of those physicians who answered the questionnaire, fifteen placed the blame on doctors, thirteen thought midwives were most often responsible, and five suggested that blame be shared equally by both. Thus, one of the vocal arguments urged against the midwife appeared not to prevail within the inner circles of the medical profession but only as a statement for public consumption. Also significant were the results of the question of whether the physician or midwife was more responsible for deaths of women in improperly performed deliveries. Here twenty-six teachers of obstetrics answered against the physician and only six against the midwife; three maintained that both were equally culpable. The survey further indicated that the average medical student witnessed only one delivery and that few professors had adequate hospital experience or felt themselves adequately prepared to handle a serious emergency.[45]

Clearly the questionnaire registered a general feeling of embarrassment, if not outright disgust, among doctors for the entire system of medical education. Williams wrote: "The replies . . . demonstrate that most of the medical schools included in this report are inadequately equipped for their work, and are each year turning loose on the community hundreds of young men whom they have failed to prepare properly for the practice of obstetrics, and whose lack of training is responsible for unnecessary deaths of many women and infants, not to speak of a much larger number, more or less permanently injured by improper treatment, or lack of treatment. . . . A priori the replies seem to indicate that women in labor are as safe in the hands of admittedly ignorant midwives as in those of poorly educated medical men." What had begun as a study to determine the status of the midwife had developed into a major indictment of medical education, a demand for better schools, higher requirements for admission, and better trained professors of obstetrics, an insistence on higher standards by state examining boards, and an overall improvement in the education of both the general practitioner and the midwife. More than anything else, the questionnaire marked a sign of approaching reform in the medical profession and signaled that the muckraking tendencies of the Progressive Era were at last beginning to encroach upon the medical profession. Heeding the progressive legislation dealing with the business community, the medical profession would eventually conclude that it was better to reform from within than submit to external guidance for change.[46]

European Regulation

By the early nineteenth century, European governments had recognized midwifery as an established profession and had taken steps to ensure that enlightened and competent midwives would continue to serve the population. Schools

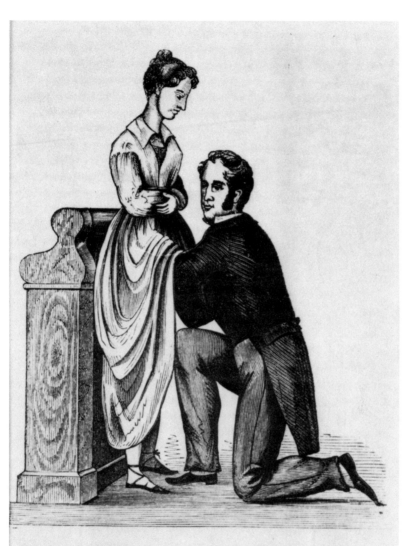

The above Plate, copied from " Magrier's Midwifery Illustrated " — edition of Dr. Doane, New York — represents some of the indelicate duties of male physicians.

Fifty thousand men, composing the medical profession in the United States, are engaged in such an occupation!

" The present practice of medicine, especially obstetrics, must be set down not only as having an immoral tendency, but as, in itself, a gross, abusive, and shameless immorality." — REV. WM. HOSMER, *in the Young Lady's Book.*

A "touching" examination. George Gregory, *Medical Morals* (New York, 1852). Courtesy of Indiana University.

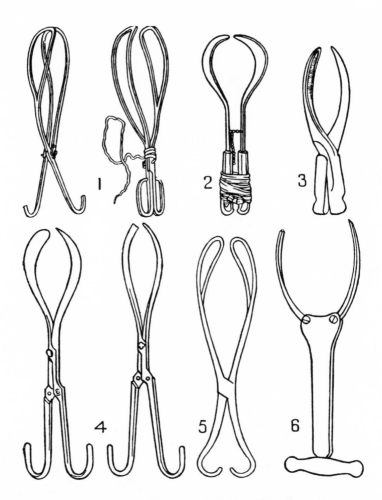

1 Forceps invented by Peter Chamberlen (the elder) about 1630, and retained as a family secret for many years (page 236)

2 Palfyn's forceps (Mains de Palfyn, 1720) ; two spoons, with handles clamped together (page 237)

3 Smellie's short wooden forceps, 1745, with the " English " lock (see page 235 and Plate XLIX)

4 Dusée's forceps, 1733 ; the first attempt to articulate Palfyn's instrument by means of the " French " lock

5 Chapman's forceps, 1733 ; the blades united by a simple groove, easily detachable (page 235)

6 Burton's forceps, 1751 ; slender blades controlled by screw handle. Burton, of York, was the original Dr. Slop of *Tristram Shandy*

Douglas Guthrie, *A History of Medicine* (London, 1945), p. 240. Courtesy of Indiana University.

for instruction in midwifery existed in most countries, with the length of training varying from six to nine months in Prussia; from one to two years in France, Belgium, the Netherlands, Scandinavia, and Switzerland; from two or three years in Italy; and three in Russia.[47] French law, dating from 1803, provided free education for midwives, with women between the ages of eighteen and thirty-five permitted to attend lectures after first producing certificates of proficiency in reading and writing. Students attended courses in theoretical and practical midwifery and also clinical lectures at a hospital. An examination was held at the end of the year's study, and a jury composed of professors of the faculty of medicine judged the competence of the student and awarded the diploma. Further regulations came in 1807 when the Code Napoleon required the midwife to seek medical assistance in every case in which the life of the mother or child was endangered. Moreover, to improve census statistics, civil authorities required midwives to report all births. In Belgium the law regulating midwifery dated from 1818 and provided for practical and theoretical courses given under the supervision of the Minister of Interior. Candidates between the ages of twenty and thirty years, able to read and write, who had an "irreproachable character," were eligible for training. Instruction lasted two years, at the end of which an examination was given by the Provincial Medical Council.[48] Swiss midwives were required to report the number of births and deaths four times a year to the medical officer of the district and to provide a detailed statement on every complicated case. The Russian law requirement that midwives study for three years included practical experience at the Polyclinic. At the end of their preparatory studies, which included instruction in venereal diseases, midwives were examined by the Chief of the Midwifery School and were given a diploma. In Sweden and Norway, with laws dating from 1810, midwives were provided free education and were subject to periodic examinations as well as criminal liability for practicing without a license.[49]

In Austria, where midwives were closely supervised, women could practice between the ages of twenty and forty-five. Before attending instruction by a professor, candidates first had to demonstrate competence in reading, writing, and elementary arithmetic. Once accepted for training, students received instruction for a period of five months, spending their days at a lying-in hospital learning anatomy, pathology, and managing a specified number of births. Under pain of prosecution, they were forbidden to undertake instrumental operations except in those emergency situations where a medical man could not be called in time. At the end of training, midwives were examined in the presence of a commission appointed by the government. Before setting up practice, however, a woman had to announce herself to the civil authorities of the area, produce documentation as having successfully completed her course of instruction, and be provided with the necessary implements, which included a tinned enema syringe, a metal female catheter, a navel-string cutter, lint, bath sponges, and strong vinegar. The law required that midwives record every birth with the registrar of the district within twenty-four hours and attend the ceremonial baptism of the child. In addition to strictures against the use of instruments, the Austrian government prohibited midwives from administering or prescribing medicines to pregnant women or children except in the most extraordinary situations.

By 1892 the German government had agreed upon an official textbook for students preparing for midwifery. Besides relating the practical aspects of midwifery, including the fundamentals of disinfection and physiology, the textbook forbade the midwife to extract the placenta by the introduction of the hand and directed her to wait one hour before using Crede's method of squeezing the fundus. Midwives were forbidden to employ forceps or perform podalic version unless the physician could not be summoned in time or the life of the mother, child, or both was in imminent danger. By 1908 forty-three institutions for the training of midwives existed in Germany: twenty-seven in Prussia; four in Bavaria; three in Baden; two each in Saxony, Hessen, and Thuringen; and the remainder scattered among the provinces.[50]

Although midwifery was common to all European countries, England was alone in outspoken criticism of the practice. There midwives and physicians battled vociferously over the issues of regulation, prohibition, male midwives, and legal status. Ironically, up to the middle of the eighteenth century, the regulation that did exist for English midwives derived from the licensing power of the office of the bishop, whose principal concern was not with obstetrical skills but with proper instruction in the baptism of infants in cases in which death appeared imminent. As early as 1303 women were performing this spiritual service along with their midwifery duties; and bishops insisted that before a license could be given, "curates must openly in the church teach and instruct the midwives on the very words and form of baptisme . . . that they may use them perfectly and none other." Eventually bishops dropped their licensing role, and women performed the duties of midwife without worrying about restrictions or licenses of any kind.[51]

From the time of Andrew Boorde in 1547 until the Medical Act of 1902, English reformers introduced twenty proposals for the teaching and licensing of midwives. The first significant effort of the nineteenth century occurred in 1813, when the Society for Apothecaries endeavored to persuade Parliament that every midwife should have a license obtained after examination by a committee from the district in which she lived and worked. The society further recommended that there be twenty-four districts, including London, each with its own board to govern the activities of its midwives. During the late 1860s and early 1870s, the Obstetrical Society of Great Portland Street in London sought an amendment in the Medical Acts to establish an Obstetrical College for the purpose of giving women access to a "registrable diploma for the practice of midwifery, and confer upon properly educated midwives a defined professional status."[52] While many considered the proposal of the Obstetrical Society an admirable improvement over the status quo, critics protested that the real motive was to eliminate midwives by demanding qualifications that would require women to be overeducated. Among the critics were the midwives themselves, who provided statistics to show that the mortality rate of the Dublin Lying-in Hospital under the supervision of medical men was several times higher than the British Lying-in Hospital, where doctors assisted only in difficult deliveries. Midwives at the Royal Maternity Charity claimed attendance at 3,666 births in 1872 with only four deaths. As far as English midwives were concerned, the Obstetrical Society justified its reform proposal only on the faulty premise of higher mortality figures among births attended by midwives when, in reality, the society clearly intended to eliminate the midwife as a competitor of medical men.[53]

James Hodson Aveling, a strong advocate of midwife reform, feared that the Obstetrical Society's proposal would create a class of medical women—not midwives—with knowledge of "obstetric science and its accessories," who would become practitioners of medicine and compete with medical men without fully qualifying themselves for practice. For all their faults, Aveling considered the English midwife a necessary evil. He wrote: "I have no wish to magnify the office of a midwife, for, judging from my experience of her in the country, I am quite sure she can never be a person having any claim to high social or scientific position. Compared with the skilled obstetrician, she is the organ-blower to the organist; still, we cannot ignore her. The surgeon has separated himself from the barber, and the apothecary from the grocer, but our relations with the midwife can never cease. In practice, we must constantly meet her, and her very weaknesses and inability to improve her position must always claim our sympathy and assistance." According to Aveling, England required roughly 11,500 midwives to serve its population, and to adequately educate such a number was beyond the capacity of any one hospital or society; rather, it was the responsibility of the state to assume direction over the matter.[54] Aveling particularly admired the manner of Prussian supervision. He observed, "How many valuable lives would have been saved had our midwives only known that an inspector was coming by-and-by to investigate, like a coroner, every fatal case occurring in her practice and that delay in sending for further help, unwarrantable interference, ignorant neglect, and all the other causes of death which may befall parturient women through their inefficiency, would most certainly be discovered and punished." For the present, England was at the mercy of careless if not "coarse and totally uninstructed women."

> In dealing with the question we have but two alternatives: We must either abolish the whole race of midwives, or we must instruct them. Licensing and registration are of great consequence, but instruction is of primary and paramount impor-

tance. We cannot feed and fatten a man without giving him food; nor can we, by licensing and registration, without instruction, make a midwife. If, then, we decide not to attempt the impossible task of annihilating midwives, we must undertake the possible but difficult enterprise of training them. It has been done in Russia, Germany, and France; and what Russians, Germans, and French have accomplished, surely Englishmen can do. It cannot be that our nation cares less about the welfare of its wives and daughters than other countries; and yet we must admit that there exists a colouring of truth in the taunt which is sometimes hurled at us when this subject is spoken about. We have our Society for the Prevention of Cruelty to Animals; but a midwife may inflict frightful tortures unquestioned. The captain of a ship may not take command of a vessel without having shown proofs of his seamanship; but a midwife, utterly ignorant, may take charge of a woman in labour, and the State cares not with what results. Dense ignorance alone can be the cause of this indifference.[55]

Because of the ambiguous nature of the Obstetrical Society's intent, as well as the divided opinion within the medical profession regarding the delicate issue of physician-patient relations, efforts during the 1880s failed to either improve the education of midwives or provide for their registration. One bill, written in 1882, never reached Parliament. Another, prepared by Fell Pease in 1890, was dropped after midwives protested that they were required to produce certificates of moral character before registration, while medical men were exempt from a similar requirement. Thus, until passage of the Midwives Act in 1902, the training and practice of midwifery remained entirely unregulated and unsupervised by the state. No recognized authority prescribed a certificate of qualification or course of training, although the Obstetrical Society did issue its own certificates in midwifery (known as L. O. S.) for some thirty-three years. In 1892 and 1893 a select committee of the House of Commons appointed to investigate the problem of registration of midwives reported that there was sufficient evidence to demonstrate the presence of "serious and unnecessary loss of life and health, and permanent injury to both mother and child, in the treatment of childbirth, and that some legislative provision for improvement and regulation is desirable." Although recognizing that midwives were necessary, the committee recommended that the government take steps to insure that the practice of midwifery be placed in the hands of experienced and qualified women; that there be a "midwife's register," which would include a system of examination and registration to be regulated by the General Medical Council; and that workhouses and lying-in hospitals provide facilities for the study of midwifery.[56]

For the avowed purpose of bringing better care to parturient mothers, decreasing infant mortality, and preventing blindness and physical defects caused in birth, Parliament in 1902 provided for legislation "to secure the better training of midwives and to regulate their practice." By its Midwives Act, Parliament established a Central Midwives Board and gave direct supervision of midwives to the County Councils of England and Wales. The board, which consisted of representatives from the principal medical and nursing organizations, was to establish rules for the direction of midwives, prepare candidates for examination, supervise examinations, issue certificates, and keep names and addresses of all midwives for the purpose of inspection. The law required that women take three months of training, which was extended to six months in 1916. The program included the personal delivery and nursing of twenty maternity cases; instruction in anatomy, physiology, and hygiene; management of labor; child care; and recognition of complications and diseases associated with pregnancy.[57]

American Registration and Regulation

In 1911 the commissioner of health for New York City, Thomas Darlington, M.D., observed, "So far as I have been able to discover, the United States of America is the only civilized country in the world in which the health as well as the life and future well-being of mothers and infants is not safeguarded so far as possible through the training and control of midwives."[58] Although states were compelling physicians, pharmacists, dentists, and even veterinarians to furnish proof of good moral character and demonstrate competence in their respective branches before practicing, American midwifery remained unsupervised. This was due in part to the midwife's having acquired her title largely through squatter sovereignty rather than a formalized educational program. Like England prior to the Midwives Act, the states never enforced any program of education, which meant those who purchased a midwife's services had to accept the limited knowledge she had acquired through age and experience. Since few laws either defined or limited her practice, little could be done to control responsibility. Where state requirements existed, boards of health merely registered all who applied, and evidence of incompetence awaited a coroner's inquiry or an indictment for manslaughter.[59] Still, physicians preferred legal chaos and incompetence to any form of official recognition through the establishment of legally chartered colleges or the appointment of examining boards with the right to grant certificates. The only law physicians would accept was one which specifically stated that midwifery, as a branch of medical practice, lay exclusively in the hands of the medical profession.[60]

In at least one area, medical men were almost unanimous in their feelings. They feared that if midwives were empowered to certify stillbirths, there would be no end to the incidence of illegal abortions. By administering drugs, such as ergot, opium, or quinine pills; vaginal douches of iodine, carbolic acid, vinegar, lysol, and turpentine and water; or by introducing crochet hooks, wax tapers, goose quills, and even hairpins attached to electric batteries, midwives could provide the criminal means to destroy unwanted pregnancies. If the midwife had the power to issue certificates, medical men argued, there would be no way to ascertain if an infant's death was natural or induced. Despite these accusations, however, fewer than five percent of the midwives were ever accused of this practice. On the other hand, the enormous number of irregular doctors and "private specialists" who practiced on the fringe of medical respectability, catering to the sexual problems of Victorian society, provided as much opportunity for criminal abortion as did midwives. Purgatives, emmenagogues, or specifics such as aloes, ergot, or savin were readily accessible, as were energetic poisons such as arsenic or cantharides. In addition, doctors and midwives gave local irritation by hand, punctured the membranes, or dilated the os and separated the membranes from the uterine walls with the aid of sponge tents, seatangle, slippery elm, and gentian root.[61]

During the 1890s New York doctors turned their attention to those midwives and "women physicians" (a euphemism for abortionists) who advertised in the daily papers as keepers of so-called "lying-in asylums." Over four hundred abortoria operated in New York in the post–Civil War decades, catering to married and unmarried women from the middle and upper classes. The New Society for the Prevention of Cruelty to Children secured the closing of several asylums whose premises had been used by out-of-state women seeking secretly to terminate unwanted pregnancies or to give their babies away. After delivery—unless an abortion was effected—the lying-in asylums discarded the children in the street or assisted in procuring adoption. Not infrequently midwives sold babies to reputable families for a modest sum (i.e., ten dollars), later to blackmail the new parents by threatening to make the transaction public. Noteworthy among these asylums were the Brown Home and Hospital for Females, the Rothkranz Home and Female Hospital, and the Winkelman Home and Lying-in Asylum. Christian Rothkranz, one of the more notorious abortionists, incorporated her home; in the papers she advertised under the title "Drs. Rothkranz; Incorporated Sanitarium for Females; thirty years' experience; treats female diseases, irregularities; positively painless; success guaranteed every case; confinements; strictly private; motherly care." Her only evidence of skill was a certificate of midwifery issued by the Columbia College of Midwifery, which was in no way connected with Columbia University, then Columbia College.[62]

Those doctors who debated the problems of midwives in the AMA's journal admitted that a large populace simply could not afford to employ an obstetrician even at a much lower cost. Conservative estimates on the number of births supervised by midwives in the United States at the turn of the century ranged from 43 percent in New York, 50 percent in Buffalo, and 75 percent in St. Louis, to as high as 86 percent in Chicago. Midwives predominated in those areas where either the black or foreign population remained high.[63] Since the midwife's normal fee of fifteen dollars included delivery as well as subsequent visits and nursing, it was difficult for physicians to compete for delivery services, especially since doctors placed such a high monetary value on their time.

Moreover, immigrants from southern and eastern Europe preferred to have a woman at the bedside of the mother. As a rule American doctors attributed this preference to the natural bashfulness of immigrant women and their reluctance to have any man, even a husband, around during the time of labor. America's new immigrants considered male attendance contrary to nature and therefore highly immoral.[64] Social workers reported destitute families who refused a doctor's attendance at delivery. When this happened, neighborhood women contributed to the payment of a midwife's fees rather than allow the woman to submit to shameful delivery by the male physician.[65] The desire to economize, combined with the immigrants' traditional aversion to masculine help, made the midwife an enduring part of urban and rural life. This tradition remained so tenacious that physicians eventually combined their desire to regulate midwives with support for some form of immigrant restriction. Alarmists argued that unless the nation initiated controls on immigration from southern and eastern Europe, the institution of midwifery would continue uninterrupted. They considered all plans for the elimination or control of midwives as impractical unless the federal government took steps to restrict the hordes of people streaming into American ports.[66]

The early regulation of midwives in the United States began with a sporadic effort by state boards of health to oversee irresponsible teaching in "midwife colleges" by specifying certain requirements for those wishing to engage in the profession. Like the proprietary medical schools, midwife colleges were private stockholding companies with motives more mercenary than humanitarian and educational. Doctors objected to the power of these institutions to confer diplomas, appalled that ignorant women could enroll for a brief course in a midwife diploma mill and graduate with a license to practice, while medical students faced increased demands for preliminary qualifications and exacting standards of medical science before being permitted to assist even a normal labor. Doctors found it equally disconcerting to compare the tightening of courses and hospital training for nurses with haphazard educational programs designed for midwives.

During the 1880s it became common practice for county

health officers in the South to call midwives together to instruct them in the management of deliveries.[67] Most of the
South's midwives were black (78 percent in Maryland), and
few had received any formal training for their work. Of the
119 midwives in Anne Arundel County, Maryland, only four
had trained in a school for midwives; the remainder were either self-taught or had first worked with a physician at the
bedside. Studies carried out in 1911 indicate that midwives of
Anne Arundel County had little knowledge of asepsis; none
used silver nitrate for the eyes, and many still lubricated their
hands and the vulva with lard. Their usual equipment consisted of a jar of lard (sometimes vaseline), a ball of twine, a
pair of scissors, and tea brewed from pepper, catnip, sweet
fennel, mint, wormwood, or tansy.[68] According to Robert
Campbell Eve, M.D., of the medical department of the University of Georgia, Negro women advanced to the position
of midwife with the barest understanding of anatomy and
carried into the lying-in room all the superstitions of their
race—as well as septic infection, tetanus, and congenital
blindness.[69] Frances Bradley, M.D., who directed the Children's Bureau, which had grown out of the Sheppard-
Towner Act of 1921, recalled one midwife who even tied a
sardine can over a child's navel to prevent bulging. Despite
legitimate criticism, few southern physicians were willing to
carry their remarks beyond obvious racial overtones. The depressed state of rural districts offered little remunerative opportunity; and, for a fraction of the doctor's fee, midwives
provided service to the South's backcountry population.[70]

   In Chicago, where some nine hundred women practiced
midwifery in 1896, the city health department received permission from the Illinois Board of Health to formulate an
Austrian-type program for governing midwives. The program provided for registration, permission to attend only
natural labor, stipulations regarding general duties and
nursing, prohibition of medicines or instruments, requirement of a casebook, provisions for reporting births, and the
management of stillbirths. To assist in these regulations, the
Chicago health department organized a staff of fifty-one
obstetricians and pediatricians to attend cases of difficult labor, inspect casebooks, and generally insure the proper ad-

ministration of the program. Although the board insisted on the registration of midwives and the various support services provided by obstetricians, the punitive aspects of the regulations remained unenforceable because of insufficient funding for proper supervision.[71]

Overall, the laws regulating midwifery at the turn of the century were confusing, if not at times contradictory and useless. In Maine, for example, the law affected only those midwives who claimed the title of physician or doctor. In Louisiana the section of the medical law relating to midwifery concluded with the statement "this section does not apply to the so-called midwife of rural districts and plantation practice who, in the sense of this act, is not considered as practicing midwifery as a profession." A similar statute in Missouri exempted all women who did not practice midwifery as a profession or who did not charge for their services. The commissioner of health in one state pleaded ignorance of the state law requiring midwives to report cases of ophthalmia neonatorum.[72] In a questionnaire sent to the boards of health in each state in 1910, S. Josephine Baker, M.D., director of child hygiene in New York City, clearly demonstrated the negligence of states regarding their own midwife legislation. By 1910 thirteen states had passed laws regulating the practice of midwifery; yet only six had any knowledge of the number of midwives in the state, and only one kept figures on the number of births. In Ohio there was no supervision for the one recognized school of midwifery; and Utah, which claimed two schools of midwifery, required a six-month course of study but had no knowledge of the curriculum taught.[73]

Advocates of prohibition looked to Nebraska, whose laws made no provision for the admission of midwives to practice. Likewise, in the state of Washington, any person practicing midwifery who was not a licensed physician was subject to prosecution. In effect the laws of both states attempted to legislate the midwife out of existence by requiring that such a person be as competent as one who had received a general medical education and had obtained a license to practice. Physician Georgina Grothan wrote, "In the present state of obstetrical science and the high standard of qualifications required therein, it is next to impossible for man or woman to obtain a knowledge of it sufficient to safely practice without first obtaining a thorough general medical education." [74]

The state of Massachusetts also looked to prohibition as a solution to the midwife problem. The 1894 law that established the Board of Registration in Massachusetts and the laws governing the practice of medicine did not specifically mention the midwife, an omission which the Supreme Court of Massachusetts interpreted as a prohibition against further practice by midwives. By curious oversight, however, the law did recognize midwives' signatures on birth certificates. Consequently, the prohibitory efforts were without effect and the practice of midwifery continued; in fact, midwives were paid by the state for returning birth certificates. [75] An inquiry carried out by the Committee of Boston in 1915 established the presence of about 150 active midwives in Massachusetts and their close association with physicians. In the Boston area, for example, Italian midwives not only attended most normal deliveries, but occasionally practiced medicine in areas other than obstetrics. [76] The study further indicated that while the public relationship between physician and midwife had deteriorated markedly in the latter decades of the nineteenth century, their personal relationships, particularly among elder doctors in the community, remained pleasant and businesslike. The same was true in other states, where few midwives lacked the ability to obtain warm endorsements from local physicians as part of their qualifications for state certification and licensing. Many became part of a physician's staff and were employed to wait upon the parturient woman before the arrival of the physician and after delivery. Some midwives were competent enough to meet almost any surgical emergency, and there were numerous reports of physicians calling upon midwives to apply forceps or to sew tears in the genital tract. [77]

Given the conflicting results of the prohibitionists, realistic reformers preferred regulation to prohibition, and commonly looked to state boards of health to secure needed supervision. Minnesota law compelled all persons who wished to practice midwifery to present to the State Medical Board a diploma from a midwifery college. If the board considered the diploma to be legitimate, it gave the midwife a license to practice for one year. If the candidate was not a graduate of a midwife college or related institution, she submitted to an examination which, if passed, entitled her to a one-year license. Midwives already practicing at the time the law was passed were required to present proof of their status to the State Medical Board before receiving a license. In addition, the board could revoke or refuse licenses for "unprofessional or dishonorable conduct or for neglect to make proper returns of births." [78]

Regulationists, in general, were willing to leave midwives in control of their age-old fiefdom, provided significant improvements were made in their education—including more accurate statistics of births and deaths—and they seek the services of the physician in cases of difficult labor. Rather than bring the power of the state to bear directly on the midwife, regulationists chose instead to emphasize the quality of education in midwife schools by forcing them to become affiliated with medical colleges which had adequate facilities for teaching anatomy, physiology, and asepsis. Regulationists sought thereby to improve the quality of midwifery through proper clinical instruction controlled by medical-school faculties. In this environment, C. S. Bacon, M.D., argued in 1897, "the midwife will come to regard the physician not as her enemy but as her counsellor and helper of difficulties, and the physician will learn to appreciate and respect the properly qualified midwife." [79]

Advocates of regulation in New York City looked to England, where problems of education, examination, licensure, and supervision seemed most analogous. As a direct result of the English Midwives Act of 1902, New York City prepared a bill under the combined sponsorship of the Medical Society of the County of New York, the New York Academy of Medicine, the New York Obstetrical Society, the Charities Organization Society and the Nurses' Settlement. The bill became law in 1907, but since there were really few institutions where aspiring midwives could receive proper training, the board of health found itself obliged to grant emergency permits in order to meet the immediate needs of the population. Given the confusion, physicians were frequently called to homes to sign birth certificates for midwives who operated without license. To make matters worse, health officials discovered that the instructional program required foreign language interpreters, since so many midwives were themselves recent immigrants who could neither read nor write English.[80]

In an effort to resolve the problems created by the 1907 legislation, the Bellevue School for Midwives, established in 1911, became the first legitimate institution in the country for teaching midwives. The school was situated on the grounds of the Bellevue Hospital, where student midwives were taught under the direction of physicians. The school required that each student observe one hundred cases and deliver at least twenty before she could graduate. All difficult cases were transferred to Bellevue Hospital. Besides its lying-in services, the school established a large community service for "outdoor patients," where deliveries were managed in the home with the midwife acting under the close supervision of a physician and trained nurse. Ironically, the creation of the Bellevue Training School hastened the elimination of midwives. The city health board made it a policy to refuse a license to any woman who was not either a graduate of the Bellevue school or of a similarly recognized European school. By 1923 the number of registered midwives had declined to 1,500, virtually half the number of a decade earlier. During the first twelve years of its program, only 410 women graduated from the Bellevue school, and it soon became evident that midwifery was a marginal institution in the process of extinction.

The problems faced by midwives in New York were not unlike those elsewhere, with prohibitionists and regulationists divided over how best to serve society's needs. In the belief that midwifery could not easily be eradicated, regulationists chose to institute strong measures of registration and supervision. Regulations did not intend to disturb the existing body of midwives but to gradually replace them with a smaller group of well-trained women. While regulationists viewed their goal as improving the delivery system to mothers through improved competence and stricter measures of supervision, prohibitionists desired to eliminate the midwife entirely by replacing her with licensed obstetricians.[81] The prohibitionists knew only too well that any effort to regulate midwives would confer upon them a legal status difficult to retract. "If midwives are licensed," one New York physician observed, "we are likely to have them in perpetuity." Licensing midwives would not only lower the quality of medical care, it would bring an end to the strenuous efforts then underway to improve medical education, standards of admission to medical schools, and the overall quality of the medical arts and sciences. The prohibitionists argued that even an educated midwife was anachronistic in an age of expanding and improving medical care. To recognize her was to support a double standard in medical delivery systems by grafting a quixotic custom upon a population demanding better trained physician-obstetricians.[82]

A significant portion of prohibitionist hostility stemmed from the overabundance of medical men and the belief that obstetric practice provided a profitable avenue for younger physicians who were beginning a practice. In New York, which had, according to the 1880 census, one physician for every 278 people, physicians believed they could well provide for the delivery needs of the state.[83] Prohibitionists reasoned that with the great number of physicians in the country, a woman could obtain the services of a reputable practitioner for almost the same price as she formerly paid to the midwife. And in the event that the fee was still too high, gratuitous aid through charitable institutions could underwrite medical costs for those women unable to afford the physician's services at the normal fee.[84]

Midwife vs. Woman Practitioner

The rationale of American regulationists and prohibitionists was not always easy to discern. Thomas J. Hillis, M.D., of New York, one of the more vocal supporters of the *sage femme*, claimed that midwifery reflected the customs and folkways of people for nearly five thousand years, and that it was "easier for a camel to go through the eye of a needle than . . . to nullify the unwritten law of the usages of the nation; in fact . . . these old customs and usages are a higher law, and one from which there is seldom any appeal." The midwife existed in every region of the globe—in both barbarous and civilized nations—wherever experience demanded her presence and abilities. The New York physician repudiated the hysterical tales of the midwife's criminal behavior endlessly recounted in the press and at medical society meetings. All things considered, midwives experienced a minimum of fatal cases, with not more than one percent of lying-in women perishing from puerperal conditions. Hillis observed that reputed deaths occurring at the hands of midwives existed mainly in doctors' fertile imaginations and that, by proceeding to legislate against midwives, the profession not only deprived honest women of a livelihood but also threw the bulk of the population on the mercy of charitable organizations because of the higher cost of physician delivery fees. By depriving the poor of their choice of a midwife, Hillis argued, the profession indirectly harmed the general practitioner, by prompting the population to look upon him as an obstacle to their free choice of medical services rather than as a benefactor of humanity.[85]

Though the state surely had the power to make and enforce laws relating to the practice of midwifery, Hillis argued that the interests of the physician and public were really not endangered by the present situation. However, should the state legislate midwives out of existence, a far more monstrous evil would emerge—the woman doctor. By destroying the midwife, the profession would open its doors to female practitioners who would feed upon the fears and prejudices of the population while providing an inferior level of medical service. "It will be noted," he wrote, "that those who take pains to find out the real sentiment of that great heterogeneous mass called the public, the women of that public in particular, will discover that that sentiment is overwhelmingly against the pretensions and prospects of the woman doctor." He advised society to allow the midwife to pursue her "useful but humble calling."[86]

In an article published in *Medical Record* in 1899, Hillis recounted how woman's natural limitations restricted her capacity as a responsible practitioner of medicine. Specifically, he considered the menstrual cycle as an uncontrollable factor that would interfere in the competition with men. He observed that during that "quarantine of nature" woman was ill of body, "morose in mind," and "altogether disqualified for the practice of her profession, for hours or days." Surely such female physicians were unequal to the daily tasks of the male physicians, let alone to the late-hour emergency calls of patients. Only as a qualified professional nurse or midwife, he argued, could woman contribute her full measure of usefulness. "To step higher is only to insure her fall, embitter her life, and show the world that there are occupations that nature did not fit her for, and that one of these occupations is the practice of medicine." By nature women were sexually, constitutionally, and mentally unfit for the responsibilities of medicine and surgical practice, Hillis maintained; yet, clearly, they had the energy, capacity, and intelligence to perform as midwives and thereby contribute to the progress of the medical arts. Women between the ages of forty-four and seventy-four were thoroughly capable of assuming the responsibilities of midwife, since by that time most had passed menopause, that Rubicon of woman's life. "Having cleared the dangerous shoals of her journey through life," he wrote, "she has a reasonable expectation of twenty-five years of good health now, as Nature has lifted her embargo and permitted her to go free." Unhindered by further "monthly tribute" to her sex, she could carry out the responsibilities of midwife without difficulty or anxiety as to her sexual and physical safety.[87]

Not only did Hillis object to women specializing in obstetrics, he feared even more their becoming general practitioners. If a woman put herself in competition with the male general practitioner, she had the responsibility of taking all patients who knocked on her door, including a man with specific stenosis of the rectum, one suffering from spasmodic or strictural affection of the urethra, or perhaps even a man with venereal disease.

> Just imagine the patient standing up, the lady physician on one knee before him, as some surgeons direct, reducing the strangulated organ. Then again, she must be ready after midnight to relieve the necessities of a toper who is suffering intense agony from a distended and paralyzed bladder after the debauch and revelry of the evening. . . . If she refers him to a male physician or to a hospital he may die before he gets there. . . . If the lady dismisses those patients with a "NO," she is cruel; she may even be a murderess and should answer before the law. If she does not dismiss them, but invites them into her consulting-room, the toper may be hilarious after he is relieved from his pain and proceed to take liberties with his fair physician. . . . We can see now the difficulties which surround the good lady and that she is on the horns of a di-

lemma. We may be able to sympathize with her and hope she will come safely through the meshes of law; but if she admitted the aforesaid man into her consultation-room for treatment, with a flush on her cheek (that is, if there was no powder there before) and a jump in the throat, she is destitute of the shame Eve felt in the garden when she clothed herself with fig-leaves, and which is ever since the glory and the pride of women.[88]

The Pittsburgh Plan

In an article written for the AMA in 1913, Pittsburgh obstetrician Charles E. Ziegler announced his opposition "to any plan which seeks to give [the midwife] a permanent place in the practice of medicine." Although he admitted there were medical practitioners as poorly equipped as midwives in aseptic knowledge and training, there was no reason for permitting "ignorant, non-medical individuals to give counsel and assistance in medical matters." Ziegler argued that it was better to educate doctors and improve standards in the medical schools than to attempt to raise the level of competence of midwives. Rather than attack the midwife directly with potentially unpopular legislation, he considered it expedient to train the physician and provide financial inducements to perform obstetric duties. "We are passing through a political, social and economic revolution," he remarked, "which is certain to result in giving to the worthy poor justice in the necessities of life, among which must be included competent medical service administered by those who are trained in medicine. They will demand it and they will get it." Ziegler insisted that such services did not mean socialism but rather an equality of opportunity that had already become apparent in the growth of savings banks, life insurance, and the increased numbers of American workers who were buying land and owning their own homes. Americans were reaching a point in their national development where most could secure the means for a good life. Judged in this light, midwifery was a relic of the past, unrepresentative of the current needs of society.

"If equality of opportunity as regards medical service is ever to come to this country," Ziegler wrote, "it cannot come so long as we train one class of practitioners to care for those who can pay, and another much inferior class to care for those who cannot." The real question before the profession and the American people was not What shall we do with the midwife? but rather How shall we provide competent medical service to the public? If all classes were included in the definition of public, it was clear that equal opportunity in the United States did not mean separate and unequal facilities in the area of maternity, since every woman had the right, as a citizen and as a mother, to proper medical care during and after childbirth. As a prohibitionist, however, Ziegler did not advocate the extinction of midwifery through outright legislation. Her elimination had to be geared to the passage of carefully planned legislation that would provide a medical system superior to the one being replaced.[89]

Of particular concern to Ziegler was the manner in which medical services were provided for the nation's charity cases; the poor in ill health were just as much the responsibility of the state as they were when being fed, sheltered, or clothed. Having physicians provide such health care without proper compensation, however, only meant an inferior level of medical attention for the poor. Ziegler argued, "Public charities of all kinds should be placed on a strictly business basis, should be well organized, thoroughly supervised and all the workers should be justly compensated." The custom of placing the burden of free medical service for the poor on the profession alone had led doctors to seek excessive fees from those able to pay, a situation which had brought harm to the cause of medicine. "The practice of medicine had been thereby converted into a trade," Ziegler reasoned, "and commercialism has destroyed much of its higher and finer side and has done untold harm in the attitude which the public should have toward the physician and the schools which educate him."[90]

Accordingly, Ziegler urged greater involvement of government in the delivery of medical services through the collection of data from charity patients to ascertain their ability to pay. He insisted that medical charity was not the sole responsibility of the profession. Surely, he argued, it was not the business of doctors "to levy tribute on individuals of means on the plea that they are serving the poor without pay." The government must be prepared to assist, through rigid investigation into the stated financial position of charity patients. If a person's income could not cover a physician's fees, then the state had responsibility to provide some form of financial assistance. In any case, the state "should pay the physician adequately for all his services to the poor and should collect by taxes from all the people their share of the money necessary to care for its charge." In Pennsylvania, for example, the state paid the difference between what the patient was able to afford and the actual cost of health care, supplemented with donations from private gifts and philanthropic societies to hospitals and dispensaries that provided health care to indigent patients. While private patients would support their own hospital care from medical payments and insurance, hospitals would service the poor with supplementary funds from philanthropic and public monies. Moreover, medical school faculties and their students could utilize tax-supported patients as clinical material for training in specialized branches of medicine. Thus all patients, both private and tax-supported, would receive the most efficient service at a minimum cost to the state. With such a system doctors in private practice were protected from plundering by staff physicians of hospitals and dispensaries seeking potential medical customers.[91]

In a roundabout fashion, Ziegler saw in this program a means of eliminating the midwife. A hospital or dispensary staff, working in conjunction with medical students, social services, and professional nurses, could replace the marginal care of the midwife. At the same time the experience gained by medical students in obstetric work would improve the overall medical capacity of the profession in an area heretofore reserved to the midwife. "If the midwife cases and such others as are dependent on public charity were used for teaching purposes," Ziegler wrote, "not only would the patients themselves receive excellent care but also sufficient clinical material would be available to give every graduate in medicine such obstetric training as would make him a safe and efficient practitioner."[92] Of course, in those rural areas lacking both doctors and hospitals, the midwife might continue her work until such time as the state provided funding for her replacement. Ziegler agreed with the findings of the Carnegie Foundation that "a sanitary service, subsidized by the state, will alone render efficient relief in backward districts without demoralizing the profession." [93]

Under Ziegler's guidance, Pittsburgh, which in the early twentieth century had one of the highest infant mortality rates of any large city in America (109 percent higher than the New York City rate for the same period), inaugurated a pilot program centered around Magee Hospital. Modeled after the Frauenklinker of Germany, Magee Hospital combined both the obstetric and gynecological wards, which previously, when separated, tended to make a midwife of the obstetrician and an abdominal surgeon of the gynecologist despite their common pathological and physiological interests. This consolidation was also in keeping with the suggestion made by Abraham Flexner, in *Medical Education in Europe*, that "consolidation avoids the necessity of drawing arbitrary lines by way of making two specialities where Nature has made but one; for obstetrics and gynecology have a single physiologic and anatomic point of departure, namely the child-bearing function." The program at Magee called for an operating and teaching amphitheater; examining, delivery, and recovery rooms; research laboratories; and a medical library. The plans even included a museum, along with special rooms for photography and X rays, hydrotherapeutic departments, and sterilizing rooms. To improve the environment, the hospital offered isolated gardens within the grounds for patients, nurses, and physicians. The medical director, with his family, resided on the hospital grounds and was paid a salary sufficient to avoid having to seek private patients. [94] The Ziegler plan of 1912 also created the Pittsburgh Maternity Dispensary, with dormitories for a dozen physicians, students, social workers, and nurses. When combined, the Magee Hospital and Dispensary formed a public-welfare and teaching unit that braved the criticism of the Pittsburgh medical profession, and in particular, the Allegheny County Medical Society, which eventually suspended Ziegler (then director of the Magee Hospital) on the charge of "acquiescing in a policy which is detrimental to the public and the profession." [95]

Eventually the free outpatient obstetrical service became an important mechanism in the elimination of the midwife.

Wherever there was a medical school, doctors advised that such outpatient services be used for teaching purposes. In the event a city had no medical school, outpatient obstetrical services could be connected with a maternity hospital. In Manchester, New Hampshire, a city of about eighty thousand, young physicians just settling in the city and looking to build a practice combined with the district nursing association to provide outpatient obstetrical services. The scheme, designed to eliminate midwives in the textile and shoe industries, which employed a large percentage of immigrant labor, required patients to pay what they were able, with the Metropolitan Life Insurance Company cooperating to pay the difference. In Boston, medical reformers created the Maverick Dispensary, a pay clinic designed to bring medical treatment to individuals who could afford only a modest sum for medical care. In obstetrical cases the dispensary charged a fee of fifteen dollars, the standard fee asked by midwives in the area. Of that amount ten dollars went to the physician, who was usually a young doctor seeking to improve his skills and build a practice.[96]

The acceptance of free outpatient obstetrical service, maternity dispensaries, and lying-in hospitals for the poor did not come easily. Advocates warned that elimination of the midwife would necessitate enormous public expenditures. Charity hospitals were relics of an older Europe, not an attribute of the American republic, and would weaken the moral fiber of the American working class. "Every hospital that is built for this purpose," one physician lamented in 1899, "proportionally increases the percent of paupers and diminishes the wealth of the state." The program to eliminate midwives through teaching hospitals would create a class of citizens who lacked self-sufficiency and who would become increasingly dependent upon government and misguided philanthropic societies.[97]

The consensus of medical sentiment was that the midwife should be eliminated along with the untrained doctor. Both were out of step with the new theories in preventive medicine and both were a danger to the health needs of the nation. With a surplus of physicians, trained midwives were superfluous. Many doctors refused to recognize the midwife as having any functional relationship to the medical profession and the community. Nor, for that matter, were they willing to sanction her customary methods of training and succession, her prior relationship with physicians, and her traditional mode of acquiring new knowledge. Medical reformers challenged not simply the midwife, but a philosophy of medicine and centuries of previous attitudes on obstetric care. And being the least organized—indeed, a social and cultural institution outside formal rules—and the least capable of making the transition into the newer scientific world, the midwife became the first fatality of medical reform.

6

Most Noble Art, Imperfect Science

HOW TO EFFECTIVELY MEET the needs of a citizenry as apt to turn to charlatanism as to seek the help of science became a major obstacle facing medical men in their relationship to the public in the nineteenth century. Medicine, neither a pure art nor a perfect science, suffered from the ignorance of those it served. Patients conceived of doctors as little more than dispensers of pills, potions, and bandages; and they turned with ease to medical sectarians who promised swift cure for dropsy, fluxes, dry gripes, ague, and fevers. In general, laymen remained indifferent to progress in pathology, new germ theories of disease, or, for that matter, primitive ideas that ascribed ills to the influence of the stars, provided they were relieved of pain and freed from the bonds of sickness. As far as the public was concerned, correct principles, safe methods, and unselfish aims were secondary to cure. And, as the profession struggled to improve medicine and its own image in the Victorian age, the ability to cure, the only tangible hold upon the patient's trust, was in danger of being lost.

Apprenticeship

America's early system of medical education developed in response to the dichotomy of a growing need for doctors and a corresponding absence of medical schools. Just as indentured servitude had been tailored from the cloth of Europe's impoverished class system and the peculiar nature of labor scarcity in the New World, so also the system of medical apprenticeship emerged from a colonial effort to provide doctors for a society unable to wait for a properly prepared and scientifically grounded physician. Seventeenth and eighteenth century youths who desired careers in medicine apprenticed themselves to a willing practitioner or preceptor who, depending on his sense of responsibility and educational background, instructed young men in his accumulated wisdom and experience. For a period of four to seven years, students joined the doctor's household, kept casebooks, and learned the art and science of medicine from close observation. In some instances students were actually bound by indenture, though this was not common. For most, apprenticeship was a less formal arrangement which consisted of an agreement based upon a monetary transaction. The normal fee for apprenticeship was one hundred dollars, which, while varying slightly from one colony to another and from rural district to urban setting, remained relatively constant from colonial days until the 1840s. In time, apprenticeship responsibilities grew from household chores to services that included mixing drugs, preparing plasters, following the doctor on his visits to patients, and taking an active part in the preceptor's practice of bleeding, blistering, leeching, pulling teeth, setting fractures, and lancing boils.[1]

Any doctor could become a preceptor and, with no supervision from any national medical organization or, for that matter, any standard by which to judge medical education at all, the quality of instruction naturally varied. Those preceptors who took seriously their responsibilities, demanded that students have knowledge of Latin and emphasized the importance of natural history, grammar, and mathematics as preparatory to a sound education. They also provided students with a variety of teaching aids, including an occasional skeleton and books such as Hippocrates's *Aphorisms,* Cowper's *Anatomy of Human Bodies* (1698), or Haller's *First Lines of Physiology* (1779). Other principal works of the eighteenth century included Boerhaave's *Institutiones* (1708), Cullen's *Institutes of Medicine* (1788), John Hunter on venereal disease, Rush's *Medical Inquiries and Observations* (1789), Pierre-Joseph Desault's *Journal de Chirurgie* (1791), Buffon on natural history, the anatomy of Cheselden and Monro, the surgery of Sharp, and the works of William Hunter and William Smellie on midwifery. Good medical libraries were a rarity, however, and those outdated texts that circulated within the medical community tended to impede medicine in much the same manner as the common law delayed more innovative legal thinking.[2]

By the time of the Revolutionary War, some 3,500 physicians were practicing in the colonies. Of this number probably no more than 350 were graduates of European medical schools, and only 51 others had received degrees from the two American schools then established. Clearly most physicians had entered the profession through the system of apprenticeship or, as was sometimes the case, by simply claiming some sort of medical skill. In effect Americans found themselves having to accept a variety of medical impostors. "Quacks abound like Locusts in Egypt," William Smith complained in his history of New York written in 1757. "To our Shame be it remembered we have no Law to protect the Lives of the King's Subjects, from the Malpractice of Pretenders."[3] American society needed doctors "before there was any way of educating them; and a method was improvised which comforted the sick with a titular doctor, who could sign a death certificate, even though he understood little of their aches and pains."[4]

Factors that helped bring stability to American medicine included the considerable number of European-trained physicians who were practicing in the colonies, the influence of European medical publications that specified treatment and unified theory, the education of American students abroad, and the concerns of high-minded preceptors like David Hosack (1769–1835) of New York and John Redman (1722–1808), who eventually became the first president of the College of Physicians of Philadelphia. In one respect European medical study offered an appealing alternative to the limitations of the apprenticeship system. Young men able to afford a more complete education supplemented apprenticeship or American medical-school training with postgraduate education at the University of Leyden in Holland; the Hôtel Dieu of Paris; Guy's or St. Thomas's Hospital in London; Dublin's Meath Hospital; Edinburgh's Royal Infirmary; or the University of Vienna, where Van Swieten's influence had set the pattern for clinical instruction. There they gained additional learning in private courses, such as William Hunter's Theatre in Covent Garden, or enrolled in the universities for a medical degree. More important, they walked the hospital wards, witnessing operations and dissections and, in general, observing and studying a greater variety of diseases than were ever seen in a preceptor's private practice. Aspiring young men packed off to Edinburgh to attend the lectures of William Cullen, James Gregory, John Brown, Alexander and James Hamilton and the Monros; journeyed to London to work with William Hewson, John Lettsom, Joseph Black, Matthew Baillie, John Fothergill or the Hunters; paid for a course on midwifery with Smellie or Colin McKenzie; worked with Morgagni of Padua; or sought the instruction of Robert James Graves and William Stokes of Dublin. In the period prior to the American Revolution, the University of Edinburgh remained the most popular mecca for aspiring American students. There William Shippen, Jr. (1761), John Morgan (1762), Samuel Bard (1765), David Hosack (1792), Philip Syng Physick (1792), and others studied for their degrees.[5]

To continue these experiences, returning American doctors offered private courses on midwifery, anatomical demonstrations and dissections, and even organized medical schools patterned on European models to serve the needs of those unable to afford study aboard. Inspired by what they saw in Europe, men like John Moultrie, Isaac Cathrall, Thomas Cadwalader, Thomas Bond, Benjamin Rush, William Shippen, Jr., John Morgan, and Abraham Chovet attempted to create a more favorable environment for health care and native medical education. By 1800 ten medical schools were organized in conjunction with hospitals and established universities (patterned after Edinburgh, Exeter, and Liverpool) and offered a level of clinical and didactic instruction which, until the 1820s and 1830s, provided the eastern seaboard states with a relatively high degree of medical competence. These schools and the year of their founding included the College of Philadelphia 1765, King's College 1767, William and Mary College 1779, Harvard College 1783, University of the State of Pennsylvania 1783, Dartmouth College 1797, Transylvania College 1799, the University of Pennsylvania and Columbia College 1792, and Queen's College 1793.[6] In general, candidates for these early medical schools were required to have served an apprenticeship; have knowledge of pharmacy; be of good moral character; possess competence in Latin, natural science, and mathematics; submit to a private examination by the medical faculty; and write a dissertation on some medical subject. As part of the degree requirement, students of the College of Philadelphia attended at the Pennsylvania Hospital for one year.[7]

The system of apprenticeship adapted readily to the early establishment of medical schools; the term of apprenticeship was shortened to three years, with the understanding that aspiring doctors would divide their time between the didactic method and the preceptor. As initially conceived, medical schools supplemented the apprenticeship by "reviewing and systematizing . . . theoretical acquisitions, while considerably extending . . . practical experience." Medical schools focused principally on the didactic aspects of medical training, providing a more intense education, through the use of anatomical rooms and chemical laboratories, than was characteristic of the bustling practice of the preceptor.[8] Courses typically consisted of anatomy and physiology, clinical and pathological surgery, theory and practice of medicine, obstetrics and diseases of women and children, chemistry and pharmacy, materia medica and botany, and medical jurisprudence. These courses were essentially the same in most schools, with anatomy, physiology, and chemistry the elementary courses and surgery, therapeutics, materia medica, obstetrics, and medical jurisprudence the more advanced courses of study. One curiosity of this divided system of medical training was that students sat through two terms of the same subject matter. The rationale for this repetitive two-year program lay initially in the limited number of textbooks, equipment, and properly trained teachers. Students who found it difficult to cover the prescribed material in the first term had the opportunity to complete their studies in the second term. To overcome the lack of textbooks, students copied lectures verbatim, and the two-year repetitive program answered the deficiencies in their writing skills. Ironically what began as a pedagogic solution for a temporary impediment soon became an institutionalized part of medical education.[9]

Despite the best intentions, medical education deteriorated in both substance and form under the divided responsibility of preceptor and school. The three-year preceptorial training period remained a prerequisite for entrance into medical schools through most of the nineteenth century, but schools neither applied these criteria consistently nor established procedures to check on the qualifications of preceptors. Physicians who desired to take on students could do so, whether or not they owned a medical book or were themselves little more than charlatans. It was not uncommon for doctors to receive a preceptor fee for falsifying a student's apprenticeship as a stipulation for admittance into medical school. "If the preceptor or student, or both of them, were lazy or careless," one physician observed, "it often happened that the student registered and then never went near his preceptor again, but spent the next two years in any way that seemed to him pleasanter or more immediately profitable than the study of medicine, and in the third year took two courses of lectures, passed an examination that was anything but rigid and then received a diploma exactly as if he had spent the whole three years in hard study."[10] Schools operated without a graded-course curriculum. To compound the problem, only a small percentage of students remained in school long enough to graduate; most entered practice without having obtained a formal degree. This meant that, while some students continued to serve only a three-year apprenticeship, some others obtained a didactic education without any accompanying experience, and still others received a combination of the two that was hardly worth the effort.[11] Provided the teacher was conscientious and competent in both diagnosis and treatment, the preceptor form of medical education gave the diligent student an opportunity for personal experience with patients and disease. Unfortunately, William Norwood commented, "the youth acquired the virtues and vices of his teacher. He perpetuated both the truth and error embodied in the corpus of medical practice imparted to him." In effect, the apprenticeship form of medical education depended on the determination of the student and the intellectual honesty of the preceptor.[12]

The Young Republic

The problems and weaknesses of the medical education system reflected those of the nation at large in the first half of the nineteenth century, i.e., how to acquire and maintain quality in a society whose democratic impulse seemed satisfied with leadership that reflected the common man. The democratization of society, begun in earnest with the Jacksonians, brought an end to the Enlightenment's healthy suspicion of human passion and the concept of an American republic built upon talent. In attacking the bugbear of elitism, Jacksonian society cast its vote for no standards at all. An uncritical faith in democracy pervaded the land and, with it, a belief in the will of the people that was grounded more in self-confidence and ideology than in experience. Lost in the scramble for equality was the Jeffersonian emphasis on education and property as the touchstones of true democracy. American society was concerned more with the origin of power than with its consequences as it forged ahead with an untested faith in democratic man, a faith that transformed the vices of disorder and decadence into the virtues of the new age. Common judgment in politics, tastes, religion—indeed, common infallibility—became a clear repudiation of the political philosophy of the Enlightenment.[13]

The ever-expanding frontier and the catalytic license it gave to groups and self-images, the effects of Jacksonian democracy and the challenges of industrialism, the immigration of peoples who were culturally, institutionally, and educationally diverse, and the self-conscious tradition of the genteel culture of the East Coast all lent to American medical development problems unlike those of Europe. These problems seriously challenged the traditional status of the doctor in society as well as the integrity of his professional-training.[14] The very expanse of the new nation contributed to the inability of doctors to control the profession in the manner of their European counterparts. Poor roads, sectional grievances, ethnocentrism, and the growing belief in regional diseases, reinforced the tendency of students to prefer medical training in the area where they wished to practice.[15] Commercial medical schools unconnected with hospitals and universities proliferated, as state legislatures granted charters to medical cliques that showed little concern for teaching facilities, medical philosophy, and curriculum. The country bristled with confidence in the common man, and, as state governments responded with legislation tuned to the voice of the new democracy, the nation faced a medical-education system that bordered on anarchy. Jacksonian Americans were open-minded toward medical irregulars and were inclined not to make distinctions that could be associated with education, European training, and orthodox medicine. In this milieu, homeopathy, Thomsonianism, and assorted sectarians plied their trade with little difficulty; and by the 1840s medicine had largely become a laymen's prerogative. In part this was due to the assertive spirit of the young republic and those "venal-minded" physicians in rural communities who thought it their right to establish an educational facility for their region. Oliver Wendell Holmes, who reflected with pride on New England's educational traditions, condemned these proprietary institutions of the South and West as inferior schools, wrongly located.[16] But the condemnation applied as well to metropolitan areas, which had witnessed the splintering of existing medical faculties as a result of petty jealousies and the subsequent creation of competing schools with inadequate facilities and ill-trained staffs.[17]

The proprietary medical schools which sprang up in the states and territories west of the Appalachians owed their genesis to the College of Medicine of Maryland, chartered in 1807. However, unlike the Maryland college, which maintained an adequate level of programmatic integrity, most imitators lacked equipment, books, and qualified teachers, a situation which, when combined with motivations that were primarily financial, gave little assurance that students would receive an education reflecting sound medical philosophy. As one historian described it, medical education took on the flavor of "amateur therapeutics and cultist practice more than orthodox medicine."[18] Characterized by the sixty-odd irregular medical colleges spawned from the botanic medical beliefs of Samuel Thomson (1769–1843), the offshoot eclectic medical institutes, the water-cure treatment of Vincenz Priessnitz, the homeopathic colleges developed by disciples of Samuel Hahnemann, and the matriculants known as Curisites and Beachites, American medical education was as much a specimen of Jacksonian democracy as it was a relic of earlier schisms that still festered as sores in traditional medicine.[19]

Those medical schools which grafted themselves onto existing colleges and universities as semiautonomous or self-constituted bodies felt the full impact of democratization. Although the grafting process allowed practitioners to organize and identify with an existing university, the faculty of the medical department usually maintained a high degree of autonomy both in terms of financial responsibility and supervision and had only nominal contact with the academic institution. In these situations a group of doctors would receive permission from a university to grant degrees under its charter; but actual control of the medical school, in terms of salaries, appointments, curriculum, and facilities, remained the prerogatives of the medical faculty, who operated a virtual *imperium in imperio*. The incomes for the medical faculty derived mainly from lecture tickets, and occasionally state legislatures permitted the use of lotteries to raise funds. Naturally this financial arrangement only reinforced the marginal caliber of medical education, since colleges were inclined to admit potential candidates for medical degrees according to their ability to pay. For the parent institution, the arrangement enhanced the image of a university that could boast a medical school; it also afforded to the medical faculty the added luster of being part of a big university. Aside from the pretence given to both parties, however, little could be said in favor of the relationship.[20]

To add to the difficulty of maintaining—or even initiating—standards in medical schools, during the 1830s and 40s various states began to abandon licensing regulations. Prior to this time, nearly every state had insured some measure of legal control over licensure (New York in 1760 was the first colony to require the examination and licensing of physicians); and this mechanism, combined with the overseeing efforts of medical societies and governing boards of the universities, insured a fair degree of regulatory control over the profession. Admittedly, state medical societies and licensing agencies viewed the license fee more as a source of income than as a modicum of quality control. In rapid succession, however, states repealed what medical legislation existed: Illinois in 1826; Ohio in 1833; Mississippi in 1834; the District of Columbia, Maryland, Massachusetts, Maine, Connecticut and South Carolina in 1838; New York in 1844; Texas in 1848; and Michigan in 1851. By mid century, fifteen state legislatures had repudiated medical licensure as class legislation and had given open access to the profession by removing the penalties for practicing without a license; and their actions—in greater or less degree—were duplicated by most other states. By the time of the Civil War, no effective medical licensing existed in any of the states.[21] Obviously there was a general confusion as to what actually defined a medical doctor in the absence of any overriding controls, since the title of doctor was attached to a host of practitioners who had no basis for the claim.[22]

Supply and Demand

From the time of American independence until 1810, 7 medical schools opened their doors. During the next thirty years, 26 more were organized; and in the thirty-five years after 1840, 47 were added. The census of 1870 listed 110 schools teaching medicine in the country, of which 77 were classified as orthodox. The same census indicated an annual production of approximately 2,000 doctors of medicine by regular schools, with 6,500 persons in attendance at lectures. Adding to that number the Americans graduating from foreign universities, immigrant physicians, and irregulars, the increase in number of physicians amounted to nearly 2,500 annually. A synopsis of a list of doctors who paid a special internal revenue tax of ten dollars for the year 1871 provides the basis for figures totaling 49,798 physicians for a population of roughly 39 million. Of the total figure, 39,070 were classified as regulars, 2,961 as homeopaths, 133 as hydropaths, 2,860 as eclectics, and 4,774 as miscellaneous and unknown. These statistics give a ratio of one regular physician to every 1,000 population, a figure considerably at variance with the U.S. Census Report of 1870, which noted 62,383 persons claiming medicine as their profession. The latter figure was 12,585 higher than that enumerated by the U.S. Assessor of Internal Revenue and was probably more accurate, since many doctors were no doubt reluctant to be counted for payment of the revenue tax. A comparison of the number of clergymen, lawyers, and doctors for the periods 1850, 1860, and 1870 in each state and territory discloses that the medical profession far exceeded the other two (see appendix).[23]

By 1902, 160 medical colleges were annually turning out

6,000 graduates, which the American Medical Association estimated to be 2,000 more than the nation could adequately absorb under the laws of supply and demand. According to the AMA, a physician required a clientele of at least 2,000 patients to earn enough to live adequately; yet only North and South Carolina, Alaska, and Hawaii provided this ratio. In 1907 the District of Columbia had one physician for every 255 persons, and even the Indian territory had a doctor for every 373. Oklahoma had one doctor for every 397 persons: Bison had a practitioner for every 16 persons; Custer, one for every 7; Meers, one for every 6; and Oklahoma City averaged out at one for every 190. New York City, with the largest number of doctors, had 5,167 for a population of 2,380,000, or one doctor for every 461 persons. These statistics, more than any other evidence, convinced the medical profession of the need to check the flow of graduates from medical schools (see appendix).[24]

The desire for an organic unity between apprenticeship and didactic education crumbled amid the avalanche of burgeoning colleges. In 1910 Abraham Flexner reported that in little more than a century 457 schools had been organized in the United States and Canada; and although many scarcely opened their doors before closing down, the impact they had on medical standards was devastating. Physicians in Illinois created 39 colleges; New York, 43; and Missouri, 42. Chicago had 14 colleges; Cincinnati, 20; and Louisville, 11. Many of these schools consisted of little more than a rented room, a few benches, a skeleton, an occasional corpse, and several physicians who were seeking to supplement their private practice with income generated from lecture tickets. "The man who had settled his tuition bill," Flexner commented, "was thus practically assured of his degree, whether he had regularly attended lectures or not."[25] In effect, medical colleges admitted and graduated students who were far below even the most generous standards. One doctor observed that in earlier years medical institutions were fewer and entrance requirements were set high, but "who ever *now* hears of even *one* [student] being rejected?" He felt that rivalry among medical colleges for patronage and the cheapening of medical education had reduced the profession to a "low and contemptible standard."[26] Medical colleges existed far in excess of public need. One critic observed, "Like the country store which doles out inferior wares at every crossroad, a so-called 'medical college' is found in almost every town of generous size; and to obtain a medical degree is within the possibility, intellectual and financial, of any youth, however lacking in mental and moral fitness."[27]

Clearly medical schools supplemented the system of apprenticeship, but they provided minimal education for American doctors—an education which proved inferior to the hospital training enjoyed by American students abroad. At a time when chemistry, thermometry, biology, surgery, and germ theory were making advances in Europe, when Schleiden and Schwann announced the cell theory, when Bichat was elaborating on tissue pathology, and when Auenbrugger and Laënnec were developing diagnostic tools, American students were being educated in institutions that provided a thirteen- to sixteen-week term and little laboratory work, few bedside opportunities, and minimal clinical experience. Even Harvard lacked microscopes and stethoscopes until well after the Civil War.[28]

Most American medical students, with the exception of those who were fortunate enough to continue their education in Europe, completed their training without stepping inside a hospital. Other exceptions were those few who found posts as house-officers in the Pennsylvania Hospital, the Massachusetts General Hospital, or the Boston General Hospital, where they observed the practices of visiting physicians. The university medical schools, which were outnumbered by the proprietary schools, maintained a semblance of standards through contact with European medical departments. Those students with incentive beyond the simple attainment of a degree continued their education in Europe under the tutelage of gifted teachers in modern dissecting rooms and hospital environments.

Although Edinburgh and London medical schools continued to attract American medical students, the pre–Civil War decades also witnessed an increasing number of Americans educated in Paris, where dissection and post-mortem examinations gave France a central role in clinical-pathological studies and the emerging science of clinical statistics. In the wards of the Hôtel Dieu, Hôtel Vénérienne, La Charité,

La Pitié, Salpetrière, and Enfants Malades, American students learned first hand the newest theories and scientific practices. Bichat's insistence on autopsy as a means of verifying diagnosis, Corvisart's use of clinical observation, Laënnec's invention of the stethoscope, Louis's deductions drawn from statistical reports, Broussais's theory of gastroenteritis, and the influence of Lisfranc, Velpeau, Andral, Trousseau, Dupuytren, and others among the Paris faculty could not but affect the intensity with which American students attacked the frailities of their own medical system and its waning English influence. Students like William Power, John A. Swett, James Jackson, Jr., John Young Bassett, Henry J. Bigelow, Henry I. Bowditch, Jonathan Mason Warren, William Wood Gerhard, Casper Wistar Pennock, George Cheyne Shattuck, Alfred Stillé, Valentine Mott, and Oliver Wendell Holmes acquired fresh ideas from their postgradute training in France between 1820 and the Civil War. Like the generations of students before them, they returned to the states and threw themselves into medicine with an enthusiasm that quickly nourished the meager fare of medical education in America.[29]

Cultivation of Nature

One factor that helped to preserve medicine from the devastating effects of its educational system was the avocation of many doctors as naturalists. Concerned with broadening their educational horizons, physicians acquired practical hobbies in natural history, a field which, although largely undefined in the nineteenth century, consisted of botany, zoology, geology, mineralogy, chemistry, anthropology, agriculture, and even gardening. There, away from the bitterness engendered by the system-builders, sectarians, and advocates of pedagogical nihilism, they browsed with intellectual pleasure, delighted in spirited discussion, and communicated across the broad, if not limitless, boundaries of nature. The country doctor found this an easy task, as he filled long miles between patients with quiet contemplation of flowers, trees, and rocks. Edward Waldo Emerson urged that his fellow practitioners relax in the mental refreshment of the pine woods and meadows rather than ride buggy wheels over tomato cans or pieces of coal along the highway. Like his father the younger Emerson encouraged his colleagues to seek out adventurous paths through the woods rather than, "like a locomotive, [become] a slave to the graded road." By leaving known highways, with their predetermined curves, grades, and landmarks, the adventurous doctor could discover the variety in nature's least known paths. "From willow-catkins and alter-tassels," Emerson wrote, "we may read if our eyes are trained, through all the sure almanac of May flower, rhodora, pink azalea, arethusa, red lilies, purple grass, rhexia, fringed gentian, to witch hazel and black-alder berries before white crystals and gleams of ice jewels must take their places. An easier study, in a book printed large on purpose that he who rides fastest may read, is, the forest trees and shrubs. You may learn them by their leaves in summer and in winter their barks will be a nicer test of your observation."[30]

John Davidson Godman (1794–1830), whose *American Natural History* (1826) and *Rambles of a Naturalist* (1833) gave testimony to the observant quality of the physician-naturalist at work, brought his medical training and naturalist's insight into perfect harmony. To read Godman's *Rambles of a Naturalist* is to feel the relaxed but observant air of one of America's earliest naturalists at work and to sense the exultation that came with every discovery. An inner peace spread contagiously from the harmony of nature to this naturalist's soul, an appreciation for nature that furnished strength for his private meditations. With a pilgrim's delight in nature, he admitted to having walked hundreds of miles simply to investigate the habits of the shrew mole, the beauty of a pine forest, the life history of the crab, and the cautious habits of the crow. Godman was enamored with the written word. He was fond of recounting his experiences with the primitive state of transportation in Ohio, observing the peculiar institution of slavery, and relating the seasons and marshes to the incidence of disease. He was equally fond of testing the observations of European naturalists against his own somnambulistic excursions into nature.[31] Daniel Drake (1785–1852) of Cincinnati described Godman, in contrast with the doctors who had become ensnared in sectarian heresy, as a man who had come to the study of nature as an investigator of facts, and not as a pupil of the schools. He was "observing," imaginative, fluent, and "graphical"; and while lacking in deep and original analysis, he made up for this deficiency with vivid and accurate delineations that marked him as much a poet and philosopher as Lucretius, Erasmus Darwin, and Good.[32]

Similarly, neurologist John K. Mitchell (1798–1858), whose interests spanned subjects from parasitic etiology to osmosis and liquefaction, urged students of Jefferson Medical College in Philadelphia in 1842 to improve their minds by going beyond the boundaries of the dissecting room and didactic education. Of all the professions, Mitchell observed, medicine demanded the greatest knowledge. A doctor could not be versed merely in the anatomical and physiological knowledge of the brain and nervous system; the human species was so complicated that the most reasoned study of the body required an extended observation that brooked everything the laboratory could offer. For Mitchell an educated doctor must also be a good naturalist. He wrote, "Our country has not been a laggard in this agreeable and useful pursuit, and here as elsewhere, the cultivators of medicine have been among the most zealous and successful of its votaries." Mitchell believed that natural history seldom seduced the true physician from the path of his professional duties; rather, it broadened his knowledge of nature—of all nature—for the greater employment of his skills. "I scarcely ever saw a professional man who made of himself a mere business hack, who was either happy or agreeable," he wrote. "Such men become usually prematurely old, and, on the whole, even in the line of the business, less for society than those who mingle judiciously in pursuits of less absorbing character." The diversity of subject matter in natural history enlivened the mind and invigorated the investigative spirit, which the capable physician turned productively to his own doctor-patient needs. With the perspective and reflective faculties enlarged by close observation of nature, he increased the chances of discovering that which the less knowledgeable physician might miss. The human species was a highly complex organism in a varied and changing environment, with every cell capable of being influenced by the interior and exterior agencies surrounding it. The study of a single disease and its relationship to causation, nature, tendencies, results, and prophylaxis, involved a study of all those varying influences on the body, a knowledge of the structure and function of each part of the human system, the factors that governed morbid action, and an intimate understanding of the nature and effects of remedial agents. Thus, to speak of medicine was to speak literally of an aggregation of materials gathered from every other science known to man—from geology, meteorology, climatology, and the laws of vegetable growth and decomposition, to anatomy and physiology, organic and inorganic chemistry, mineralogy, natural history, and mental philosophy.[33]

Mitchell urged his fellow physicians to enlist in the investigative pursuits of the Franklin Institute or to cultivate the exhibitions of agricultural and horticultural organizations, where they could observe great public cabinets of minerals and useful displays of nature. In addition, he suggested that doctors form library associations and collect specimens for their own or their society's cabinets of natural curiosities. From these endeavors early medical schools established museums for anatomical specimens and botanic gardens for pharmacology; Solomon Drown, professor of materia medica and botany at Brown Medical School, for example, grew and prepared most of the herbal medicines used by the college. Mitchell remarked: "Do not suppose that in thus improving your minds beyond the common precincts of medicine you will make a worse doctor, while you compound a better citizen. Our noble art takes advantage of every idea."[34] Mitchell's son Silas followed his father's footsteps into medicine and likewise appreciated "the play of the mind" in natural history that seldom failed to improve the powers of observation. Silas wrote, "One man goes to and from the bedside, or talks to a chronic case, and sees and hears no more than the bare symptoms; another is curiously wide awake as to all his senses; by mere habit nothing escapes him, and some day he gets out of all this results when other men fail."[35]

Perhaps no other pastime included as many serious minded amateurs and ready-made savants as natural history. From David Hosack's *Hortus Enginesis*, Thomas Say's work on entomology and conchology, and Hare's study of atmospheric storms to Joseph Leidy's *Fresh Water Rhizopods of North America* (1879), the lectures of Dunglison on the instincts of animals, and Horatio C. Wood's botanical collections, the curious mind of the physician-naturalist roamed from man, beast, and bird

to the most obscure vegetable mold. Despite the undisci-
plined nature of many of these endeavors, medical educators
insisted that early training in the observation of external
phenomena and the exercise of reasoning faculties were of
foremost importance to the new generation of doctors. The
want of such curiosity and scientific habits of mind had permitted the phenomena of mesmerism, electro-biology, spiritualism, and their kindred spirits to gain adherents from
among those whose training should have taught otherwise.
The lack of mental discipline and adequate interest in scientific pursuits left doctors susceptible to the defective claims of
mountebanks.[36]

European physicians and surgeons and American medical
students educated abroad provided the major source of naturalists from colonial times into the nineteenth century. Historian George H. Daniels observed, "This predominance of
physicians followed naturally from the fact that leading medical schools, such as the ones at Padua, Edinburgh, and
Leyden, offered the best scientific education of the day as a
regular part of medical instruction." Their experiences in
botany, chemistry, and anatomy affected generations of doctors and encouraged a continuing interest in natural history.[37] They were thus responsible in part for preserving the
integrity of the medical arts from the snares of a disintegrating educational system and the siren appeals of the sectarians.
Natural history served as conservative ballast to Victorian
medicine as doctors steered amid the gusty winds of sectarian claims and educational bankruptcy. In John Warren of
Harvard, David Hosack and Samuel Latham Mitchell at the
College of Physicians and Surgeons of New York, Benjamin
Silliman at Yale, and countless amateurs, American physician-
naturalists offered examples of high-spirited, educated men
anxious to expand the limitations of their formal education.
In a certain sense they were librarians of the earth who en-
camped in natural history to secure it from the intrusions of
capricious destruction; what they preserved for future generations of naturalists they likewise achieved for medicine by
bequeathing to the savants of the new age a critical eye and an
uninterrupted medical tradition.

The link between medical practice and natural history
tended, over the course of the eighteenth and nineteenth

centuries, to create a conservative common sense that outlasted the dogmas and pathies of the age.[38] President Eliot of Harvard recognized this tendency when he noted that the special studies which fell under the category of natural history had proven excellent preparation for medical school, since "the mental constitution of the physician is essentially that of a naturalist." Until embryology, botany, geology, chemistry, physics, mathematics, psychology, foreign languages (Latin, French, and German), and principles of drawing became standard preparatory courses that students mastered prior to formalized medical school training, he argued, natural history would remain an invaluable aid in understanding anatomy, histology, and pathology. It disciplined the mind to perceive accurately and to attend patients with more than a genial smile, a box of tools, and an assortment of theories.[39]

Initial Reform Efforts

In seeking causes for the proliferation of medical colleges in the years before and after the Civil War, doctors often blamed depressing wages and the widening distance between worker and employer that forced young men to seek a career in medicine in the mistaken belief that "the doctor is never out of a job and can never fail of steady living." The resultant multiplication of schools with notoriously inadequate training degenerated into a fratricidal struggle among medical graduates to make a living. "Is it then to be wondered at," physician Emil Amberg wrote, "if every year sees, added to the medical profession, hundreds, nay, thousands of young men who are designed by nature and prepared through training and inheritance to be farmers, tradesmen, and mechanics rather than physicians? Furthermore, is it a matter of surprise if these doctors inheriting commercial instincts and unaffected by the modifying influences of a university training yield to the pressure of competition and descend to common business methods?" The outcome of this unbridled commercialism the critics of medical education described as survival of the shrewdest rather than of the fittest as was suggested by hardy evolutionists.[40]

Out of fear of the unwholesome effects of competition upon the profession, doctors began to attempt to control the tendency toward commercialism. Physician R. H. Babcock commented in the *Journal of Sociologic Medicine*:

> We cannot restrain the forces in the body politic that are impelling young men and women to study medicine, but we can help build up barriers that will keep out undesirable students. The first step in this direction is toward a higher medical education. Existing institutions for medical training must be forced on to a higher plane, and the establishment of low-grade schools must be made an impossibility; as a college or university education broadens a student and generally develops the best there is in him, teaching him that success depends on individual merit and hard work, and consists of something more than mere money-getting, it should be made impossible for any but college-bred men and women to obtain a degree in medicine. That the people may be made to appreciate the evils of quackish and ignorant medical practice the people will have to be properly instructed lest in our attempt to protect them they legislate against their own best interest from the mistaken notion that we are endeavoring to establish a physicians' trust. Only by restricting the accession to our ranks of individuals with grossly commercial methods, can we hope to see our inherently noble profession stand upon that lofty plane that will force respect even from a commercial people in a commercial age.[41]

In keeping with the outlook of the small business and professional men in nineteenth-century America, physicians were, at first, reluctant to organize to improve standards, fearing their endeavors would be looked upon as monopolistic. Quality control in the granting of medical degrees was discouraged by opposition to special privilege, by fears of bigness, and by the belief that the professions should be an open frontier for all and not be proscribed by class limitations. Thus in 1839, when the Georgia legislature reorganized the Board of Physicians and gave it the power to examine medical candidates and grant licenses, the law carried a provision that nothing "be so construed as to act against the Thomsonian or Botanic practice or any other practitioner in the state." As one disgruntled physician observed, the law had the effect of "acting the play of Hamlet with the part of Hamlet left out."[42]

There were those, of course, who had no fear of competition and actually encouraged its growth within the profession. The Reverend Henry H. Tucker told the graduating class of the Medical College of Georgia in 1867 that by making oneself necessary to the community through diligent work and dedication there was no way that one's merits would remain undiscovered. "Have no fears of competition," he advised. "It is unmanly to fear competition. Never run from it. Rather court it; and the more able it is, the more it will develop your own manhood, and add to your mental power and professional ability."[43] Tucker was not alone in his views; hundreds like him resented the outcry against proprietary schools and their yearly crop of graduates. For them the desire to reduce the number of practitioners by improving medical-school standards would simply turn aspiring medical students to the schools of the irregulars. Rather than lament the crowding of schools, they appealed to the laissez faire philosophy of William Graham Sumner of Yale and urged the medical profession to rejoice, since "every young graduate will displace some less competent man, or will set up a lively competition, that will put each opponent on his mettle. If medicine ceases to be a desirable pursuit as compared with other careers, men will cease to engage in it, and thus the law of supply and demand, left to its unhampered operation, will regulate our growth."[44]

Many also believed that a cheap medical education enabled ambitious and talented youths from the "humbler classes" to enter a profession otherwise "crowded with the more indolent and inefficient offspring of wealthier people"; from those humbler classes would come brains and energy to advance medical science. "Poverty is a stimulant to exertion greatly needed in so laborious a profession as medicine," G. E. Frothingham, M.D., remarked in 1886, "and not only will those who have this stimulus be most likely to properly qualify themselves for the practice of medicine, but will likely be most sympathetic and humane to those who are actually poor and need their services."[45] The efforts of Frothingham and others to delay stricter medical standards, however, were drowned out by those demanding change. Reformers dismissed as specious the ratiocination that raising standards was no more than the effort of a pernicious aristocratic clique to oppress the poor and control entrance into the profession. Rather, they felt that those who opposed higher standards were simply protecting their own sheepskins and medical licenses.[46]

Unlike European medical organizations which were national in authority and aristocratic in design, the American Medical Association evolved through a process that was democratic in design, national in authority, and elitist in practice—much in keeping with many other developmental aspects of American society.[47] The initial calls for such an organization came not just from individuals but from colleges and medical societies concerned with the erosion of the physician's economic and social status. The medical societies of Vermont and New Hampshire invited delegates from the New England states and New York to discuss educational problems as early as 1827. Similar efforts were undertaken by the faculty of Bowdoin College in 1828, Milton M. Antony of the Georgia medical faculty in 1830, Ohio physicians meeting in Columbus in 1837, New Hampshire physicians in 1838, and resolutions put forward by John McCall, Alexander Thompson, and Nathan Smith Davis of the Medical Society of the State of New York in 1838 and 1845 that the teaching and licensing of doctors become separated. These efforts culminated in a national convention held in May 1846 in the hall of the medical department of the University of the State of New York. One hundred nineteen delegates from medical societies and schools from as far away as Louisiana attended. At a convention held the following year, many of these same delegates adopted the name American Medical Association.[48] The organizing zealots behind the AMA included Richard Arnold of Georgia, Edward Delafield of New York, Jonathan Knight of Yale, Nathaniel Chapman of the University of Pennsylvania, Nathan Smith Davis, Alfred Stillé, and Isaac Hays. From the very inception of the association, these men viewed the AMA as a vehicle for higher standards for preliminary education and improved medical training. Within a year of the AMA's founding, they were instrumental in establishing committees on medical education, medical sciences, practical medicine, surgery, obstetrics, medical literature, and publications. The establishment of other standing committees soon followed, including anatomy, physiology, materia medica, chemistry, forensic medicine, vital statistics, hygiene, and sanitary measures.[49]

Advocates of tightening medical standards commonly looked to the Army and Navy Boards of Examiners for Surgeons as precedent for their own concerns. Regardless of diploma, candidates for surgeon's appointments in the military were required to undergo an examination. From 1841 to 1849 only 55 out of 170 applicants managed to pass the Army Medical Board examinations. During the same period only 77 out of 175 passed the Navy Medical Board examinations. According to H. S. Heiskell, M.D., the acting surgeon-general of the United States Army, the most striking causes for failure were "insufficient preparatory education, a hurried course of pupilage, want of proficiency in practical anatomy, in pathology and in clinical medicine." In the *Transactions* of the American Medical Association in 1847, Navy surgeons William Maxwell Wood and Ninian Pinkney remarked that a medical student who appeared before one examining board could not identify the freezing and boiling points of water, contending that such knowledge was useless; another identified castor oil as the oil from the animal castor; and still another located the solar plexus in the sole of the foot—yet all three individuals were graduates of respected medical schools. Between 1900 and 1909, 45 percent of the doctors who applied for positions with the naval medical corps failed the qualifying exam; in roughly the same period, 81 percent of the applicants failed the Marine Hospital Service examinations; and between 1888 and 1909 the Army Medical Corps flunked 72 percent of its applicants.[50]

Beginning in the mid-nineteenth century then, several forces converged to bring about medical reform, including the founding of the AMA and mounting dissatisfaction with medical standards, licensing, and sectarianism. In 1848 the AMA recommended that medical education be founded upon clinical and demonstrative teaching, that medical colleges and hospitals cooperate in a concerted effort to provide students with greater experience, that hospital appointments be decided on the basis of merit, that greater quality control be obtained through a lengthened period of study as well as demanding requirements for admission, that a minimum of five case studies either replace or augment the medical thesis, that more impartial medical examinations be conducted by visiting examiners from outside the institution, and that faculties of the various medical schools provide the AMA with a roster of faculty and list of requirements for medical degrees. In 1849 it suggested additional reforms, including replacement of the repetitious two-year program with a more structured course of general and specialized studies and the establishment of general examining boards under the aegis of the AMA, which would confer certificates.[51] Through the early part of the nineteenth century, the length of the medical term varied from thirteen to twenty weeks; only after the AMA recommended a six-month term in 1847 was an effort made—albeit slowly—to accept the longer term. The University of Pennsylvania and the College of Physicians and Surgeons were the first to comply. Finally, the AMA began to compare European educational standards with those of medical schools in the United States. The publication of these comparative analyses was, Morris Fishbein remarked, "one of the most potent factors in raising the standards of medical education in the United States."[52]

Additional efforts to restructure the system of medical education came in 1852, 1858, and 1860 with proposals from members of the AMA to separate medical schools from licensing practices. In each instance, however, the medical schools proved too powerful a lobby and the proposals met with defeat. Efforts to encourage state societies to examine (i.e., license) doctors who wished to practice in the state came to a similar end. Not until 1874 did the AMA turn the corner in its fight to upgrade standards in the profession. In that year the national organization terminated its close association with the proprietary interests of medical colleges by excluding their representatives from its meetings. Despite this change, however, the AMA was not immediately able to capitalize on its strength; instead, it looked to the creation of independent licensing boards in each state as the medium for upgrading standards.[53]

Those physicians vocal enough to express opinions in the medical journals stressed that the country was in dire need of better trained doctors—not simply with more thorough training in medical skills, but also with more preparatory training in the liberal arts before entering medical school. Reformers thought it odd that the profession which touched

important areas of life and death as a whole had less understanding of the collateral arts than did the normal bachelor
degree graduate. A report submitted to the National Medical Convention in Philadelphia in 1847, for example, concluded that "no standard of preliminary education was en-
acted in any single state in this Union; but that the whole
matter was left to the decision of the Practitioner, who was
asked to receive a pupil into his office."[54] The situation had
deteriorated to the degree that many young men who commenced their medical studies were constantly embarrassed
by their inability to understand the technical words in their
manuals. In 1869 Henry S. Hewitt, M.D., remarked, "We do
not hesitate to say that unless our culture is improved, our
relations with the intellectual and cultivated classes re-estab-
lished, unless medicine proclaims herself the ally and cham-
pion of learning and intellectual authority, we shall not only
cease to advance in the direction of pure induction, but shall
lose even the splendid results of sound empiricism."[55] A good
preliminary education, reformers argued, developed the
mental qualities in a physician, who needed to be as skilled in
his understanding of the human mind, the foibles of temperament, and the requirements of discerning the true etiology of disease as in the ability to wield a scalpel or prescribe a
drug. Richard D. Arnold, M.D., president of the Medical Society of Georgia, observed that, "Wherever in our profession
we have had a careful, educated, judicious, and sensible observer of the phenomena of disease, there we have had a
good physician." But he went on to say that individuals of
that caliber were rarely conspicuous outside those schools
which had adopted a higher standard of admission. In effect,
reformers encouraged the bachelor's degree as a worthy substitute for the pleasing but more individualized study of natural history.[56]

In a speech delivered at the annual meeting of the Association of Medical Editors in 1871, Horatio R. Storer, editor of
the *Journal* of the Gynecological Society of Boston, reflected
the thinking of the association by insisting that a competent
and improved medical profession demanded a good liberal
education as a prerequisite to medical school training. "Unless early education be well laid and solid," he observed, "the
most elaborate after-structure will prove easily shaken and

unsafe." An admirer of President Charles Eliot of Harvard (1834–1926), and, in particular, the educator's famous essay on "The New Education," Storer could not help but despair of statistics indicating that only a small proportion of the law-yers, doctors, and ministers in the country were actual hold-ers of bachelor's degrees. On the average, a professional man received less education in the liberal arts and decidedly less culture than those who held a bachelor's degree.[57] Figures available for 1900 indicate that only 50 percent of the the-ological students, 20 percent of the law students, and 7 per-cent of the medical students had received an academic de-gree before attending their respective professional schools. As late as 1906 the AMA was recommending a minimum of one year of college preparatory to medical school.[58]

Some doctors believed raising admission standards or im-proving curricula a distant goal and sought immediate re-form in several areas. Many encouraged physicians to be-come more active members of their local medical societies, and some advocated preparation of a thesis at stated inter-vals in their career as a test of their medical knowledge.[59] Doctors also urged careful supervision of medical students by the preceptor, who was to make sure the student had a good preliminary education before receiving him as a charge. In addition, the preceptor should insist that his students enter only those medical colleges where courses of instruction were thorough and dissecting rooms were supervised by compe-tent teachers. Provided the preceptor was vigilant in his tu-toring, carefully supervising instruction in the materia med-ica, and providing counsel in operations, a medical student would acquire a practical experience that would then carry into the lecture hall. "If such studies have been diligently pursued in the office of the Preceptor," a Georgia practi-tioner remarked in 1851, "the student will go off to the lec-ture room prepared to understand all that the lecturer may demonstrate or expound, and thus make a full use of his short course of lectures."[60]

Many of the advances made in medical education during the second half of the nineteenth century came from doctors who had returned from Germany bringing with them ideas on hospital and clinical teaching. Although the traffic of American students to Germany did not really begin until after the Civil War, the ouput of German literature in the 1840s indicated a perceptible shift from the clinical medicine of Paris.[61] The German influence also marked a move away from structural pathology to histology and physiological research. Despite the brilliance of François Magendie (1783–1855), Claude Bernard (1813–1878), and Raspail, French hospital medicine gave way to the cellular pathology of Virchow and the German schools. American medical students who sought to supplement their meager education at home went to Das Allgemeines Krankenhaus, Vienna's great General Hospital, where the important instructional doctors included Heinrich Bamberger and Friedrich Schauta in obstetrics, Joseph Kauders and Ernest Fuchs in ophthalmology, Theodor Billroth in surgery, Emil Zuckerkandl on surgical anatomy, Victor Urbantschitsch on the ear, Schrötter on nose and throat, and Isidor Neumann and Moritz Kaposi on the skin. At the University of Strasbourg, Friedrich Recklinghausen taught pathological anatomy, and Wilhelm Waldeyer histology. The superiority of the work of men like Johann Muller in physiology, of Theodor Schwann, Jacob Henle, Justus von Liebig, Karl Rokitansky, Wilhelm Valentiner, and Hermann Weber eclipsed the work being done in the English schools and, as a result, began drawing increased numbers of American students.[62] Eventually some fifteen thousand American doctors were educated in Germany and Austria between 1870 and 1914, and their awareness of salaried professorships, clinical teaching, licensing examinations, academic prerequisites for medical training, and laboratory experience served to reinforce efforts to improve medical education in their homeland.[63] First in England, then in Paris and Italy, and finally in Germany, American students found the opportunity to learn what their poorer colleagues would never learn at home; it was this group of European-educated students who became the teachers and medical reformers of the late nineteenth century. Out of their experiences emerged a new era of medical education in America.[64]

Curriculum Reform

In remarks published by editors of medical journals across the country, there appeared to be genuine unanimity that the

profession needed to raise its standards of medical education. Although states like Minnesota and Kentucky passed
stringent legislation regarding the practice of medicine
within their jurisdiction, nevertheless other states, such as Illinois, were overburdened with "medical riffraff" to the extent that they became "the dumping-ground for all the medical refuse and parasites of the profession." There cancer
quacks, faith-cure apostles, Indian medicine men, root and
herb sharks, and countless specialists from hair restorers to
sexual advisers, fed upon the delusions of the public.[65] Some
editors were so disenchanted with the existing state of the
medical arts that they urged the formation of state medical
schools and even a National Medical School to be supported
by congressional funds. Supporters of the latter reform idea
even urged the creation of a national hospital that would
provide at least six months of postdoctoral training for all
graduates of regular medical schools. This school and hospital complex, according to its supporters, would eliminate
both the uneven nature of medical education and the multitudinous problems of reciprocity laws. After completion of
training at the National Medical School and Hospital, physicians would be issued a diploma that would entitle them to
practice anywhere in the United States. Implicit in the proposal was the suggestion that by dictating the number of
medical graduates accepted each year for certification, the
school could effectively control the quantity as well as quality
of those practicing medicine.[66]

In 1859 the medical department of Northwestern University took the initiative to improve conditions of medical instruction by instituting a three-year graded program. This
reform effort was not repeated until 1871 when Charles Eliot
overrode the opposition of Harvard's medical faculty with
his insistence upon graded instruction, the replacement of
the two-year (total of eight weeks of lectures) program with a
three-year extended teaching term, and the requirement of
an academic degree for admission into medical school. In
1874 the Harvard catalog urged those who were intent upon
a degree in medicine to focus special attention on the study
of natural history, chemistry, physics, and the German and
French languages during their undergraduate years. Eliot
remarked: "It is fearful to think of the ignorance and incom-

petence of most American doctors who have graduated at American schools. They poison, maim, and do men to death in various ways, and are unable to save life or preserve health." It was not until after 1910 that the four-year program of thirty-two weeks of instruction gained acceptance.[67]

While Harvard's decision to raise standards had the immediate effect of causing a decline in enrollment, the university counteracted the financial problem by substituting salaried professorships for the school's previous dependence upon student fees. Though other universities were slow to follow, eventually they too employed procedures similar to those initiated by Eliot. The Universities of Pennsylvania and Syracuse upgraded the curriculum and introduced clinical training in 1877; Francis Delafield and William H. Welch opened clinical laboratories at the College of Physicians and Surgeons in New York and Bellevue Medical College in 1878; and Yale and the University of Michigan followed in 1880 with laboratories in the experimental sciences.[68] The University of Pennsylvania added yet another innovative idea when Provost William Pepper founded the University Hospital, which was directly supervised by the medical faculty. With the development of clinical teaching, the hospital became an essential part of the medical school and functioned for the care of patients as well as for the education of doctors. When the medical department of the University of Wooster in Cleveland made hospital facilities available in 1885 for the bedside teaching of its students, Frank J. Weed, M.D., the school's dean, noted the significance of the innovation. Previously students were forced to travel about the city to hospitals, where they viewed operations from perches in the amphitheater; now, with a hospital under the exclusive control of the school's medical faculty, students had "all possible opportunity for actual bedside teaching and medical and surgical clinics."[69]

These efforts were complemented by the equally exacting standards demanded by the newly established Johns Hopkins Medical School, which was founded in 1893 out of the philanthropic generosity of Baltimore railroad magnate Johns Hopkins and organized on the principle of the German university clinics. The school's first president, Daniel Coit Gilman (1831–1908), not only insisted upon an academic degree as a prerequisite for admission into the medical program (Johns Hopkins became the first American university devoted principally to graduate education), but also instituted a broad series of financial, curricular, and clinical reforms. As Abraham Flexner later remarked, Johns Hopkins "was the first medical school in America of genuine university type, with something approaching adequate endowment, well equipped laboratories conducted by modern teachers, devoting themselves unreservedly to medical investigation and instruction, and with its own hospital, in which the training of physicians and the healing of the sick harmoniously combine to the infinite advantage of both." [70] Under the careful tutelage of William S. Halsted, Howard A. Kelly, John J. Abel, Mary E. Garrett, John Shaw Billings, William H. Welch, Franklin P. Mall, and William Osler, the Johns Hopkins Hospital embarked upon an educational program which soon became a catalyst and model for other innovative undertakings in medical education. [71]

The upgrading of medical education did not come without criticism. Doctors complained that medical school clinics undermined "the sense of economic independence and self-respect in the community" by providing free medical service without questioning ability to pay. Young doctors seeking to build their practices accused the clinics of pushing them to the brink of starvation. [72] Yet, as medical historian R. H. Shryock remarked, it was this clinical program, "superior in most respects to the old single-preceptor relationship, which led to the abandonment of apprenticeships during the 1870s and the 1880s." [73] Other critics remained, however. Henry J. Bigelow, who was among the ranks of those urging improvements in the medical instruction system in the United States, objected to reformists with quick solutions. Bigelow was particularly skeptical of Charles Eliot's elective system; he believed that few students were competent to decide which subjects were most applicable to their needs. A well-balanced medical education demanded the highest level of supervision and guidance. "You cannot turn out medical men with the uniform perfection of Ames shovels or Springfield muskets," he reminded the Massachusetts Medical Society in 1871. "The popular and specious cry for raising the standard of medical education comes often from those who know little of its difficulties, and it is notorious that those who clamor loudest accomplish least." For Bigelow the quality of medical education depended in the last analysis on the individual student and conscientious teacher.[74]

Above all Bigelow admired the Horatio Alger attitude of young men who came from impoverished circumstances. Too often those who were "born to education" settled into insignificance "while the whole land is full of heroes who have fought their way to usefulness and eminence . . . by sheer force of will and determination." Despite imperfections in the existing system, it nevertheless succeeded in producing eminent men in the sciences, furnishing capable teachers and distinguished practitioners of medicine. "Most eminent men are in a large degree self-made," he observed, "and have pursued their subject from the attraction before them, and not from a stimulus behind. The material out of which philosophers are made is largely supplied from their own intrinsic and determined will. Genius is talent with a strong driving power, whether versatile in all directions, or more profitably guided by taste or circumstances in one direction. You cannot create this talent or compel this taste. You may, indeed, give it opportunity, but you cannot force it."[75] These fears of elitism that Bigelow expressed extended back through the formative years of the AMA to remarks made in 1846 by Professor Martyn Paine of the Medical Department of New York University when he accused the association of playing aristocratic politics behind a masquerade of curriculum reform. "There is an aristocratic feature in this movement," he warned. "It is oppression toward the poor for the sake of crippling the medical colleges."[76] Men like Bigelow and Paine feared the general thrust of reform legislation would limit the upward mobility of competent but impoverished young men.

Despite the appeal of Henry Bigelow, the concern for more thorough liberal arts education as preparation for medical school had become public currency among medical educators in the nation's better universities. Arguing that knowledge was an indispensable factor in the extension and preservation of free institutions and that, to achieve this end, society must consider a means for repressing the "hoards of imposters" who traded on public credulity, reformers sought

both internal and external regulations to ensure the maintenance of a high standard of medical education. Behind the
shibboleths of elitist versus democratic education lay the
more pervasive concern that the law of supply and demand
had been grossly violated by the annual production of inadequately trained doctors. Under suspicion in this regard were
those medical schools organized in rural areas in the western
states where educational and clinical advantages suffered for
lack of population and qualified medical teachers. To deal
with the problem, reformers urged that any city with less
than 75,000 inhabitants be prohibited from organizing a
medical college. These same individuals also urged the creation of state laws to control the issuance of diplomas by medical colleges; and when state legislation proved unreliable,
they sought to convince medical colleges to emulate the four-
year requirements of Harvard, the University of Pennsylvania, and Jefferson Medical College as reliable alternatives.
Reasoning that quackery would find it difficult to gain recruits from among thoroughly educated physicians, reformers demanded not only preliminary educational qualification but also stronger and tougher standards in medical
schools, a lengthened period of training with clinical experience before graduation, and the creation of independent
boards of medical examiners in each state to check the cre-
dentials of medical graduates. It was not the desire to improve medical knowledge by diluting it that sparked the
strong sentiments of reformers; rather, it was their intention
to give direction and competence to medicine by keeping it
in step with the intellectual achievements of the age.[77]

Yet another sign of reform from within the profession was
the formation of the American Medical College Association
in 1876 under the leadership of J. B. Biddle, Nathan S. Davis,
and Samuel D. Gross.[78] The association's insistence on three
years of medical education forced its breakup in 1882 following the withdrawal of eleven schools. Eight years later, in response to a call from the medical schools of Baltimore (University of Maryland, Baltimore Medical College, College of
Physicians and Surgeons, Baltimore University, Woman's
Medical College of Baltimore, and Johns Hopkins University), the American Medical College Association reorganized
under the name of Association of American Medical Col-

leges (AAMC). With sixty-six medical schools participating in its first year, the association expressed renewed interest in a three-year course of six-month sessions, a graded curriculum, written and oral examinations, preliminary examinations in English, laboratory instruction in chemistry, histology and pathology, and uniform standards for those seeking membership in the association.[79] Although the majority of medical colleges in 1901 and 1902 belonged to the AAMC, the fact that the association possessed no licensing power prevented it from exercising more than an ancillary role. Membership in the association was little proof of quality education. "This could only be the case," a Michigan doctor wrote, "if a permanent joint committee (of the AMA and AAMC) would continually inspect the colleges." But so long as there were forty or fifty different examination boards, many of whose members were appointed for political purposes, the results would inevitably prove negligible.[80]

One significant sign of change was a return of the state licensing boards that had died prematurely during the Jacksonian Era. Under increased prodding from the AMA and AAMC, thirty-five states either established or resurrected some form of licensure system for medical graduates by the 1890s. In 1891 the National Confederation of State Medical Examining and Licensing Boards was founded; and it, along with the AAMC, urged minimum entrance requirements for medical schools, a standardized curriculum, and a three-year program. So extensive was the popularity of examining boards that by 1898 only the Alaskan Territory existed without licensing regulations. Most of these boards were created in the 1880s and 1890s; and although many simply required the registration of a diploma or a certain number of years in practice, others had already begun to demand both a diploma and a state examination regulated by the state board of health. In fourteen states licensure extended to graduates of only certain approved (i.e., reputable) schools. Overall, licensing boards provided a minimal level of control over the worst types of medical schools; but, clearly, the criteria for licensing were neither uniform nor rigidly enforced.[81]

The immediate effect of the state licensing boards was more pretended than effective reform. Most boards were apathetic to educational requirements and, while some faced strong political pressure not to injure the graduates of local institutions, others were the object of political spoils and fell far short of meeting their legal responsibilities. Unfortunately, since many states simply required a medical diploma as a prerequisite for licensing, a lucrative market for bogus degrees developed. Unscrupulous medical merchants, such as John Buchanan, William Paine, and Rev. T. B. Miller of Philadelphia; Rufus King Noyes of Massachusetts; Fred Rutland of Milwaukee; and George Dutton, Horace W. Bailey, and W. S. Cowan of Vermont, operated flourishing diploma mills, granting diplomas by mail in the latter half of the nineteenth century. Buchanan admitted having sold 60,000 diplomas over a forty-year period. For fees that ranged from ten dollars to several hundred dollars, individuals could purchase diplomas that met the licensure laws of the various states. Until the states insisted upon an examination as a prerequisite to medical licensing, diploma mills like the Independent Medical College of Chicago, Trinity University of Medicine and Surgery, Excelsior Medical College, the Wisconsin Eclectic Medical College, and the Druidic University of America exploited the intent of state law by continuing to grind out "doctors" for American society. Twenty-one of these mills were selling diplomas in 1894. Despite their profiteering, the very existence of state licensing boards set in motion the gradual extinction of marginal schools by indicating that their degrees did not meet the requirements of the Progressive Era's demands for reform.[82]

Not until its reorganization in 1901 was the AMA able to exert a sizable influence on medical education. In cooperation with state boards, the AMA's Council on Medical Education (formed on a permanent basis in 1904) made a number of recommendations, which included improved educational standards, hospital training, and financial restructuring of medical schools. In effect, schools that depended upon tuition alone for support could not provide adequate medical faculties, clinical training, and other services necessary to produce competent doctors. Only through a combination of tuition, endowment, and state aid could a medical school create the type of doctor required by the new age. Just as big business had begun to trim competition through internal efforts aimed at bringing stability to the economic system and avoiding potential radical reform by state and local regulatory agencies, so too the council undertook in 1904 to expose and destroy the multitude of inferior medical colleges by publishing the poor showing their graduates made on state medical exams.

Under the influence of Arthur Dean Bevan of Chicago, Nathan P. Colwell, William T. Councilman, and others, the Council on Medical Education insisted upon reforms that eventually led to the closing of a number of marginal schools. It inspected 161 schools and found 82 acceptable, 47 doubtful, and 32 unsatisfactory. Between 1906 and publication of the Flexner Report in 1910, the Council's activities were responsible in part for the closing of 29 schools. In 1905 the AAMC Committee on Visitations and Inspection initiated studies of several member colleges, and by 1906 the AMA had launched a school-by-school survey under the direction of N. P. Colwell, M.D. In 1907 the Council on Medical Education began classifying medical schools on an A (worthy), B (acceptable), and C (hopeless) basis. The following year evidenced still greater changes with the AMA exercising proprietary rights over medical schools through insistence upon school inspection, publication of the results, and the decision of the National Conference of State Medical Examining and Licensing Boards to adopt the medical-school equipment list devised by the AAMC.[83] Recognizing the need for change, yet facing hostility within its own ranks, the Council on Medical Education in 1908 urged the selection of an impartial outsider to conduct a study of medical education.[84]

The Flexner Report

In 1908 the Carnegie Foundation for the Advancement of Teaching authorized a comparison of medical education in the United States and Canada with that of Great Britain, Germany, and France. Henry S. Pritchett, president of the foundation and former professor of astronomy at Washington University in St. Louis, expressed concern that medical education had become a commercialized institution in America, with the public largely ignorant of the skills required of trained doctors. Indeed, public awareness of medical education had deteriorated to the point that patients could make no "discrimination between the well-trained physician and the physician who has no adequate training whatsoever." Given the developments in medical science and education since the 1870s, Pritchett's remark was perhaps exaggerated; nevertheless, it emphasized public ignorance of the nation's medical education system as well as the lack of internal professional awareness of the future needs of America's medical schools. "One of the problems of the future," Pritchett remarked, "is to educate the public itself to appreciate the fact that very seldom, under existing conditions, does a patient receive the best aid which it is possible to give him in the present state of medicine, and that this is due mainly to the fact that a vast army of men is admitted to the practice of medicine who are untrained in sciences fundamental to the profession and quite without a sufficient experience with disease."[85]

The task of carrying out the Carnegie Foundation's assignment went to Abraham Flexner (1866–1959), a graduate of Johns Hopkins and a schoolmaster in Louisville. Flexner made visits to each medical school in the country; and although his visits seldom lasted more than one or two days, he had little difficulty in abstracting the information needed for his study. More often than not, he discovered schools that were not much more than commercial enterprises under the control of cliques of local doctors and with little or no hospital connection. When the foundation published its now famous bulletin number four in 1910, Flexner became a byword in the medical community, and his influence over medical education in North America was immediate and pervasive.[86]

In the foundation's published report, Flexner was by no means reluctant to suggest the power of the state as an agent of reform. He wrote: "The physician is a social instrument; and as disease has consequences that immediately go beyond the individual specifically affected, society is bound to protect itself against unnecessary spread of loss or danger. It matters not that the making of doctors has been to some extent left to private institutions. The state already makes certain regulations; and it can by the same right make others. Practically, the medical school is a public service corporation." With this in mind, Flexner considered it wrong for the state to maintain a laissez-faire attitude.[87] Like many progressive thinkers of his day, Flexner preferred social control to drift. He supported the Jeffersonian tenet that the capacity of a truly democratic people was dependent upon education and protection of property rights; but he appealed to a broader definition of property which aimed at raising the social and economic status of the medical community. The democratic aspect of the educational system was no small item either in Flexner's perception of medicine's coming of age or in the thinking of opponents of reform. As late as 1911, a member of the Judicial Council of the Association of American Medical Colleges condemned the educational prerequisites for medicine as "distinctly un-American and undemocratic" and stated that they "should not be tolerated." It seemed to him ludicrous that "a man can hold any of our public offices without having seen the inside of a college, and yet we are demanding that before he is even qualified to study medicine a doctor shall have a B. S. degree!" Evidence of this strong egalitarianism extended deep into American society and required the most carefully reasoned response to avoid a patriotic reaction to the nation's democratic faith.[88]

Like Tocqueville, Henry Adams, and Edwin L. Godkin of the *Nation*, Flexner feared the social consequences of a society unable to distinguish between the problems and prospects of democracy. Opening the profession to all who desired to be doctors, he warned, not only denied the rights of society to a high level of medical competence, but also allowed the facade of personal liberty to endanger the well-being of the greater society. Controls or restrictions on medical education were not only in the social interest but, in the end, strengthened the liberties of all citizens. "Has democracy, then, really suffered a set-back?" he asked. "Reorganization along rational lines involves the strengthening, not the weakening, of democratic principles, because it tends to provide the conditions upon which the well being and effectual liberty depend."[89]

Flexner left his harshest criticism for the commercial aspects of medical education. Overproduction and low standards had given rise to the cruel exploitation of youths "caught drifting at a vacant moment by an alluring advertisement or announcement, quite commonly an exaggeration, not infrequently an outright misrepresentation." Flexner urged a concerted effort to reduce to 31 the total number of medical schools in the United States, which by 1904 had reached as high as 166. Actually the process had already begun before the publication of his report. From 1904 to 1909, 10 percent of the medical schools had either closed their doors or had merged with more substantial institutions. Although this brought a corresponding decrease, from 5222 to 4442, in the annual number of new doctors, Flexner intended that the number should continue to diminish to about 3500.[90] The Flexner report sufficiently influenced the profession so that by 1933 the number of degree-granting institutions decreased to 66. To improve the quality of those that survived, Rockefeller's General Education Board, inspired by the reasoning behind the report, invested $50 million in the upgrading of the nation's medical schools.[91]

Flexner intended that the ratio of physicians to population would eventually stabilize at about one for every thousand persons. Although this figure was well below the ratio of physicians to population in Germany (1:1912) and Austria (1:2120), it was comparable to that of the United Kingdom (1:1007) and would, he believed, adequately maintain the financial position of the physician. Moreover, it was much improved over the current national ratio of 1:568—a figure that was frequently even worse in urban areas. To arrive at the desired ratio, Flexner suggested that the number of physicians graduating from medical schools be adjusted to 1:1500. This, when combined with replacing every two medical vacancies due to death with only one new physician, would eventually achieve the desired ratio. "The country needs fewer and better doctors," Flexner wrote, "and the way to get them better is to produce fewer." To help achieve this end, he urged that state boards reject applicants who could not pass minimum medical standards and that enormous pressure be exerted upon marginal medical schools to close their doors. Along with improving the quality of medical education, Flexner intended his reform ideas to improve the social and economic condition of the average doctor.[92]

The Flexner report marked the culmination of several generations of reform thinking in America. Although Flexner himself had called for the wholesale extinction of schools, the actual results corresponded more with earlier recommendations of the Council on Medical Education, in that between 1904 and 1920 the number of medical schools declined to eighty-eight, the number of students to 14,088, and the number of graduates to 3,047. In effect, Flexner did not so much instigate reform as provide a rationale for what should be, as well as what already existed in the form of improved medical instruction and the gradual elimination of marginal schools. His report produced a landmark policy statement that served as a catalyst for medical reform in the years ahead. In effect, Flexner warned the profession to set its affairs in order or face the regulatory efforts of state and federal governments. In response to Flexner's warning, planning organizations such as the Committee on Medical Legislation, the Council on Medical Education, the National Confederation of State Medical Examining and Licensing Boards, and the Association of American Medical Colleges, pursued their goals in much the same manner as the informal trade associations of big business. Recognizing that the educated American doctor had been virtually eclipsed by the changes in medical science, these planning councils looked to a reorganization of the profession that would allow innovation at a self-directed pace, thereby removing the possibility of potentially destructive outside reform pressure. The Flexner report provided the profession with an outsider's look at itself and, with it, a recognition that corrective legislation by external agencies (i.e., the states) would either be lacking in uniformity, thereby sanctioning inequalities, or be far more extensive and perhaps even more destructive of existing institutions. Fearful of outside interference and believing in the right of autonomous reform, American doctors were persuaded, albeit reluctantly, to accept an organizational structure carrying the same capacity for internal reform that industrial corporations had already achieved.

Flexner's report did not come as a surprise to the medical colleges or the profession in general. Countless schools simply closed their doors following the report; others merged or reorganized in the hope of achieving the improved standards demanded by the report. In addition, schools began to uniformly insist upon a bachelor's degree prior to admission into medical school, a three- or four-year graded curriculum, clinical instruction, and hospital internship. Despite the implications the study had for marginal schools, many were good-natured enough to swallow the bitter pill with grace and dignity. Such was the response of J. F. Stevens, M.D., dean of the medical school affiliated with Nebraska Wesleyan University. In his letter to the president of the university, published in the *Journal* of the AMA in 1909, Stevens gave full recognition to the forces at work to upgrade medical education.

We would respectfully call your attention to the fact that educators and physicians throughout the United States, recognizing the inferiority, on the whole, of the American medical schools, as compared with those of Europe, have determined to raise the standard of medical education to such a point that our colleges will command the respect of the world. While academic training and opportunity have grown into magnificent and commanding proportions, the professional schools, with the exception of a small minority, have remained essentially elementary or even worse. The spirit of progress has at last become supreme and on all sides may be seen the work of destruction, reorganization, and rebuilding. The American Medical Association is doing a splendid work in securing and digesting statistics, and reflecting the strengths and deficiencies of our institutions. The Carnegie Foundation, in a different manner, lends its words of wisdom, and a multitude of smaller bodies and societies, including state examining boards, are working together with hardly a discordant note, for the same purpose. Standards of entrance requirements have been raised to such a point that one full year's work in an accepted college or university is required for matriculation. Soon it will be two years, and later a bachelor's degree will, without a doubt, be the sine qua non. Small colleges that have found it impossible to stand the strain of such requirements have been forced to step from the field altogether, or to merge with some other school. In several states nearly, or quite, all of the small schools have been blended with the state institution. At the same time the requirement is going forth that schools shall have at their disposal a dispensary and hospitals sufficiently patronized to permit of a very wide study of disease. These requirements cannot be met in a small city. Again, with the rapid advancement in medicine has come the need of costly laboratories, under the direction of highly cultured men. Subjects, too, that once belonged to the 'mere mention' hour in the course of study, have developed into great fields with divisions and subdivisions, each demanding a special training for its comprehension and most certainly for its proper teaching. None of these requirements insisted on by educators and the medical profession generally is in excess of what it should be, and this institution is in full harmony with that view. . . . We fully realize that to maintain our standing and dignity as medical teachers, in the continuance of our college, it will be necessary to add to our working force a goodly number of trained instructors. This we cannot do, and because of this, and for the reasons easily deduced from the above discussion, it has been decided that it is best for our institution voluntarily to close its doors, in the interest of higher medical education.[93]

In abandoning the parochial views of the proprietary colleges and the states' rights arguments of county societies, the committees of the AMA and the AAMC thus became a recognized part of America's medical reform. To the credit of these national planning councils, they recognized the capacity to internalize reform needs. In achieving a corporate image, however, both the AMA and the AAMC relied upon the grass roots nature of the professional organization and recognition by the practitioner that his future social and economic status depended on his belonging to the AMA and cooperating with it to make himself more efficient, more humane, and more educated. In mobilizing a common set of goals, the medical profession enabled its membership to rise quickly in economic security, quality of practice, and social prestige. Ohioan Charles A. L. Reed, chairman of the AMA Committee on Medical Legislation, insisted that the social position of doctors keep step with the scientific revolution then occurring in medicine. This implied that doctors must be willing to keep abreast in their education. Only then could the profession "guard its prerogatives and conserve its status in a democracy presumably founded on the principles of equality."[94]

There were two distinct perceptions of the AMA held by its membership, which at times intersected to reinforce a specific problem or issue and which on occasion stood at cross purposes. Doctors with marginal medical training tended to view the AMA as a democratic instrument for their integration into the mainstream of professional life and acceptability. For them the AMA was not a vehicle to challenge the existing medical education system but simply a mechanism by which they might identify with other doctors and reap the recognition they considered their due. On the other hand, doctors whose educational training had been completed in the older university medical schools or abroad perceived the AMA as a lever of reform, and they sought to obtain for medicine many of the same ends corporate leaders had already achieved through successful manipulation of the business world. Accepting the existence of continued growth of the large corporation as both natural and inevitable (that trusts were the reality of the future), this element hoped to establish a similar corporate environment for medicine. In effect, they sought to turn the professional outlook away from the laissez-faire environment of the small businessman and mold medical education and health care into a well-disciplined image similar to that of the more stable corporate order. To achieve this, however, reformers sought to convince the practitioner by speaking not to the corporate image, which he feared, but to the necessity for greater participation of all doctors in the association to improve the social and economic status of the profession.

By maximizing its strength, the AMA influenced medicine in much the same way as the corporate world had earlier affected its relationship with the free market. The views of the leadership in the profession coincided with the views of big business and especially with philanthropic organizations, such as the Carnegie and Rockefeller foundations, which financed their studies and helped upgrade the quality of the surviving medical schools. The directors of these foundations endorsed the concept of self-regulation, claiming, as they did for their own parent industries, that only the medical profession had the informed intelligence sufficient to meet its managerial problems. The AMA and its leadership chose to align with the corporate idea in the late nineteenth century, and through the strength of corporate management was able to move quickly to reform itself. Once achieved, the corporate ideology of the AMA remained dominant and largely unchallenged until the mid-twentieth century, when its aims ran counter to the "welfare capitalism" of the new democracy. Unfortunately today's new democracy has little appreciation for the process that had occurred earlier. Like Rockefeller and Carnegie, the early history of the AMA had virtues which were largely ignored, let alone understood. To appreciate the coming of age of both business and medicine is to recognize the nature of the American environment from which the Progressive reform movement evolved and the growth and stability that replaced the insecurity of an earlier age.

7

The Business and Ethics of Medicine

"CHANGES IN SOCIAL CONDITIONS are always insidious, usually unnoted til long after they are evident, and in time, often seemingly explosive," Charles Phelps, M.D., remarked in his presidential address before the New York State Medical Association in 1897. In this statement Phelps reflected one of the overriding concerns of nineteenth-century medical men as they pondered the impact of the financial and industrial revolution upon their profession.[1] As a group, doctors generously applauded the heroic achievements of their age and the ruthless spirit from which emerged the "fittest." Industrial statesmen spoke highly of the benefits of competition and the need for a laissez-faire environment, yet few doctors were aware that monopoly and the lack of competition had allowed the giants to thrive. Indeed, the nineteenth-century business community appeared to exist on two distinct levels. On the upper level industrial entrepreneurs spoke the language of the marketplace, but their actions clearly revealed a concerted effort to eliminate the competition. Beneath them struggled the broad mainstream of small shopowners, business, and professional men—the middle class—who, believing in the rhetoric of nineteenth century capitalism, unsuccessfully attempted to act out an ideology that had meaning only in the backwashes of the emerging corporate world. As part of this lower level, doctors found themselves in a situation strikingly similar to that of their business and professional contemporaries who felt threatened by the growth of specialization, the limitation of individual enterprise, and the subsequent loss of financial and social standing in Victorian society. The internecine feuds over fee bills, patents, consultation, and proper advertising were symptoms of this malaise. Only after pursuing the course of successful trusts and monopolies did physicians ultimately stem the destructive tendencies of oversupply and unwieldly competition that threatened their financial integrity. Not by continued competition, but rather through a concerted effort to control it, were doctors finally able to bring stability, long-range predictability, and economic security to their profession. Although it was not until the early twentieth century that a dramatic change was accomplished, nineteenth-century doctors established a national organization with a code of ethics that served as their first line of defense and as a catalyst for more substantive reform.

The National Code and Its Aftermath

The National Code of Medical Ethics developed largely in response to the crisis in medical standards and education in the early decades of the nineteenth century. Concerned physicians met the emerging crisis initially through the promotion of professional libraries and journals, and later with the creation of medical societies invested with licensing powers. Weak as these early efforts proved, they nevertheless represented a latent desire among the profession's more outspoken doctors to effect some form of control over the chaotic scenery of quacks, pretenders, and poorly trained regulars who entered medicine with ever-increasing ease. With the expansion of medical schools and spread of sectarianism, a feeling prevailed that a written code of medical ethics, more than rules of etiquette, would help establish uniform standards among medical men and provide the basis for mutual support—an esprit de corps—among the regulars of the profession. Forerunners of this thinking included the New Jersey and Massachusetts state medical societies, which first incorporated ethical principles and etiquette into their constitution and bylaws in the 1760s. The *Law, Oath, Precepts,* and *Decorum,* as well as the first chapter of *Physician,* written by Hippocrates, provided a common funding source for these ethical concerns. Early American codes were also influenced by the popular Edinburgh physician John Gregory, whose *Lectures on the Duties and Qualifications of a Physi-*

cian (1772) became a popular inspiration, and by Benjamin Rush's 1794 lectures on ethical duties and medical jurisprudence, which received frequent praise in medical circles. More important, however, was the influence of Thomas Percival (1740–1804), an English physician, whose interest in medical ethics during the 1770s culminated in a code published in 1803 under the title *Medical Jurisprudence, or Code of Ethics and Institutes Adopted by the Profession of Physic and Surgery*. Curiously, American physicians showed little concern for the fact that Percival had written his code as an effort to sort out the competing interests of physicians, surgeons, and apothecaries in mill-town hospitals, such as the Manchester Infirmary, which he helped to organize—circumstances that were fundamentally different from American medical realities. Nearly all early ethical regulations in New Hampshire (1819), the District of Columbia (1820), Cincinnati (1821), New York (1823) and Maryland (1832) reflected Percival's influence.[2]

Another catalyst of medical reform was Samuel Brown (1769–1830), professor of theory and practice of medicine at Transylvania Medical School in Lexington, Kentucky, who suggested that the regulars in each county form a secret society governed by Percival's code of ethics; only those who accepted the code would share in the society's brotherhood. The result was the code of Kappa Lambda Society of Aesculapius (also variously known as the Kappa Lambda of Hippocrates or Kappa Lambda Association of the United States), which was founded in Lexington in 1819. Two years later, a Philadelphia chapter became active and exerted a strong influence for reform during the 1830s. Eventually chapters existed in nearly all major cities. Although the societies as conceived by Brown were intended to become national in scope, public and professional reaction to their policy of secrecy and exclusiveness in the late 1820s destroyed the potential for good they had once manifested.[3]

In 1832 the Medico-Chirurgical Society of Baltimore developed a code that borrowed liberally from Rush, Gregory, Percival, the Kappa Lambda Society of Philadelphia, and the New York State Medical Society. All of these sources, with additions from James S. Stringham, professor of medical jurisprudence of the College of Physicians of New York City;

Ryan's *Medical Jurisprudence* (1832); and Theodoric R. Beck's *Elements of Medical Jurisprudence* (1823), laid the groundwork for the national code of ethics that was to be adopted unanimously by the AMA convention held in New York in May 1847. The national code, written by a committee headed by Isaac Hays (1796–1879) of Philadelphia, marked the culmination of earlier efforts to arrive at a system of ethics setting forth the high aims of the profession. The AMA code of medical ethics differed structurally from the Percival code, which had focused principally upon hospital conduct, apothecaries, and jurisprudence; the major thrust of medical discontent in the United States, unlike the experiences of the English medical profession, occurred in private practice rather than in hospitals, which were few in number. Moreover, the English distinction between physician (university-trained) and surgeon (apprentice-trained) did not exist in the young republic.[4]

The Hayes committee arranged the AMA code into three chapters, with each chapter subdivided into numerous articles and sections. The first chapter treated the duties of physician to patient and the obligations of patient to physician; the second, the duties of physician to other physicians and to the profession at large; and the third, the duties of the profession to the public and the obligations of the public to the profession. Of the three chapters, the second provided the fabric out of which the first and third were written. Dealing with such matters as how to maintain dignity and honor, the problems of quackery, advertising, specialism, disingenuous meddling at the patient's bedside, and consultation, the second chapter became the heart of the code and the source of the profession's subsequent troubles during the nineteenth century.[5]

Following publication of the code in 1847, articles in medical journals across the country supported and elaborated upon its principles, particularly in the areas of quackery, consultation, patent medicines, and the need for a truly scientific foundation in medicine. Doctors from Massachusetts to Texas drew from the code themes for innumerable speeches and lectures before their societies, graduating medical classes, and public lyceums. If repetition was the key to education in the Victorian age, medical students should have possessed an uncommon knowledge of medical ethics. There were those, for example, who enthusiastically claimed the code to be the most noble production of man since the Declaration of Independence. On the basis of its initial popularity in almost every region of the country, the AMA in 1855 required adoption of the code as a prerequisite for membership in the national organization. Countless state, county, and district medical societies adopted the code and thus became affiliated with the national association.[6]

However, the code did not receive unanimous approval from the nation's doctors. From its inception, some doctors questioned its articles, jurisdiction, potential sanctions, and intended purpose. Opponents like the medical societies of Rhode Island and the District of Columbia were reluctant to disregard their own codes, and the Medico-Chirurgical Society of Baltimore chose to adopt only selected portions of the national code. The Special Committee on Medical Ethics created by the State Medical Society of Ohio, which had long been a proponent of improved licensing procedures for physicians and an advocate of greater professional unity, considered the national code no more than a book on good manners. The committee denounced the code as "luminous with simplicity" and suggested that it be transferred to the pages of Mother Goose's melodies. Despite the committee's strong opposition, however, Ohio practitioners approved the national code.[7]

Alfred L. Carroll, M.D., and John C. Peters, M.D., editors of the *Medical Gazette* of New York, were similarly caustic in their opposition; they likened the code to the Articles of Religion printed in the *Book of Common Prayer* which few took the trouble to examine, let alone follow or obey. The code, Carroll and Peters claimed, was full of romantic sentiment and trivia, made unctuous by its "milk-and-water morality." Clearly it suggested rules of conduct or etiquette rather than principles of ethics.[8] In effect, it ignored "a personal sense of honor among the members of an honorable profession" by legislatively enacting articles that "are in themselves so manifestly improper, that no man with a spark of gentlemanly feeling, or even of common honesty, would be guilty of them." If it was necessary to remind members of a liberal profession of the evils of intrigue and artifice, and of de-

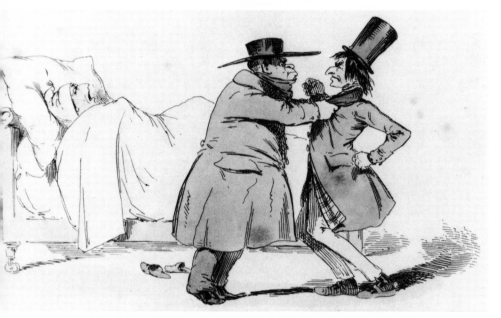

Henri Monnier. The homeopath and the allopath, in the presence of dear Mr. Gobard, treat each other as blackguards, grab each other by the throat, and the sick man dies for want of help. Lithograph. Courtesy of National Library of Medicine, Bethesda, Maryland.

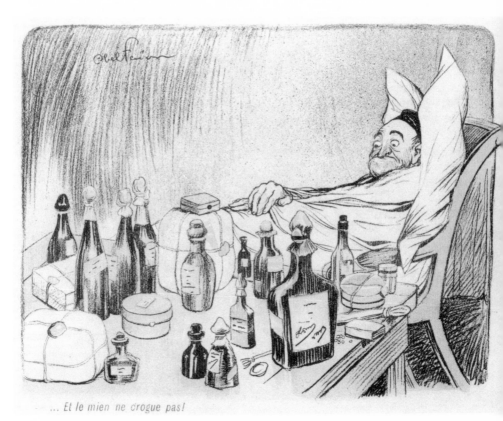

... Et le mien ne drogue pas!

Jules Abel Faivre (1867–1945). . . . *And mine doesn't medicate!* Lithograph (1902).
Courtesy of National Library of Medicine, Bethesda, Maryland.

frauding fellow members of the profession, then, the editors wrote, additional clauses should be inserted to prohibit forgery, arson, rape, pickpocketing, and other purely criminal deeds. It was the intention of both Carroll and Peters to place ethics "on the plane of common sense," suggesting that the implied necessity for a written code lowered the public's estimation of the profession.[9]

Critics of the code were quick to point out that many sections were blatantly pompous, while others were careless and negligent. The article (ch. 1, art. 1, sec. 1), which stated that the obligations of each physician were "deep and enduring" because there was "no tribunal other than his own conscience to adjudge penalties for carelessness or neglect," failed miserably to recognize the reality of malpractice suits.[10] Another article, which referred to the obligations of patient to physician, was criticized for legislating in an area where the profession could exercise little, if any, control. As one doctor remarked in 1891, he had "never yet met a layman—except a proof-reader—who had read the code, or who would recognize its authority if he had."[11] For some the code seemed designed to protect the established practitioner against the young physician, who, to abide by its provisions, was forced to "grow strong in modesty, like the violet beneath the grass"; to yield to the judgment of "ancient colleagues"; to avoid social contact with families having a physician; and, in general, to "assume the demeanor of Uriah Heep at the expense of dignity, self respect and individual independence."[12]

The code's basic failure, opponents maintained, was in its refusal to recognize the essential business relationship that existed between doctor and patient. In this relationship, the *Medical Gazette* editors argued, the doctor was no more than one half of a mercantile transaction, which despite lofty pretense was governed by the common laws of supply and demand. If dissatisfied with a doctor's services, a patient had the legitimate right to purchase services elsewhere. "This may be a humiliating view of our practical status in the community," the editors reasoned, "but it is undoubtedly the true one, and we do not act upon it voluntarily, the public does, and we are forced to accept matters as we find them." Under such circumstances they thought it ludicrous for doctors to appeal to the "sacrifices of comfort, ease, and health," which

they voluntarily assumed and their "right to expect and require" reciprocal duties of the public.[13]

What particularly irked opponents of the code was the
manner in which the AMA attempted to dictate policy to
state societies. Although itself created by an affiliation of
state and local organizations, the AMA demanded conformity to certain specifics in the code. By utilizing the threat
of expulsion over its member organizations, the AMA raised
the issue of state rights versus national authority; and the
subsequent feud had all the markings of a Webster-Hayne
debate on the source of true sovereignty. In the opinion of
the Ohio Medical Society, the national code of ethics had
been adopted merely as a recommendation and was never intended as an "imperative law." The adoption or rejection of
the code by individual societies was thus a question of expe-
dience, to be determined by societies within their own organizations. The Ohio society charged that the AMA, at the
time of its origin, had given no indication that it would dictate policy to the state societies. But it now sought to reduce
all state organizations to the same cast; and under such restraints, the state and local organizations were becoming little
more than "acknowledged cripples." If the AMA had even
hinted at the outset that it possessed such a power, the Ohio
society concluded, it "would have lived but to die."[14]

Patents

Although there were malcontents who objected to the code
from the very beginning, significant opposition did not
emerge until the 1870s, when the association began taking a
more forceful legislative attitude toward irregularities. One
of the first indications of this opposition occurred in 1876,
when J. Marion Sims, M.D., president of the AMA and
founder of the Woman's Hospital in New York, asked the
profession if it was not time to revoke the code, as it had out-
lived its usefulness and had become unjust in its demands.
Sims had experienced first-hand the code's punitive nature
when in 1869 the New York Academy of Medicine tried him
for unethical advertising and betraying the secrets of a patient. He was particularly concerned with the code's condemnation of proprietary patents. As the designer of several

gynecological instruments, including the uterine elevator, speculum, tenaculum, and button sutures, he thought it altogether proper for an inventor to receive just compensation for research and development of new techniques.[15]

Sims was not alone in his objections. Two other forceful opponents of the code, the Ohio Medical Society and the New York *Medical Gazette*, made similar appeals to rescind or revise the prohibition over rights of invention. Though they had no objection to the code's prohibitions regarding patent medicines, whose mystery of composition had been gilded with bold deception, the same proscription could not apply to the physician who designed and patented a tool for surgical use. Unlike the nostrum peddler, inventors of surgical instruments did not put their articles into the hands of the laity or make the instrument a secret. In a speech read before the Medical Society of New York in 1873, Ezra Hunt observed, "When a physician patents an instrument, he merely offers it to the profession as a tool to be tried by them without secrets, but only protected as to its authorship. . . . But when a man puts up a patent medicine, it is as a secret compound to be used by persons without medical advice."

The prohibition on medical patents countered the very principles of the nation's capitalistic ideology. Hunt noted that, "Where an inventor invents an apparatus which proves to be new in principle, or in the application of a principle, we see no reason why a benefit therefrom should not accrue to the inventor." By patenting the instrument an inventor did not necessarily increase the price of the article unduly; he protected himself and distinguished his work from that of imitators. Hunt claimed that instruments not patented by physicians were all too often plundered by manufacturers, whose changes or lack of quality control made them dangerous or worthless.[16]

The Special Committee on Medical Ethics of the Ohio Medical Society reported that the surgical instrument was constructed "to give occupation to genius, and to add to the skill and renown of the surgeon." It was not the society's intention to advocate the propriety of obtaining a patent for every surgical instrument, but rather an attitude of liberality that would allow every physician to judge for himself the means at hand. If an individual invented or perfected a

useful instrument, he should have the option of presenting it
to the profession by means of a patent, since those who
worked for the perfection of surgical instrumentation did so
at enormous cost in time and money to themselves. Despite
the vocal support given the cause of medical patents, the
AMA in 1854, 1866, 1895, and 1909 successfully defeated resolutions to liberalize the restrictions set forth in the code.[17]

Fees

The rise of the industrial middle class, the changes brought
about by finance capitalism, and the broad expansion of medical services to the working classes brought corresponding
changes in the manner of payment to physicians. For one
thing, the ancient custom of rewarding physicians with voluntary offerings or honorariums before treatment occurred
with less and less frequency. In their place, doctors erected a
standardized schedule of payment, which, as defined, was not
pay for services rendered but a fee—an arbitrary amount that
in no way compensated the physician for his knowledge and
skill.[18] Regardless of definition, however, doctors arranged
fees on the basis of time consumed, degree of skill required,
and nature of the particular disease. Although cautioned
never to extort higher fees from the rich or slight fees from
the poor, the social and economic condition of the patient almost always determined the amount of variation used in the
final settlement. Books and articles on physician's fees urged
that charges for medical services be the same for all "whether
it is the mouth of a poor patient or a rich one, for a friend or
for a stranger." The difference, if any, could be adjusted at
the time of settlement; "but let it be understood that it is a
deduction, and not that . . . charges are variable according
to the patient."[19]

The substitution of fees for voluntary offerings or honorariums came as a mixed blessing to the medical profession.
As one doctor wrote in 1900, "the gratitude of some patients is
properly described as an acute symptom, showing greatest
prominence during the height of the illness, subsiding quickly
during convalescence and quite disappearing as recovery is
reached."[20] Benjamin Rush advised his medical students to
equip themselves for practice with two pockets: a small pock-

et for fees, and a large pocket for insults.[21] A poem that made the rounds of medical societies in the nineteenth century appeared to strike a common chord.

I. VERY ILL

"Name, oh doctor, name your fee!
Ask—I'll pay what'er it be!
　Skill like yours, I know, comes high;
　Only do not let me die!
　Get me out of this and I
The cash will pay you instantly.

II. CONVALESCENT

"Cut, oh doctor! cut the fee!
Cut, or not a dime from me!
　I am not a millionaire
　But I'll do whatever's square;
　Only make a bill that's fair
And I'll settle presently.

III. WELL

"Book, oh doctor! book your fee!
Charge—I'll pay it futurely,
　When the crops all by are laid,
　When every other bill is paid,
　(Or when of death again afraid)
I'll pay it—grudgingly."[22]

Part of the difficulty stemmed from the reluctance of the medical profession to employ the same methods used by businessmen in fee collection. "The ideal collection is cash at the time of services rendered," one physician observed, "and that this ideal is not oftener realized is due to simple neglect or fear on our part." Failure to insist upon this method created any number of embarrassing problems, least of which was the actual collection of fees. Few doctors, for example, kept accurate accounts of their professional services; and when bills were presented to patients, they were sometimes sent five or six months after treatment. Having long ignored the business aspects of the profession and obligingly extended credit far beyond the most reasonable bounds, doctors found themselves in the awkward role of having created an environment hostile to more businesslike procedures. To correct this, medical societies established business bureaus designed to instruct their members on bookkeeping and bill collection. Some societies even urged members to require a written acknowledgment from the patient regarding the correctness of the bill and a promise to pay within a certain time period. If payment was not forthcoming, the doctor could then use promissory notes with interest clauses attached and, as a last resort, employ collectors to settle the delinquent charge. Medical societies also made available to members lists of individuals in the community who did not pay their bills.[23]

"Medical men show more financial failures, when judged from a commercial point of view, than any other class," J. J. Conner, M.D., wrote in the *Journal* of the AMA, "but this is not because the members of the medical profession are incompetent men, or do not earn a living, but because they have inherited a faulty system of doing business."[24] Advocates of more businesslike procedures advised physicians never to become so absorbed in their scientific interests as to neglect the means which made it possible for them to pursue their vocation. In 1900 one doctor reminded his colleagues, "We do not, in these days of definitely specified terms in the business world, depend upon the patient's sense of gratitude, or expect an honorarium simply as a fee for services rendered, but we arrange before or after the service for a stated fee, much as is done in the commercial world."

Despite encouraging signs, doctors continued to lament their depressed financial state, claiming that fewer than 25 percent of the medical graduates managed to make a living in the profession—the remainder finding it necessary to supplement their incomes with other forms of work. The realization that the average income of physicians was under $1,000 in 1900 gave added impetus to the need for standardized fees as well as a precautionary directive that the profession should not become embroiled in the competitive market, seeking to steal another's patients with cut-rate fees.[25]

The code of ethics of the AMA took special note of the distressing economic problem when it encouraged the medical faculty in every town and district to adopt uniform rules for the payment of fees and stressed the need for adhering to those rules with as much uniformity as varying circumstances would admit. By the 1850s medical societies in many of the larger cities had established fee-bills, and by the end of the century the practice had extended to smaller towns. Only the rural practitioner tended to ignore the fee-bill. Doctors who appealed for improved business practices within the profession were unanimous in their support of uniform fee-bills. They also urged doctors to establish protective associations to weed out persons who would not pay their bills and to devise better means of fee collection. Two such organizations that proved particularly successful in this endeavor were the Detroit Physicians' Business Association and the Physicians' Protective Association of Jackson County, Illinois. In both instances, physicians established uniform fee-bills and abated the nuisance of nonpayers by maintaining lists of persons known to have defaulted on medical payments and refusing to attend them unless paid in advance.[26]

Advocates of greater professional unity were quick to admit that doctors were their own worst enemies in economics. Despite efforts to rally to each other's support by insisting on the use of standardized fees, many physicians, fearing that their efforts would be interpreted as monopolistic, chose instead to compete for the lowest fees, hoping to make up the difference from increased volume. In numerous cities, doctors made house calls for as little as fifty cents and office consultations for twenty-five cents. "If the loss by competing for cheap fees could be restricted to those who indulge in the practice," E. L. Hayford, M.D., observed in 1900, "the trouble would soon correct itself, but the entire body feels its effects. No greater mistake is made by a physician than in cutting rates. A community will promptly accept the value that the doctor places on his ability."[27]

Contract System

While the AMA, through its state and county medical societies, succeeded in bringing limited regulation to the marketplace through the encouragement of fee-bills, its efforts proved altogether useless in controlling the practice of contract work. The contract system had thrived in the South from colonial days to the Civil War, providing cheap medical care for plantation families and their slaves. In the latter half of the nineteenth century, benevolent societies throughout

the nation negotiated for collective medical service and received it, largely because of the unwholesome competitive
nature of medicine and the overabundance of doctors.

Collective, or group, medical service was popular in the
railroad and manufacturing centers of urban America and in
the coal, quarry, timber, and mill towns of the backcountry.
There doctors made special arrangements with companies to
provide medical service to employees at a specified monthly
fee that was deducted by the company from the employees'
paychecks. A typical fee was fifty cents a month for an unmarried man and seventy-five cents for a married man and
his entire family. Since the employee had no choice of doctor,
this system created a virtual doctor's trust, which sometimes
degenerated into political chicanery with physicians competing with one another for the contract and facing kickback demands from employers. Despite these impositions physicians
preferred to work out their contracts with company management rather than with the workers themselves or their
unions. During the anthracite coal strike of 1903 in Pennsylvania, for example, contract physicians identified with the
company position and refused to accept payments from
union treasuries. What made the system appealing to the
contract physician was that it ensured payment for medical
services from individuals who, in different circumstances,
might choose charitable hospitals, dispensaries, anatomical
institutes, home remedies, or promises of quick cure from
medical sectarians.

Regardless of its temporizing appeal, the contract system
did not prove to be a satisfactory financial relationship for
the medical profession. For one thing, it forced physicians to
attend to ailments not worthy of medical attention. It also
necessitated a lower fee-bill for extra services, such as surgery or obstetrics, not included under the contract. While the
system brought medical services to the laboring classes at a
lower price, to the chagrin of the profession, it also provided
a cheap substitute for those who were capable of paying regular professional fees. Doctors could always point to an afflu-
ent merchant or professional man who, having once worked
in the quarries or timber country in youth, continued to pay
a small monthly fee for medical services.[28]

In an analysis of questionnaires sent to 138 physicians in

the city of New Orleans in 1896, 41 percent of them served 55,000 people in contract practice and received an average payment per family amounting to $1.19 per year. A 1908 report indicated that in over one hundred cities across the country, approximately 3 percent of the population belonged to companies, fraternal lodges, or organizations that hired doctors through the contract process.[29] In cities where the contract system became popular among fraternal societies and trade unions, young doctors seeking a financial foothold in the competitive world were never lacking. Although the contract system was considered unethical by established doctors, it represented a clear reflection of the ruthless competition and continued impoverishment that plagued the profession. State and local medical societies refused to enforce sanctions despite the AMA's efforts to identify contract work as a form of irregular practice.[30]

Advertising

Given the competitive nature of the profession, medical men in the nineteenth century used both direct and indirect methods of building a clientele. Callous types, for example, were not above puffing their way to success through any means available. The medical pharisee, as G. Frank Lydston, M.D., described him to the Chicago College of Physicians and Surgeons in 1892, could be recognized in either of two forms: a lean, cadaverous misanthrope "who would make an excellent understudy for an undertaker" or a fat, sleek, unctuous doctor, "on whom the cloak of religion rests ever so lightly, especially on fast days." Whether lean or fat, both were cast from the same mold: their materialistic theory of life centered around the ability to turn a fast dollar. Both were members of the church (preferably two or three); and from those churches, they regularly employed hirelings with resonant voices to call them out during services to attend a serious case. This contrivance made even the most drowsy backslider sit erect in his pew and admire the compelling dedication of the doctor. Both of these pharisees, Lydston observed, were great believers in ethical codes and used their mighty voices and flaunting reputations to attack young doctors who dared set foot in their neighborhoods. Lydston de-

scribed the medical pharisee as a noxious weed in the broad
field of city practice, whose bearing, unfortunately, was food
for the masses who crowded his offices and wept at his
passing.[31]

Doctors who were desperate for patients sometimes employed drummers to frequent fashionable business or resi-
dential areas, where they would contract for business or
spread stories of their successful cures and famous patients.
Still others exploited popular delusions or errors (particularly sexual disorders or diseases of women and children), impressing patients with the belief that they were
worse off than they really were; substituting fear and anxiety
for hope and cheerfulness; deprecating fellow practitioners;
approaching invalids without invitation; "slipping up on the
blind side of man's political, religious, or sectional bias, and
soliciting favor," or puffing themselves and their achievements before the public press.[32]

The relationship between the advertising physician and
the press proved one of the more troublesome problems facing the profession. In effect the advertising physician had to
preserve the image of a liberal professional and at the same
time utilize the newspapers as a medium for improving his
financial status. Unfortunately mountebanks had used the
press for years as their advertising channel, wreaking havoc
among the gullible, filling their own pockets through countless schemes. With few exceptions the press in America, as in
Europe, was immune to the protests of medical societies and
continued to sell space to charlatans who guaranteed cure
for the entire list of human ills. For those doctors who
believed the press would provide the proper medium of
communication between themselves and the community, the
problem of preserving the dignity of the profession became
more than just an exercise in semantics. Some, for example,
chose to advertise themselves indirectly by circulating letters
from patients (both real and contrived) that praised their
particular skills. Others circulated handbills and pamphlets
containing notice of reputed cures and praises from known
public figures. A physician whose practice had been lauded
by a professor or whose name was followed by a degree was
far more impressive than one whose praise was generated by
a mere tradesman.[33]

In general, doctors condemned the fantastic claims and preposterous advertisements for quack medicines that filled the newspaper columns; they also objected to specialists' shingles swinging in the breeze like tavern signs. "The man who goes about seeking patients," one critic remarked, "proves, by that very fact, that patients do not seek him, and that is the very best evidence that he is not worth seeking."[34] In general the profession felt that the only legitimate way in which physicians could publicize their names was through the presentation of scientific papers in local societies, distributing reprints of articles to the profession but not to the public, editing and contributing articles to journals, teaching in medical schools, and working in clinics. As one doctor explained, "the lay press has no part in the life of physician save to record his obituary." Although a doctor should be allowed to advertise in medical periodicals meant only for professional eyes and to insert his name and specialty "where custom has established a precedent," he should avoid the daily press. Reports of the proceedings of medical societies, successful operations, curious cases, cures, and all the other medical items that served the interests of quackery were to be excluded from newspaper columns. "Restrict our medical opinions save when pertaining to public health and hygiene," one doctor remarked, "and let the other and disreputable methods of advertising mark as a quack the one who indulges in or allows it."[35]

Medical societies were notoriously lax in enforcing advertising restrictions and began to tighten their rules only in the early decades of the twentieth century. Some limited advertising to business cards, while others forbade the mention of a doctor's name in news accounts on the suspicion that doctors furnished the press with information for articles lauding their work.[36] Although medical societies recognized the need to prohibit overt advertising, they also realized that the press was the greatest potential educational medium in society and sought ways to turn it into a "cheerful companion" for true medical concerns. State and county medical societies thus encouraged the AMA to establish a bureau of education to disseminate information on matters of public health and hygiene. "With the friendly aid rather than the opposition of the press," one concerned doctor wrote, "more could be accomplished in a short time in the way of creating public sentiment in favor of certain reforms and in matters of legislation than can be accomplished by medical journals in the next twenty-five years."[37]

Internal Feuds

Jealousy and envy had long been rife among American doctors, who in their relations with each other were capable of the grossest insinuations and slanders. The pretensions of the medical man who "garnished and larded" his speech with mellifluous uses of the personal pronoun had turned many a medical society into a bear garden.[38] To make matters worse, doctors had carried many of their quarrels into the public arena. The feuds between Daniel Drake and John Moorhead of the Ohio Medical College, between Benjamin Rush and William Shippen, Jr., between Shippen and John Morgan, and the conflict between the editors of the *American Medical Recorder* and Jefferson Medical College were just a few examples of controversies that spilled into the public forum to the detriment of the profession.

William B. Lyman, M.D., remarked that this incessant backbiting had created much of the public's criticism of the profession. The effort "to build ourselves up by tearing down the confidence in others," he wrote, was responsible for the public's lack of confidence in the scientific achievements of medicine and led directly to the prosperity of quackery and sectarianism. Unless a spirit of mutual courtesy and fair-dealing developed within the profession, he warned, the instinct for self-preservation would breed such destruction that no effort could ever establish the position of trust in society.

Part of the problem, Lyman said, was that the ranks of the profession had been recruited "from the toiling, laboring classes of people, amongst whom the instinct and consequent emotions of self-preservation are yet in their full ascendancy." Unlike the European doctor, whose profession had long "been tempered by the effect of generations of affluence and protection of wealth," the American medical man reflected a competitive environment that led him to seek a more individualistic approach to success. Another part of the problem was the lax requirements for medical education, which had encouraged "cheaply and inefficiently educated doctors" who "robbed the justly deserving of the fruits of their labor." Then too, the government, in failing to subsidize scientific inquiry, had turned many investigators from the field of honest scientific investigation. Thus, Lyman wrote, the spirit of commercialism had given license to petty emotions rather than a more generous spirit or broader reason.[39]

The success of the doctor depended, in the last analysis, upon the confidence the community reposed in the profession. Medical men were quite aware that this confidence was irreparably lost when the profession lacked harmony of purpose or, as occasionally happened, when professional feuds became public issues. When that occurred, the public turned instead to quackery, which had always pretended to own truth. Medical feuds were destructive to all involved, since "the mind of the community is very apt to begin with distrust of the one charged, and to end by disgust of the assailant, and in its double condemnation to feel a general sense of contempt for the whole profession." To improve its image, the profession must remove differences of opinion from the "mire of public highway." Neglecting the spirit of mutual consideration caused a distrust of the medical community upon which quackery was "building its enormous superstructure."[40]

The Power of Expulsion

According to Ashbel Woodward, M.D., president of the Connecticut Medical Society, the establishment of a national society ushered in an era of progress for the medical profession and medical science. Until the AMA was created, doctors had "no adequate medium through which the enthusiasm of the earnest and the ardent could be brought to bear upon the spirit of others." For too long the isolated and independent medical community, by turning inward toward its own local societies rather than outward toward national concerns, had stifled legitimate reform. But all this changed with the creation of the AMA, whose annual meetings drew together medical men from all parts of the country and whose code brought order and a common set of principles to the profession. Woodward was careful, however, to distinguish between the power inherent in the code of ethics and the binding nature of laws that defined the relationship between man and state. "The force inherent in the code is wholly of a moral character," he observed, and instead of "acting upon the fears, [it] appeals to the noblest sentiments of humanity." Its only recourse to improper conduct was to expel an errant member from the association.

> .The right to exclude from the association a member who openly violates its laws, no one will question. In this quiet method of purification a society possesses a great advantage over the state. Governments have successfully tried the most varied expedients, ranging between extreme lenience and extreme cruelty to secure obedience from subjects. Success has always been partial because punitive measures fail to eradicate evil propensities. Fear may restrain from overt crimes, yet malcontents remain within the national borders, and if chance gives them power, may strike a parricidal dagger into the heart of their country. . . . When, on the other hand, a voluntary association removes a member, the separation is complete. By pruning the branches the symmetry of the tree is preserved. Disaffection, the fruitful arm of discord, departs, leaving behind harmony and united strength. Efforts are not distracted by jarring councils, nor is time lost or thought consumed in applying remedies to domestic wounds.[41]

Not all physicians willingly shared Woodward's opinion. According to some critics, the great benefits designed by the founders of the AMA had failed to accrue, and the expulsion power of the national organization had degenerated into a "Thirty Years War" among its membership. Rather than harmonizing the various needs of the profession, the code had become "a fireband, a disorganizer," at least in the eyes of those who became the object of its scrutiny. Critics, such as Louis Bauer, M.D., of St. Louis, blamed the power of expulsion for having transposed the code into an engine of oppression within the medical profession—because "men jealously, maliciously intent upon persecuting a fellow member, may distort the meaning of the Code to suit their malign purposes, thus enter into a regular conspiracy to blacken character, and that under the sanctity of the Code's provisions." Bauer condemned the code as an unscrupulous tool for those avaricious physicians who used it for persecution, injustice, and malice against true medical fellowship. In effect, the code had driven some of the most capable men out of the profession, "leaving the field to a class which feast on bicker-ings as maggots on decomposing cheese." In contemplating the various unsavory features of the code, Bauer thought it time to end its mischievous use as an instrument of tyranny and injustice. His remarks were not those of a disinterested observer, since he himself had been censured by the St. Louis Medical Society for interference with the medical treatment of another physician and felt, perhaps justly, that the society had not only accused him wrongfully of the charge, but used unethical procedures to carry out its vengeance.[42]

In another notable case, the AMA expelled Julius Hom-berger, M.D., of New Orleans in 1866 on grounds that his newspaper advertisements violated the code of ethics. De-fending himself against the charge, Homberger reasoned that the code had been created at a time when many who called themselves specialists did so on the pretense that they had discovered a new cure. Quite correctly, the AMA looked upon such charlatans with disfavor. But the code, he argued, had been framed under circumstances that no longer ex-isted; and it now extended to those legitimate members of the profession who, practicing largely in cities, found it nec-essary to advertise themselves both to other physicians and to the public. In essence, Homberger said, the code had forgot-ten the true specialist in much the same manner as the fra-mers of the Constitution had forgotten the interests and rights of the Negro.[43]

Specialism and Fee-Sharing

Medical journals in the latter half of the nineteenth cen-tury abounded with articles on the passing of the family phy-sician, the decline of the general practitioner, the rise of the specialist, or on specialization in medicine. This tendency was not brought on by the changing preferences of patients so much as by the increasingly complicated nature of medi-cine itself. Specialism had been a natural outgrowth of gen-eral medicine, which in company with developments in the sciences over the course of the century had matured to the degree that no one mind was capable of fully grasping every portion of the discipline. With advancement in the art and science of medicine, surgery had become the first general specialty, with doctors in this field performing abdominal op-

erations at a time when the generalist seldom ventured into
the body's cavities except for emergency cases of strangu-
lated hernia or appendicitis. Similar specialties developed for
the genito-urinary organs, throat, eye, ear, skin, heart, lungs,
and nervous system. Since specialists treated a clientele that
was temporary at best, they chose a variety of techniques to
ensure regularity in their remuneration. Traveling specialists, for example, announced their coming through the columns of the local press and sometimes employed advance
agents or "cappers," who combed the rural districts to drum
up cases.[44] In addition to these questionable methods, specialists insured the regularity of referral cases from generalists through the payment of a commission or fee-sharing.
With no official AMA position on fee-sharing, physicians
pursued a financial course that had grown from the day-to-
day relations of generalists and specialists in a period of rampant competition and difficult times.[45]

As the practice of fee-sharing matured, doctors who par-
ticipated in the transaction regarded it as in no way conflicting with the demands of highest moral conduct. The test of
its ethical measure, they reasoned, was not in the presump-
tion that it interfered with previous practices or even that it
enabled certain commercial advantages to accrue to both
parties; rather, the true test was whether the practice was in
accord with the good of the patient. Those who supported
the practice had no doubt that consultation with another specialist or the referral to a more capable doctor would bring
patients into contact with those best qualified to treat their
particular problems. Arrangements of this sort were common among professionals, particularly in law, where attor-
neys used eminent jurists in difficult cases.

Doctors argued further that a fee-remuneration contract
between themselves and specialists was preferable to a well-
meant courtesy or an occasional present. One generalist
wrote: "I believe that there ought to be a business relation so
perfect that the check would not come as a surprise but simply as a business incident. There is a mutuality in the work—
why not in the fees?" Since physicians would continue to be
feeders of specialists' offices and hospitals, the system would
work for the betterment of medicine as well as the needs of
the patient. The referral system not only met the financial

needs of doctors, but succeeded in improving their mutual relations as well.[46]

Although practitioners were able to ensure reasonable remuneration adjustments with specialists, they found it difficult to obtain fees in cases referred to hospitals, since in most instances they did not participate in operations and took part only occasionally in postoperative treatment. In several cities physicians sought to skirt these difficulties by assuming responsibility for the patient's time in the hospital. In these situations the physician would employ a specialist to treat his patient at an agreed upon fee, and the specialist would then leave the aftertreatment entirely in the hands of the generalist. The patient thus remained under his doctor's care throughout the course of hospital confinement. As an alternative, generalists would employ surgeons or specialists who were willing to share a combined fee.

For their part, specialists were often reluctant to discuss the issue of fee-sharing for fear of appearing too obliging and of giving recognition to a fee structure that might prove difficult to change. Those whose skills, location, and circumstance put them in the center of a thriving practice had no need to divide fees with the general practitioner. According to them, their skills were essential, and any fee paid for important work should not be subject to extortion by an unskilled generalist.[47] Besides the insistence of successful specialists that the practice of fee-sharing had outgrown its usefulness, there was also the formidable opposition of those who, like G. Frank Lydston of Chicago, denounced it in the most vehement terms, accusing both parties of unethical conduct. Both the surgeon and generalist, Lydston argued, were as dishonest as a man could be without violating statutory law. The participating parties in fee-sharing were a menace to the general prosperity and respectability of the profession. They were advertisers "on a lower plane than a common quack," who had no ethics or code, but acted as a common businessman.[48] Lydston later rescinded his position and suggested several instances where fee-sharing might be practiced.

> 1. A general practitioner and surgeon may form a co-partnership out and out, and announce the fact, presenting joint bills for services.

2. The specialist may present a joint bill which openly claims a fee for combined services, the general practitioner and surgeon each receiving his fair and just proportion of the fee—adjusted according to the service actually rendered by each.

3. The general practitioner may conduct all the financial negotiations with the patient, call a surgeon in to operate and pay him whatever sum is agreed upon between the two physicians. Here the general practitioner presents a bill which is understood by the patient to be a bill for joint services. If the patient is satisfied with the total amount he is not likely to concern himself with the arrangement that his physician has made with the operator. If the surgeon is satisfied with his own fee, it is a matter that concerns nobody else.

4. There are cases in which the general practitioner may render honest and competent assistance to the surgeon. Here a joint bill should be rendered.[49]

Despite the clarifications advocated by Lydston, the revised Principles of Medical Ethics accepted by the AMA in 1903 did not approve of fee-sharing. It was not until the 1912 revision in the code that the AMA softened its position, conceding most of the exceptions noted by Lydston.

Consultation with Irregulars

The code bore evidence of careful work in treating the troublesome problem of consultation with irregulars. As clearly stated, "no one can be considered as a regular practitioner, or a fit associate in consultation, whose practice is based on an exclusive dogma, to the rejection of the accumulated experience of the profession, and of the aids actually furnished by anatomy, physiology, pathology, and organic chemistry." This notwithstanding, the profession had long given lip service to the consultation clause, preferring financial rewards to the rancor of yet another thorny issue. This was particularly true in the large metropolitan areas where both regulars and irregulars knowingly split consultation fees with one another. This association was due in part to the fact that many urban irregulars not only demonstrated more than average medical competence, but their patients often came from the socially prominent and educated classes. In rural areas, where sectarians were less powerful and less educated than their urban cousins, consultation was far less frequent.

Those favoring consultation argued that few of the sectarians continued to practice in strict accordance with their original beliefs. H. M. Lymann, M.D., commented in 1878, "A living dodo or a moa would hardly excite greater enthusiasms in ornithological circles than would now be aroused among scientific men by the production of a genuine believer in the dogmas of Hahnemann or Thomson." Lymann believed that the code should be revised to reflect this. Although he doubted that many regulars would like to meet on equal terms "the hoary knave whom they have known since youth as a villain past redemption," still, he felt moral character more than scientific opinion should be the governing principle, and the AMA should consider framing a new article that would reach out to the "liberal" homeopath.[50]

The proponents of consultation thought the practice no more heretical than the earlier consultations between Brunonians and Rushites. Opposed as these two systems were in their pathology and therapeutics, they conducted a mutual intercourse nonetheless; and over a period of time, their party lines fused under a banner of a broader orthodoxy.[51] But the compatibility once evident among the Rushites and Brunonians was not apparent among the regulars and irregulars in the second half of the nineteenth century, despite evidence that many openly ignored the code. The fears engendered by the loss of licensing power, the surplus of doctors, ruthless competition, and poor medical schools had led the AMA to shore up the foundations of orthodoxy.

Although the AMA had attempted to portray homeopaths as unschooled in the true art and science of medicine, homeopathy had blossomed as a respectable alternative to orthodox therapeutics among the highest levels of American society. Americans of German extraction remained the core of its practitioners and patients, and from that element emerged a broad spectrum of enthusiastic converts. Many parents who accepted the heroic therapeutics of the regulars for their own diseases preferred homeopathy for their children. By mid-nineteenth century growing numbers of the professional and intellectual classes, especially the clergy, had deserted to its doctrines. "Whether attracted by the idea of the 'spiritualized essence' of the drug or repelled by the 'poisoning and surgical butchery' of regular practice," one historian remarked, "many clergymen were zealous propagators of homeopathy."[52]

In large measure the AMA's resentment against homeopaths stemmed from the economic edge they often experienced in their communities. Not only did homeopaths receive higher than average incomes, but their patients were more apt to pay their bills. The combination of economic competition, frustration, mounting resentment at the loss of patients, and anxiety regarding the inroads homeopaths made into traditional therapeutic practice helped to swing the AMA to a more forceful stance in its position on consultation.[53] Eventually, the national organization insisted that local societies not only purge irregulars from their lists but that they also enforce the policy regarding consultation. To achieve this the AMA began to take more determined action with regard to the code's interpretation. Unfortunately, its successes were achieved at the expense of public opinion—not so much because the public favored the sectarians as because they objected to the AMA's efforts to restrict freedom of the marketplace and the independence of sectarian believers. A nation that could boast a multitude of denominational and sectarian religious creeds could only look disparagingly on the strident efforts of the AMA to reduce similar trends in medical science.[54]

In 1870, on objections raised by physicians J. L. Sullivan and Horatio R. Storer, efforts were undertaken to exclude the Massachusetts State Medical Society from representation at the annual AMA meeting on grounds that the society had allowed irregular practitioners to become members. When faced with expulsion the Massachusetts society quickly passed a resolution excluding irregulars from membership. The resolution was without effect, however, since the society's constitution provided that no member could be expelled without a trial and conviction. Furthermore, the statutes authorizing the society as a licensing agency required it to admit all applicants with degrees from Harvard Medical School. Since several of Harvard's graduates had converted to homeopathy, the society faced a troublesome dilemma. To resolve the problem, the Massachusetts society relinquished its power as a licensing agency and created in its place a trial board, which during a period of seven years expelled the irregulars, a situation which brought public sympathy to the side of the sectarians. At a grand fair held in Boston, $100,000 was raised to organize a medical department under homeopathic control at the recently established Boston University (which had among its founders Isaac Rich, a patient of the prominent homeopathic physician J. T. Talbot).[55]

Notable efforts were also made to include homeopathy within the system of medical education at the University of Michigan at Ann Arbor. Reputedly the popularity of homeopaths in the state had resulted from their success in treating malaria and Asiatic cholera during the 1840s; there were even unfounded allegations that the university regents were themselves patrons of homeopathy.[56] Actually the regents had opposed the state legislature's efforts to include homeopathy in the academic program. In May 1875, however, fearing that continued refusal would imperil the financial existence of the university, and accepting the position of the state medical society that a special school within the university would not be objectionable to the profession as long as there was a common Board of Censors, the regents withdrew their objections and accepted a grant to establish a college of homeopathy at the university.

The Michigan legislature provided funds to suport the cost of two homeopaths (who were paid five hundred dollars more than the regular medical staff), but a complete faculty and a full complement of courses was not funded. In effect, homeopathic students were obliged to take part of their instruction from the regular medical faculty in the university. This arrangement, however, provoked the state medical society, which threatened to destroy its connection with the school by proposing a resolution that "no person shall be admitted to membership [in the state medical society] who practices or professes to practice in accordance with any so-called 'pathy' or sectarian school of medicine, or who has recently graduated from a medical school whose professors teach or assist in teaching those who propose to graduate in or practice irregular medicine." Although the state society ultimately rejected the resolution, its intent was clear—to threaten the University of Michigan into creating separate facilities for educating its sectarian students.[57]

The debate over the proposed resolution quickly reached

the AMA meeting at Philadelphia in June 1876, where delegates of the State Medical Society of Michigan attempted to
have the medical faculty of the university excluded from
membership in the AMA. A vicious verbal battle ensued between the school's faculty and the state medical society, including accusations of unprofessional conduct, violation of
the national code with respect to relations with irregulars
(brought against the state medical society for advocating a
mixed board of medical examiners), and a number of personal accusations. A resolution put forward by J. M. Toner of
Washington, D.C., and adopted at the national meeting read,
"Members of the medical profession who in any way aid or
abet the graduation of medical students in irregular or exclusive systems of medicine are deemed thereby to violate the
spirit of the [code of] ethics of the AMA."[58]

The matter was also referred to the judicial council of the
AMA, which in 1878 concluded that "while deprecating the
practice of aiding or abetting in any way the teaching and education of students known to be supporters of singular and
exclusive dogmas in medicine as beneath the dignity of right-
minded teachers of an honorable and liberal profession," the
constitution, bylaws, and code of ethics of the AMA contained no clause under which the charge could be adjudi-
cated. Rather than have the dispute end on such an indeci-
sive note, Nathan Smith Davis proposed an amendment to
the code of ethics that stated, "hence it is considered derogatory to the interests of the public and the honor of the public
for any physician or teacher to aid in any way the medical
teaching or graduation of persons knowing them to be supporters and intended practitioners of some irregular and exclusive system of medicine."[59]

In speaking against the amendment, Edward S. Dunster,
M.D., professor of obstetrics and diseases of women at the
University of Michigan, argued that the proposed amendment conflicted with articles already in the code and that,
since medicine was a liberal profession, its members should
share knowledge with others, and enlighten the public so
that quackery and all similar evils might be suppressed. Dunster charged that the proposed amendment "virtually denied
the right of a medical education to all except believers in our
own system" and prohibited the dissemination of truth to
those who were in particular need of it.[60]

Surely no man in his sense for one instant can entertain so monstrous an idea. Establish the principle embodied in the proposed amendment that the physician shall not teach the truth to those who believe in irregular or exclusive systems of medicine, and it would prevent mankind from teaching truth or science of any sort to skeptics or unbelievers. It would prevent the professor of astronomy from teaching the Copernican system if among his students there were unbelievers who held the Ptolemaic system; it would prevent the professor of physics from promulgating the undulatory theory of light, if among its auditors there were skeptics still clinging to the Newtonian theory of the emanation of material particles. Nay, more, it would forbid the Christian clergyman from preaching the truths of the Gospel of Christ, if perchance in his congregation there were atheists, or heathen or miserable sinners, who were 'supporters and intended practitioners' of free love or polygamy, or any other abstract or concrete form of deviltry of any name or nature whatsoever.[61]

Since the public insisted on recognizing homeopaths, Dunster believed homeopathic physicians ought to be educated as thoroughly as possible, particularly when this could result in an improved standard for all medical education. What made the amendment ludicrous in Dunster's eyes was that it could not be enforced without at the same time closing nearly every public clinic in the United States with homeopathic attendants. To further demonstrate the absurdity of the amendment, Dunster argued that the dictum would fall most heavily upon writers of medical textbooks, whose texts were used to teach homeopathic students. This meant that even the former president of the AMA, Samuel D. Gross, as well as Dalton and Flint, Sims and Thomas, Emmet and Barker, Wood and Stillé, Da Costa, Loomis and Bartholow, Van Buren and Gouley, and Hamilton and Sayre faced censure from the association for not prohibiting the use of their works in homeopathic colleges. Whether intended or not, these men, the most orthodox of the regulars, were teaching sectarians and would continue to do so long after they themselves had died.

The assumption implicit in the amendment that sectarian creeds would be strengthened if their adherents were taught by regulars was another cause of dismay to Dunster. He urged that his medical colleagues look to Europe where homeopaths had first to graduate from a regular medical

school and to Canada where all practitioners of medicine, regardless of sectarian belief, were required to pass a standard
examination before entering practice. As the editor of the
Canadian *Lancet* had reported, "We in Ontario have discovered that the true way to crush out 'pathies' and 'isms' is
to educate all up to the same standard; to adopt a leveling-up
process, instead of the antagonistic one."[62] This was why,
Dunster observed, homeopathy existed in a state of disarray
in Canada and Europe while continuing to flourish in the
United States. With the exception of two chairs at the University of Pest in Hungary, not a homeopathic college or
professorship remained in all of Europe by the late 1870s.
"Their practice, stripped entirely of the Hahnemannian vagaries and absurdities," Dunster reported, "is so closely allied to that of rational medicine that it differs but little
from it." As a result, regulars and homeopaths associated
without restriction or condemnation and even met together
in consultation.

Dunster stated that rational medicine would eventually absorb that which was good and useful in European homeopathy. This absorption process had been noted at the World's
Homeopathic Congress in 1876, when European representatives observed that only in the United States, where independent schools could still be established, did homeopathy have
any future. In Europe there was little hope, since homeopathic students could not develop except under the influence
and traditions of the old-school regulars. This, Dunster said,
was an open confession that homeopathy could not survive if
forced to work within the restrictions of the regular schools.
He concluded: "Let us encourage all such teaching. Let us in
every possible way bring their methods and results face to
face with ours, content to abide by the issue. For if rational
medicine cannot triumph in such a contest, she deserves to
fall and be buried in oblivion."[63]

Dunster's remarks circulated widely through the profession. As a result, a substitute amendment was adopted at the
1881 AMA meeting in Richmond. It stated that no teacher
could examine or sign diplomas or certificates of proficiency
for the students of an irregular system. In effect it permitted
the Ann Arbor medical faculty to continue teaching homeopathic students, provided they did not sign the medical di-

ploma given by the college. The AMA thus compromised its official position by recognizing the wishes of the Michigan electorate. As evidence of the compromise, Ann Arbor's medical class of 1879 contained 63 homeopathic students out of a total of 386. Moreover, the school remained a bastion of homeopathic education until the end of the century. The issue was thus resolved, not by a heroic purge of orthodoxy, but by a mild, almost homeopathic dose of expectant therapeutics—the AMA's hope that Michigan's homeopathic problem would ultimately resolve itself *vis medicatrix naturae* through gradual absorption by the regulars.[64]

The revision of the code of ethics of the New York State Medical Society in 1882 brought the sectarian feud to a head by signaling a victory for New York City practitioners, many of whom were specialists who benefited financially from consultations or referrals from homeopaths. The substitute code was briefer than the national code of the AMA, omitting as immaterial those portions concerning duties of physicians to patients, obligations of patients to physicians, duties for the support of professional character, and obligations of the public to physicians. The rule governing consultation was amended to read, "Members of the Medical Society of the State of New York, and of the medical societies in affiliation therewith, may meet in consultation legally qualified practitioners of medicine. Emergencies may occur in which all restrictions should in the judgment of the practitioner, yield to the demands of humanity." In effect "legally qualified practitioners" meant all persons who had received a license from the state board, whether they called themselves hydropaths, eclectics, homeopaths, or some other name. The second major deviation from the national code stated that "in case of acute, dangerous or obscure illness, the consulting physician should continue his visits at such intervals as may be deemed necessary by the patient or his friends, by him, or by the attending physician."[65] Despite these changes, the membership of the state medical society insisted that they could have their revised code and still remain bona fide members of the national organization. This departure was championed by the New York *Medical Record*, the reputed birthplace of the liberal doctrine.[66]

Not all homeopaths were pleased with the decision of the

New York State Medical Society to permit consultation. This was particularly true among the "highs," who remained strict adherents to Hahnemann's principle of attenuated drugs.[67] Exemplary of this attitude was the Homeopathic Medical Society of Lancaster, Pennsylvania, which opposed the "gratuitous" action of the New York society, warning that no good could come of consultation between the schools. To complicate matters further, the action of the New York society precipitated a revolt among its own membership, when conservative dissidents, including the prominent pharmacist Edward R. Squibb, attempted to reverse the society's action of the previous year and return to the national code. When the motion for reversal failed, the conservatives withdrew to form a rival New York State Medical Association.[68]

Overall, the decision for a revised code represented the preponderant influence of New York City physicians in the society. The *New York Herald,* for example, reported that advocates of the new code had received the support of only 1,265 of the 3,827 members of the rural medical societies in the state; and according to the *Medical News* of Philadelphia, a poll of the medical profession in New York State taken by the council for the New York State Medical Association indicated that 20 percent of those canvassed chose to adhere to the revised code, 7 percent wanted no code at all, and 73 percent desired to return to the old code.[69]

Opponents of the revised code refused to recognize the emergence of "highs" and "lows" among the homeopaths. Instead, they saw an impassable chasm separating homeopathy from regular medicine. A regular argued in 1882, "Believing homeopathy to be wrong, how is it possible for a man to countenance it or in any way endorse it?" There was no sense in the argument that the enemy be embraced that he might be crushed. On the contrary, any recognition given the homeopaths as consultants merely reinforced the medical delusions they practiced on the public. "If your attending physician is to still treat his case with infinitesimal doses, and that is certainly what we are led to suppose from the language used, I would like to ask what possible difference it would make to the patient so far as treatment is concerned by having had a regular consultant?"[70] It was not who was correct and who was wrong, but the impossibility of harmonizing the views of two such totally divergent schools that made consultation fruitless, the regular observed. He continued, "Such an effort can have no other aim in view than pecuniary interest for the one or both of the consultants, as such consultations can in no manner be of benefit to the patient—provided both consultants were honest." Hahnemann's theory must either be admitted as valid, conservative regulars argued, or rejected out of hand, for the two schools were as impossible to mix as it was for a minister to preach just enough Presbyterianism, Episcopalianism, Methodism, and Catholicism to satisfy a mixed congregation. Either the principles defined in Hahnemann's medical system were correct and proper or else the system had to be regarded as fraudulent.[71]

Despite the inner consistency of their argument, old-code supporters failed to account for changes made in homeopathy over the decades. Moreover, the fact that legitimate consultation existed between allopaths and homeopaths was evidence of reforms in both camps. As indicative of this new reality, leading doctors—e.g., Abraham Jacobi, St. John Roosa, Fordyce Barker, and Francis Minot—appealed to a greater liberalization of the code. As a token peace offering, Henry I. Bowditch of Harvard Medical School and former president of the AMA suggested that "every State Society follow the lead of New York and let the members be allowed without injury to their status in those bodies to consult with members of other legally constituted medical societies." The members of all medical sects should be allowed to join the state societies of the regulars, provided they passed an examination on their medical knowledge.

Toward this end, Bowditch urged the creation of a single medical licensing board, with allopaths maintaining a majority, which would judge the competence of applicants from homeopathic, eclectic, and regular schools. When sectarian candidates proved to this state board of examiners or censors that they had studied medicine for the proper length of time and could pass an examination, they would then be entitled to the same rights as regulars. The fight between regulars and homeopaths, he observed, had gone on for too long and would continue only to the detriment of medicine and the rights of individual conscience. Bowditch chided the regulars for their intolerance, reminding them that the tyranny of medical orthodoxy had been responsible for the infinitesimal dosages of the homeopaths in the first place. In 1890, however, the New York legislature voted by wide margin to create three separate licensing boards, clearly demonstrating the strength of the irregulars in preserving their right to independent existence and also the division that continued to plague the regulars.[72]

Changes in both allopathic and homeopathic practice over the next several decades tended to dissolve differences and provide for more peaceful coexistence. During the 1880s the Cook County Hospital in Chicago placed every fifth medical case and every fourth surgical case under homeopathic treatment. Comparative mortality statistics indicated a difference of roughly one percent, with the allopaths reporting a 7.2 percent mortality and the homeopaths 8.2 percent. Also, in the 1880s homeopaths were permitted to use Boston City Hospital for clinical instruction. In 1888 the Massachusetts Medical Society reversed its earlier stand by admitting the graduates of homeopathic schools into their fellowship, provided they renounced their beliefs. Although such an admission was a "heroic" pill for any homeopath to swallow, the offer actually marked a significant concession by the allopaths, since, in effect, it recognized the legitimacy of a "low" homeopathic medical education as sufficient preparation for a medical career.

By the turn of the century, both the AMA and the two competing New York societies were seeking ways to resolve their differences. A major breakthrough occurred in 1902 when Frank Billings, the president of the AMA, informed the two New York societies that the national code was no longer binding upon the AMA membership and that, in its place, an "advisory document" accepted in principle the position of the New York State Medical Society. With this major concession the society's exclusion from the national organization ended, and by 1904 the medical profession became unified in a broader orthodoxy. Only after the reorganization of the AMA in 1903, however, did the national organization consent to changes in the medical code. While the AMA did not attempt to return to a prohibition against consultations with irregulars after the 1903 and 1912 revisions in its ethical code, nevertheless, in 1924 an understanding was adopted which forbade voluntary association with cultists.[73]

Despite appearances, the concessions of the AMA had not been forced by a position of weakness. By 1900 the organization had successfully achieved national prominence due in large part to notable successes in sanitary science, pharmacotherapeutics, germ theory, and aseptic treatment. Moreover, Abraham Flexner's famous study of medical education in 1910 demonstrated the clear and present need for stricter entrance requirements, more clinical experience, expanded curriculum, and lengthened course time. His report, an excellent example of reform consciousness in an age of Progressivism, marked a significant watershed in the history of sectarian medicine. The code itself began to slide into the backwaters of medical concern as schools faced the more substantive problems raised in the Flexner report. Homeopathy suffered a sharp decline, to the extent that by 1923 only the New York Homeopathic College and Philadelphia's Hahnemann Medical College remained of the many institutions dedicated to the sectarian system. Even the homeopathic program at the University of Michigan, once a seedbed of support, succumbed to a reorganization plan that merged the homeopaths with the regulars in 1922.

Druggist and Dry Goods Grocer

Although the AMA's 1847 code of ethics referred to the abusive nature of patent medicines (ch. 3, art. 1, par. 4), it failed to recognize the deteriorating relationship between the doctor and the retail druggist. From the standpoint of the medical profession, the apothecary had degenerated into little more than a "dry-grocer" who availed himself of the physician's patronage only as an accessory to dispensing his patent medicines, cosmetics, and garden seeds. In 1887 a Minnesota doctor remarked, "It seems to me that we are to a certain extent in bondage to those who ought to be our servants; that we are being used largely as a convenience." Druggists, hoping to enlarge their business enterprises, embarked on a course that had taken them far beyond the role of dispensing drugs. While this new direction brought prosperity to the somewhat depressed financial state of pharmacy, it nevertheless caused the druggist to regard the physician "in much the same light as he does his cigar case or soda fount, simply an annex to his business."[74]

Some of the largest transactions took place at the patent-medicine counter, where—ethics aside—the pharmacist became a "dispensing physician," preparing his own specifics and selling proprietary drugs of dubious value. In 1881 one doctor complained that pharmacists had "so industriously and energetically wedged themselves between the 'dear public' and the professional province of the physician" that before long they would monopolize the field of medical practice. Druggists were closer to the public ear than the doctor and were increasingly sought for advice in therapeutic matters. Medical men, cajoled into passiveness by "the friendly allurements of pharmaceutical convenience" had drifted farther and farther from "the fundamental wisdom of guarding and garnering their professional knowledge." Unwittingly doctors had allowed their professional knowledge to come "under the caprice and manipulations of persons of acute business instincts," who had undermined "the purpose and province of physician to continuous and damaging trespass." Once having obtained the confidence and patronage of the physician's former patrons, the druggist developed "a continuous undercurrent of medical practice over the counter . . . either with or without the aid of the physician's prescriptions on file." Unauthorized renewals of prescriptions often resulted in patients' making prolonged use of potentially dangerous remedies, such as calomel, tartar emetic, nux vomica, the iodides and bromides, chloral, morphia, opium, and alcohol.[75]

In responding to medical criticism, pharmacists replied that, while the ideal situation might well allow the pharmacist to live entirely on his business with the physician, few were able to exist on prescription sales alone. Profits from prescriptions were not as great as seemed and the proliferation of drugstores had caused a further dwindling of profits. There were also increasingly heavy overhead expenses. In many instances druggists were forced to enter into agreements with doctors, rebating to them amounts ranging from

25 to 50 percent of the prescription price for sending patrons to them.[76]

Moreover, the pharmaceutical profession accused physicians of exaggerating the public's use of patent medicines, complaining that profits from the nostrums were not nearly as large as doctors seemed to believe. In defense of their business, pharmacists claimed to have little control over the patent-medicine trade, since the nostrums were nationally advertised and people requested them irrespective of the pharmacist's own particular feelings. "It does not necessarily follow," one pharmacist argued, "that because we have them on our shelves we must push them, and such is not the case."[77] In any case, almost every patent medicine on the market could claim certificates from doctors recommending its wonderful properties and healing virtues. The real hypocrites of the patent-medicine trade were the doctors themselves who brazenly encouraged the nostrum business with their own recommendations. The long list of patent medicines—from Pond's extract and Radway's Ready Relief, to Holman's Liver Pad and Swain's Panacea—were testament to the nature of the problem.[78]

In its committee report on medico-pharmaceutical relations in 1880, the Philadelphia Medico-Legal Society placed blame on the physician for delegating too much responsibility to the druggist in the management of therapeutic drugs. "By permitting himself to depend on the druggist more and more," the committee report stated, "the physician has at length realized that the druggist has well nigh got not only the compounding, but the dispensing lines into his own hands, and is practically driving the medical team for himself." By patronizing druggists through the system of prescription writing, physicians had all but removed themselves from control over their patients in choice of remedies. As one solution to the problem, the committee suggested that doctors make agreements with druggists to remove the endless shelves of quack nostrums and rely solely upon doctor's prescriptions. Physicians could then develop lists of cooperating druggists and send their patients only to those specified on the lists. If these remedial efforts failed, the committee then urged the physicians to cut all relations with the pharmacist and dispense their own drugs.[79]

Knights of the Pill-Bags

Those who objected most strenuously to counter-prescribing druggists urged physicians to conceal from patients information regarding the nature and content of the prescription drug. Only this would prevent patients from requesting the medicine again when the symptoms reappeared and also from communicating knowledge of the remedy to friends. The "loose way of speaking of remedies before patients," one doctor remarked, "conveys the impression that the remedies are not of much account, can be used by any one, repeated as often as necessary, and that the science of therapeutics is nothing more than the fitting of pegs in holes already made for their reception." Given these difficulties, numerous physicians decided to dispense their own medicine and thereby keep the knowledge of drugs from the ears of both patients and pharmacists.[80] One doctor who had lost many of his patients to counter-prescribing druggists decided that he could survive only by moving his practice to another district and dispensing his own medicines. "I do not make any profit out of my medical stores," he wrote. "In fact, I am willing to throw them in with the advice, preferring to lose my medicines rather than my patients." This way, however, he was no longer annoyed by having his prescriptions repeated without his consent.[81]

The idea of doctors dispensing their own drugs had actually been borrowed from homeopaths, who, following the advice of Samuel Hahnemann, prepared their own dilutions so as to circumvent polypharmacy, heroic dosages, and impure drugs prepared by the retail druggist. Another catalyst for the practice derived from the nineteenth-century development of the wholesale drug manufacturer, who was able to supply the physician with pills manufactured cheaply yet with precision, with the formula and dose printed on each bottle. A third incentive came with the development by William Brockedon of London and Jacob Dunton of Philadelphia of the tablet triturate and the compressed tablet which allowed the physician to provide medicine that was cheap, uniform in strength, easy to carry, in a form acceptable to most patients, and easily absorbed into the system.

Doctors found it convenient to rely upon wholesale houses, which could manufacture medicines cheaply and in mass quantity and had the technology to maintain uniform strength, purity, and freshness in drugs. Doctors found they could at last carry a sufficient supply of medicines in their own handbag, thus keeping patients from what they felt were the snares of the retail druggist. They now had a weapon that would work for their own interest and that of their patients, who all too often felt cheated at being supplied with only advice and a prescription by the physician. The goodwill incurred by diagnosing illness and filling the prescription—all paid for in one visit—appeared reasonable and efficient to both physician and patient. Then, too, when the physician filled the prescription himself, there was less chance of the prescription being misread, or an improper remedy supplied. It also lessened the evils of self-doctoring, the nefarious system of commissions paid by druggists to physicians, counter-prescribing, the dangers of refilling without authority, and drug substitution. "If the patient is compelled to come to the physician when his medicine is exhausted," one doctor observed in 1896, "it gives the physician additional opportunity for examining him and effecting a radical cure, which is often lost by prescription practice."[82]

Pharmacists responded to the prospect of dispensing doctors by arguing that nothing could be gained by either profession's taking an antagonistic position. In a paper read before the Illinois Pharmaceutical Association meeting in Peoria in 1881, pharmacist V. H. Dumbeck observed that doctors had made broad and sweeping charges, which on close inspection were unproved and poorly contrived. Both the physician and pharmacist were co-laborers in the advancement of pharmacy. When, therefore, a physician "considers us unworthy and incompetent to compound his prescriptions, and ignores the pharmacist and puts up his own prescriptions, is it then to be wondered at that he loses the respect the pharmacist had for him." Doctors who ignored the specialized abilities of the pharmacist by dispensing their own medicines only antagonized the goodwill of the pharmaceutical profession. According to Dumbeck, the majority of pharmacists opposed counter-prescribing as unprofessional and believed, somewhat optimistically, that all would be well again if only physicians promised not to dispense their own drugs. "If physicians wish to prevent encroachment on their domain," he warned, "they should avoid invading others' property."[83]

In the last quarter of the nineteenth century, Adolphe Burggraeve (1806–1902), a professor of medicine at the University of Ghent, attempted to reform both pharmacy and therapeutics by suggesting a solution to the divisive feud then raging between the homeopath and allopath. Burggraeve insisted that both schools were products of the uncertainty of the Galenic pharmacopoeia and that each bordered on medical heresy—homeopathy by moving to infinitesimal doses that lacked the power to cure and allopathy by using massive doses that literally drowned the patient in dangerous medicines. Between these two rivals were those hopeful souls who practiced "armed expectation," preferring to stand by and allow disease to run its course, acting only against complications. These tendencies in medicine induced the Belgian physician to introduce the science of dosimetry, a pharmacotherapeutic theory based on a twofold premise: that medicines were to be administered in small doses measured mathematically, and that they were to be given in accordance with the law of gentle stimulation, prescribed with the idea of sustaining the vital powers, combating fever, and restoring the bodily functions to their normal condition.[84]

In his effort to discover a more rational ground between the schools of homeopathy and allopathy, Burggraeve claimed that French pharmacist Charles Chanteaud had achieved the first major breakthrough in pharmacodynamics by manufacturing alkaloids in doses of mathematical precision. In place of the illusory infinitesimal dose prescribed by the homeopaths, Chanteaud had developed a process for producing precise chemical quantities (centigram, milligram, or demimilligram) of pure active drugs.[85] Burggraeve believed that homeopaths who administered their triturations and dilutions in only a quadrillionth or quintillionth of a gram justified the witticism: "What is homeopathy? It is to throw a milligramme of substance somewhere in the Seine at the point where it enters Paris, and to drink a few drops of the water, taken where it goes out." Furthermore, according to dosimetrist Albert Salivas, "the proportion of the homeopath's elements is never exactly known to the manufacturer even if he is the most careful and conscientious in his work." Besides, the properties of the plants used by the homeopath lacked uniformity—drugs varied according to the country of origin, the time of harvesting, the method of preservation, the condition of freshness or drying at the time of processing, and the method of preparing the plant.[86]

Despite Burggraeve's ostensible purpose of finding a therapeutic alternative to the claims of both homeopaths and allopaths, he expressed little faith in the pharmaceutical profession as a whole and, in all the journals dedicated to the advance of dosimetry, he recommended and advertised only the products of Charles Chanteaud. Ironically what began as an effort to revolutionize pharmacy and therapeutics degenerated into a massive advertising campaign for the manufacturing company of the French pharmacist. In effect Burggraeve sought to eliminate the local pharmacist by suggesting that doctors prepare and sell their own drugs from dosimetric granules manufactured by Chanteaud and sold wholesale by Burgoyne, Burbridges, Cyriax and Farries of London.[87]

Physician T. Trudeau of New Orleans, editor of the *Dosimetric Medical Review,* introduced dosimetry into the United States and was soon followed by a number of imitators. Physician Wallace Calvin Abbott (1857–1921) of Chicago, editor of the *American Journal of Clinical Medicine* ("The Alkaloidal Clinic") and founder of Abbott Laboratories, became one of the more successful imitators of Burggraeve's dosimetric pharmacy and therapeutics in the United States. Like Burggraeve, his alkaloidal company stood in opposition to the -isms and -pathies of nineteenth-century medicine. There was but one true medical man, Abbott maintained, and he was the doctor who chose to use small and regulated doses of the most active remedies. Borrowing his thunder from European dosimetrists, Abbott campaigned to replace "promiscuous" formulas, nauseous drugs, and "problematical" remedies with soluble granules given in precise and effective doses and produced by his Chicago laboratory. In his *Alkaloidal Digest,* first published in 1893, Abbott listed five essential reasons for the use of alkalometry.

1. It cures—where it is possible to cure—*cito, tuto et jucunde.* Its chemistry is done outside the sick body. It never produces "drug sickness."

2. It gives maximum results in the shortest possible time, with absolute safety and with no possibility of overdose, or cumulative effect.

3. It enables the practician to give the most potent medicines to the youngest infant, the most squeamish invalid, or the aged, without the aid of scales, measures or menstrua.

4. It enables the doctor to push a remedy exactly *to effect* without leaving him to wonder if he may not have poisoned his patient.

5. It makes it possible for the practician to have always with him sufficient standard medicaments of unchangeable strength and consistency for every possible emergency, and to practice the most certain, safe and sure method of medication at small cost. It eliminates "chance" and makes medicine as nearly "an exact science" as it is possible for it to attain.[88]

By the turn of the century, increased numbers of physicians were dispensing their own medicines. In the origins of dosimetry and its imitators rose one of the early movements for unifying the goals of chemist, druggist, and physician in a singular pharmaco-therapeutic program. Despite its many deficiencies, dosimetry initiated a trend toward standardized quality in products, an increasing concern for exactness in dosage, and an attempt to improve the image of the pharmaceutical industry in the absence of outside regulation.[89]

The deteriorating relationship between druggist and physician was tangential to a much larger controversy that was emerging within the pharmaceutical profession itself, between retail druggists and large industrial companies that were producing drugs cheaper and of more standardized quality than those compounded by the corner apothecary. By the nineteenth century, much of the scientific and investigative initiative of the individual pharmacist had been overshadowed by research done in the large manufacturing houses. Pharmaceuticals prepared by industrial drug companies, distributed in a form ready to dispense, meant the retail druggist's professional skills were no longer required. Ironically, while the retail druggist's educational and professional abilities improved through the century, his actual status declined to that of a salesman for miscellaneous articles. The commercial aspect of the job carried greater weight than his scientific qualifications. The retail druggist was fast becoming a dealer in ready-made drugs rather than a compounder of medicines. For its part, the medical profession was unaware of the economic forces causing this change, although it was partly responsible for this situation because of its choice of ready-made compounds advertised by the industrial pharmaceutical companies. Doctors preferred that the druggist purchase tablets compounded by a manufacturing house rather than have the patient wait for him to measure and stir a simple prescription, particularly if the ingredients required a specified freshness.[90]

Yet, for all of that, the relationship between physician and pharmacist over the centuries had never really matured beyond one of sibling rivalry. In 1711 Bernard de Mandeville remarked: "A Physician is brought up among Gentlemen. He has the advantage of passing his Youth, where Whit, Learning, and good Manners are in greater esteem, and the base thought of Lucre, more dispis'd than where else, and . . . he is ever taught to direct his Labours to a noble end, the God-like office of restoring the afflicted." The apothecary, on the contrary, Mandeville wrote, commenced his profession with "the servile drudgery of a Foot-boy, is bred in a paultry Shop, which by his Labour he is first made to clean, and afterwards to furnish." Before long, he learns, "all the insinuating Tricks and other vile Artifices" of retailers and, "imbued with the Barbarous, as well as sordid Craft of pinching on the one hand the industrious Wretch, that, for want of Employ, attempts to live by Simpling; and squeezing on the other an unreasonable profit from the pittiful Halfpenny of the most Necessitous."[91] This bad feeling enabled doctors to blame their traditional rivals rather than search for internal weakness as the cause of their own social and financial distress. To be sure, the chaos within the medical profession contributed significantly to the manner of condemnation they accorded to the pharmacist. Rather than admit publicly that the unnecessary mushrooming of medical colleges, questionable medical degrees, improper licensing, therapeutic nihilism, and sectarian feuds had helped to aggravate their own financial and social problems, doctors preferred to seek identifiable scapegoats outside the profession on whom responsibility could lie.

A Search For Ideals

From the protection of their offices and societies, doctors voiced alarm at the spreading materialism of the new industrial society. Like Ralph Waldo Emerson, the conscience of America in mid-century, they felt that with the coming of machines and assembly-line techniques, men would lose sight of the inherent value of labor and would seek instead to create subsidiary values from the comforts money could produce. Every energy seemed bent on money-getting; and despite warnings that this new spirit was a detriment to the individual by its "loosening [of] his moral and spiritual tone and dulling, if not deadening, [of] his finest sensibilities," men appeared content with "being enveloped in this great maelstrom." According to V. M. Reichard, M.D., president of the Cumberland Valley Medical Association, each physician had a responsibility to stem the currents of commercialism in the profession by holding firm to a high ideal. Only by clinging to the best in human nature could doctors avoid the cynical pessimism spreading through society. Those who went through life with neither ideals nor hopes, with little care for their fellow man aside from the material benefits obtained, would find their lives barren of love and joy. The world owed man nothing. "The debit," Reichard reminded, "is all in the other column. It is a privilege to be allowed to live in the world, and every man who comes into it comes bearing a load of debt." From the pioneers who hewed the forests to the men who harnessed steam and electricity, to the dedicated souls who worked for civil and religious freedoms, men and women were making out of their lives something infinitely more than a "mere sordid wish to get all possible gain out of life and no proper spirit of service."[92]

In speech after speech before medical societies and graduating medical classes, doctors like Reichard recounted the dignity of the vocation and the gravity of its responsibilities. Much as a young lord of a feudal estate, who on attaining his inheritance must carry the burden of his possessions, each

doctor carried into every sickroom the rigors of his education, the tools of past medical achievements, and the heavy
responsibilities of maintaining life and health. Doctors were
fond of recounting this inheritance—the unselfish labors of
Vesalius, Harvey, Jenner, Laënnec, Hunter, Pasteur, and a
host of predecessors. The achievements in ascultation, thermometry, hypodermic medication, vaccination, microscopy,
and antisepsis could not be judged simply as aids to mon-
eymaking but as milestones on the road to human progress.[93]

In the last analysis, the future greatness of medicine depended upon the capacity of the profession to satisfy the aesthetic rather than mercenary needs of medical men. Success,
material gain, and the plaudits of society were of little value
to the true physician unless his training had been obtained
honestly and his skills improved both the patient and himself. "What I do eagerly desire to place irrevocably in your
hands," Silas Weir Mitchell remarked to a graduating class,
"is the belief that the means must be such as your best moments will approve. For then, whatever comes, you will at
least be secure that your defeats or your victories are but a
part of the loftiest education and a preparation for the
higher evolutions of the other world where, as I trust, the life
of effort may still go on with yet nobler aims and more secure
results."[94]

Not only must the doctor in his youth form an ideal for the
conduct of his life and discover moral laws to mold and guide
his conduct, but he must also carry that ideal and those
guides into every aspect of his professional life. For the physician the proper principles which guided life's conduct were
priceless treasures—an "inward light thrown forward on the
paths of duty, making all action easier." Although man would
sometimes fail in his work, such principles lightened the burden. "Surely no man who in time of doubt has made up his
mind to abide by the loftiest moral purpose can have failed to
feel the relief, the illumination, which such decision casts forward on the way of purpose."[95] To view medical life as simply
a business with commercial aims was to fall into the trap of so
many professional men in the century who had forgotten the
value of their labor and looked instead to the end of their
service, the fee obtained. Those medical men who were en-
thralled by material wealth, Mitchell warned, transformed

their patients into things and failed to notice, or enjoy, their essential humanity.

Yet, try as they did to steer clear of the pitfalls of the marketplace, doctors discovered that the combination of mushrooming medical schools, an excess of physicians, and the growth of specialism within the profession tended to create an environment that fell easily within the parameters of the competitive age. Despite their efforts to the contrary, doctors resembled so many other small business and professional men who found themselves searching for alternatives to the ruthlessness of an uncontrolled market. Their concern for old American values, like Emerson's, was a genuine reaction to the prevailing thrust of a materialistic culture; but they ultimately failed to understand the real nature of the business world. Their fear of spreading materialism dissipated their energies on the unwholesome effects of the financial revolution and did little to correct the causes of their own situation.

Throughout its stormy history, the AMA's code of medical ethics had never really been more than a sideshow—or at best a skirmishing ground—demonstrating professional intent. As one critic described it, the code was a "hodgepodge of ethics, etiquette and tradition delivered with a senile sententiousness."[96] While the code had unquestionably served a useful purpose during the organizational years of American medicine, its confusion between ethics and etiquette had marked it for extinction by the time the AMA had achieved most of its professional objectives. The code had been conceived as a panacea to the diverse needs of the profession; yet, as a monolithic cure for its many ills, it proved as fickle as Jaynes's worm lozenges.

> The efficiency of the code as an irritant is due in a measure to its mistaken mode of application. To swallow it as a whole would be erroneous polypharmacy. It should be disposed of section by section. One portion is designed as a tonic to good resolutions; another as a stimulant to flagging industry; another as a food for the construction of moral purposes; another as a cataplasm to allay the inflammation of misunderstanding; another as a lubricant to diminish the friction of jealousy; another as a collyrium to lessen the congestion and reduce the ocular tension occasioned by real or fancied professional wrongs; another as a cylindrical lens for the correc-

tion of mental or moral astigmatism, to enable one otherwise oblivious to vertical truth or horizontal justice to recognize the beauty of both in clear-cut lines without penumbra. But so habituated are we to prescribe the inclination is well-nigh irresistible to tip this . . . down every other man's throat, while we feel his pulse and await results.[97]

For those who wished to graft high social position on their commercial instincts, the code became an arrogant taskmaster to be either rigidly adhered to or given lip service to in everyday practice. For others it became a subtle amusement employed to disguise punitive intentions under the transparent cloak of moralism. Some, too, in their deontological zeal reduced the code to the form of a breviary—an intellectual testament to their apocalyptic visions of the profession. For them it became a source of continuous meditation, almost unearthly in its neural dreams and spotlessness.

Despite many deficiencies, however, the code did prove responsible to the martial needs of the regulars in their efforts to suppress the sectarian tendencies of the age. At the time of the code's composition, the profession had been annoyed by the "pestilent little group" of homeopaths, Thomsonians, and other similarly styled sects; and the accumulated indignation of the regulars to their claims and misrepresentations transformed the code into a catapult for their expulsion from medical societies and from any claim to legitimate knowledge of the healing art. The code also served as a catalyst to the profession's hopes and a prophetic warning to those recalcitrant heretics whose commercial or ideological habits remained resistant to the pressures of orthodoxy.[98]

8

Evolutionary Medicine

DOCTORS, ALONG WITH CLERGY, entrepreneurs, and academics, served as moral philosophers for Victorian society. Noted practitioners like Oliver Wendell Holmes, Silas Weir Mitchell, Hiram Christopher, Lawrence Irwell, Edward Waldo Emerson, and Lawson Tait were at home in poetry, ontology, science, morals, and practical wisdom; and out of their speculations came ideas that are still debated by philosophers today. With the publication of Charles Darwin's *Origin of Species* in 1859 and *Descent of Man* in 1871 and the resulting plethora of scientific and philosophical digressions, doctors found themselves faced with a theory that intersected life—and their profession—at almost every angle. It was not enough simply to dismiss any possibility that Darwin's theory was true or to accept it with indifferent acquiescence. Doctors were disposed, by habit and temperament, to study nature; and their perceptions of Darwin's hypothesis—its concept of time, species, force, law, justice, and causality—indicated a deep and abiding concern for every imminent point in evolutionary speculation. Commentaries began appearing in medical journals soon after publication of Darwin's thesis; and while practicing doctors generally looked on as Louis Agassiz, Asa Gray, Thomas Henry Huxley, Presbyterian theologian Charles Hodge, or Reverend Enoch Burr heatedly debated the issues, they were not in the least hesitant to take sides in the ensuing battle, since most understood how profoundly it affected life. As highly esteemed confidants of middle-class society, doctors both fed and reflected secular culture; the ubiquitous manner with which the theory encompassed nature caused them to react in a variety of ways.

Their delight for the written word brought wisdom, wit, and indignation to the fore, making them fiery partisans of the evolutionary feuds that so dominated the age.[1]

Christian Medical Scientists

Nineteenth century physicians were very much aware of their influence within the family circle. Perhaps it was because they stressed the importance of this direct relationship with patients that they had ear to the most closely guarded family secrets and found themselves in a more confidential relationship than many a spiritual advisor or confessor. But to the degree that physicians became confidential friends within the family circle, they also exerted a wide and effectual influence over social decorum. Doctors occupied a "commanding" station in Victorian society, where they not only observed the sufferings and joys that existed in each family but also brought to their relationship with the family a stock of experience, authority, and intimacy which patients willingly admitted into their personal lives. "What responsibility then rests upon the physician!" Worthington Hooker remarked in 1850. "How careful should he be in the expression of his opinions! How important that he should be right upon the great moral questions which agitate the community, and that his morality should be strictly that of the Bible!"[2] Those original thinkers who most thoroughly enlarged the boundaries of human knowledge were the same who in their personal lives and public work shone "with the lustre of the Christian faith." The true medical scientist imitated the life of "him who once walked the earth, the embodiment of heavenly benevolence, at whose touch the sick were healed, and at whose command diseases and death fled away." In effect the prescriptive and proscriptive aspects of nineteenth-century medicine were most often rendered in the name of the Christian God.[3]

In his address to the graduating class of medical students at Yale University in 1898, Clarence J. Blake, M.D., of the Harvard Medical School elaborated upon a common nineteenth-century theme of a medical priesthood. "You have a great service before you," he told the class. "You are going out, as each one of you realizes, to a ministry,—a ministry to which you cannot be equal, of which you cannot be worthy, unless you hold it to be, each to yourself, in your own estimation of it—a priesthood." The true doctor was one who showed reverence for the body, of which the patient was a "tenant" at the will of the Creator, and who also demonstrated an appreciation for the moral value and use that accompanied the body through life. Foremost in the very essence of a physician was the obligation to extend understanding beyond the microscope and the materia medica. The practicing physician was a man "in whom the weak trust, to whom the sinking look for help, and the sorrowful for such mede of consolation as the truth can bring." In no other work was an individual given the opportunity to see and study life so closely, to analyze human needs and motives, and to provide counsel to both body and mind. The doctor assumed the very tasks performed by the minister—a responsibility that could only be considered a privilege of the greatest magnitude.[4]

Doctors were thus encouraged to look beyond simple intellectual ascent by demonstrating true piety and "a cordial reliance" upon the merits of Jesus Christ as the only ground of acceptance with God.[5] No physician was thoroughly educated until his intellectual and moral faculties had been submitted to the purifying influences of Christianity. The physician needed Christian faith not only to sustain him amid anxieties, cares, and responsibilities, but also to provide the soothing balm of faith for patients. As friend and confidant of the sick, he in his labors intersected both the spiritual and physical side of humanity; he had open access to the soul's hidden recesses when he carried with him a Christian understanding of man.[6] Like the minister, the physician worked with "the common degeneracy and ruin of the race" and carried into each sickroom the potential for spiritual salvation.[7]

One doctor remarked: "The grand, subtle and mysterious union of body and spirit—mind and matter—neither Socrates, Galen, Hippocrates, nor Aesculapius, could comprehend, tried they ever so earnestly. But we, who stand in the resplendent blaze of Christian civilization, know that they were feeling darkly after the Great Physician of all humanity, and failing to find Him in His infinite power and beauty, they paid homage to the science of medicine itself. Does it not seem fitting and possible that the profession should arrive at that pure and elevated plane, where all its representatives shall be Christian medical scientists?"[8] Physician Ezra Hunt expressed this reliance of the physician on Christ in a poem written in 1859.

> Deep are the wounds which sin has made,
>   Where shall the sinner find a cure?
> In pain, alas! is nature's aid,
>   The work exceeds all nature's power.

> Sin, like a raging fever, reigns
>   With fatal strength in every part,
> The dire contagion fills the veins,
>   And spreads its poison to the heart.

> And can no sovereign balm be found!
>   And is no kind physician nigh,
> To ease the pain and heal the wound,
>   Ere life and home for ever fly?

> There is a great Physician near,
>   Look up, O fainting soul, and live;
> See, in his heavenly smiles appear
>   Such aid as nature cannot give.

> See, in the Saviour's dying blood,
>   Life, health, and bliss abundant flow;
> 'Tis only this pure sacred flood
>   Can ease thy pain and heal thy wo.[9]

In both their public and private lives, nineteenth-century doctors viewed themselves as physicians of both body and soul; it was precisely this dual responsibility that demanded a Christian spirit in medicine. The healing art was to be administered with the idea of elevating every man to the final glory of the Redeemer's kingdom. Medicine was eminently a Christian calling, and no practitioner could fully meet his responsibilities without such Christian principles governing his actions, chastening his judgments, and sustaining his everyday work. Without religion few physicians could resist the tendency toward skepticism and materialism, and none could reap the rich harvest for God from the chambers of the sick and dying. Religion enlarged the physician's capabilities of usefulness. A true religious spirit blended well with scientific endeavors, fostered principles and habits conducive to professional success, qualified the physician for work with the dying, and brought comfort to the bereaved. Never, the argument went, had the physician schooled in proper Christian mental and moral qualifications failed to sustain the honor of the profession against the assaults of materialism and skepticism.[10]

Medical writers warned frequently of the temptations of skepticism, of working too closely with inductive reasoning, and of avoiding more general questions, particularly those that led the mind to affirm purpose and final causation. They noted, moreover, that those physicians who excluded God from the universe, believing that matter was self-propagating, self-governing, and self-originating, became hardened and indifferent to the exposures of pain and suffering, the shadows of death, and the secrets revealed in the dissecting room. In becoming a "hard mental machine' the medical skeptic destroyed that essential ingredient whereby he could influence the moral nature of the patient. Materialism tempted doctors to lose sight of their patient's entirely. Silas W. Mitchell of Philadelphia wrote, "It is the fear lest you drift into this materialistic conception which makes me eager that you shall not quite lose touch of the feeling that the soul of a man dwells in this house of clay and that forever you are dealing with an immensely complicated and ethereal thing, which thinks as well as feels." Rather than causing the physician to become immune to the mysteries of man, the experiences in the dissecting room should provide a growing sense of the "awfulness" of life. Out of those experiences should emerge a keener perception of life, its riddles, man's limitations, and a sense of intellectual humility.[11]

Initial Reactions

During the early years of the Darwinian controversy, roughly from 1859 to the death of Louis Agassiz in 1873, few practitioners were sufficiently trained in morphology and physiology to defend or otherwise question the evidences of evolution. At best, doctors had pursued anatomy for practical medical purposes rather than for speculative philosophical deductions. Thus, during the initial years after the publication of Darwin's theory, the majority of medical men preferred to discuss the theory along paths already traveled by theologians, cataclysmic geologists, and metaphysical Platonists who were intent on judging science against the truths of philosophical rationalism and Biblical literalism. The editor and proprietor of the *Richmond and Louisville Medical Journal*, E. S. Gaillard, who was also professor of the principles and practice of medicine in the Louisville Medical College, accused Darwin of being in league with atheists, skeptics, and all the other "unworthy children of science" who endeavored "to subvert or destroy . . . the description of creation as given by the inspired Moses." Gaillard believed that the tools of true science were simply additional supports for the revealed word of God and not deadly matériel for combat over a proper interpretation of creation.

True science only confirmed in different language and with newer instruments what religion already understood through revelation. Had not the fundamental unity in language discovered by philologists vindicated the truth of the Mosaic record regarding the dispersion of man following the confusion of tongues? Did not ethnography and physiology demonstrate that despite variations in complexion, color of hair and eyes, contour of skull and facial angle, it was possible to reconcile the diverse races of man with the essential unity of origin? Was the same not also true of the vegetable and animal kingdoms which, despite climate, domestication, and isolation, maintained distinguishing characteristics of the original types? And, after admitting that the first two verses in the book of Genesis had no immediate connection with the verses that followed (i.e., that millions of years might have lapsed between the creation of the heavens, the earth, light, and man), was it not possible to reconcile the Bible with geology? While the writings of Moses were only "aggregations of historical fragments, chronologically not immediately consecutive," did not the heaps of gravel, remains of bones, pinnacles of granite, deposits of sand, and rolled masses of rock give evidence of the great Deluge? For Gaillard and others like him, who paid obsequious attention to the religious symbols of the day, philology, ethnography, physiology and geology simply confirmed what revelation had long before ordained as true.[12]

Those doctors who were enamored with the philosophical heritage of Plato and Aristotle rather than with Biblical literalism found it difficult to throw off their ontological and teleological biases. Despite the appearance of change, and a universe perforated by a million channels, all life forms existed as on a ladder—a great chain of being—where the distance from the top to bottom symbolized a stable world order, where each species illustrated a relation with every other species, where all forms were in an ascending scale toward perfection, and where faith in Divinity was ontologically necessary and constituted the ground for all existence. In an article published by the Massachusetts Eclectic Medical Society in 1872, John S. Andrews, M.D., remarked: "We still affirm that the grand law of life and its history is stability. From generation to generation, and as far as our proofs can reach, there has been no suspension of this law, so far as to allow the introduction of a new species. Natural history stands on the immutability of types." The concept of mutability of species was judged contrary to the very basis of western science and Christian philosophy.[13]

Camped within this group of believers were the ardent admirers of the Swiss-born Louis Agassiz (1807–73), professor of natural history at Harvard, whose work revealed an organic conception of life in which man was not just an extraneous result of a chance meeting of particles, but the benefactor and servant of the Divine Plan. Agassiz found an intellectual and holistic significance in the divisions of the animal world and in the appearance of organic development in the divisions of life.

> If we put a material interpretation upon [organic changes] and believe that even Man himself has been gradually developed out of a Fish, they are repugnant to our better nature. But looked at in their intellectual significance, they truly reveal the unity of the organic conception of which Man himself is a part, and mark not only the incipient steps of its manifestation, but also, with equal distinctness, every phase in its gradual realization. They mean that when the first Fish was called into existence, the Vertebrate type existed as a whole in the creative thought, and the first expression of it embraced potentially all the organic elements of that type, up to Man himself. To me the fact that the embryonic form of the highest Vertebrate recalls in its earlier stages the first representatives

of its type in geological times and its lowest representatives at the present day, speaks only of an ideal relation, existing, not in the things themselves, but in the mind that made them.[14]

Medical partisans of Agassiz listened gladly to his Platonic metaphysics and in his reassuring words found resistance to the skepticism and materialism of their age. They rejected the tendency of modern science to repudiate teleology by following the road of Lucretius and the French Encyclopedists into materialism. Emotion and intelligence were not latent in a "fiery cloud"; neither, for that matter, were philosophy, poetry, science, and art from Plato and Shakespeare to Newton and Raphael the work of blind matter. Physical forces were not in themselves capable of producing all that existed.

Though evolutionary protagonist Thomas H. Huxley (1825–95) and morphologist Ernst Haeckel (1834–1919) believed that species had resulted exclusively from the chance molecular arrangement of the cosmic vapor, most American doctors relied on the writings of Agassiz to confirm that all species constituted a continuous and graduated series under the guidance of the divine idea.[15] Agassiz found a parallelism running between the types of past and existing life forms and also between extinct species and the embryonic development of living species. "The leading thought which runs through the succession of all organized beings in past ages," he wrote, "is manifested again in new combinations in the phases of development of the living representatives of these different types."[16] For Hiram Christopher, M.D., of St. Louis, this circumstance described by Agassiz could not have occurred by the action of blind forces. "Is it not rather unquestionable evidence of the presence and action of a creator, who, in all these differentiations, of the entire system of organized beings, is working toward the idea of his mind, to which all these various types of structure are but the phases of the development of that ideal?"[17]

Those enamored with Agassiz's Platonic typology viewed the advocates of the developmental theory as unthinking worshipers at the shrine of materialism who had bridged an immense hiatus of proof with a dearth of facts and a host of probabilities. They accused the evolutionists of concealing their motives under the guise of physiology and endeavoring to spread materialistic philosophy into all realms of society—

from the nation's economy to the motives of human action, the nature of ethical conduct, and even the very existence of man's soul. In claiming that physiology sanctioned evolution, that anatomy and embryology demonstrated it, that comparative anatomy and paleontology confirmed it, and that only ignorance or prejudice could deny its truths, the new materialism had begun to analyze man as if he was not different from a piece of animal tissue and not better than a brute "indulging in a dream of immortality, and breathing aspirations as baseless as the chase of a dog who barks in his slumber." It was from the pretentious claims of biology, one practitioner lamented, that human lives and hopes were reduced to chaos, "leaving no ambition but the blind struggle of the mightier trampling upon the weaker, and no end but an infinite wreck and waste, like the scarred face of the moon in its awful stillness and desolation."[18]

The Antimaterialists

Critics of materialism were convinced that future historians would look unkindly at Darwin's impact on science and society. They accused the Darwinian protagonists of making evolutionary theory coextensive with the life of the universe, of welcoming Darwin as the long-awaited messiah, and of replacing the hidden God with the mechanical process of natural selection. Medical critics of evolution did not always quarrel with Darwin's evidence of the continuous developmental succession of organic beings; but they did refuse to admit the spirit of materialism that overshadowed the process and, through the efforts of men like Haeckel, ventured to ignore the relationship between man and God, the existence of the soul, the Natural Law, and man's moral imperatives. From the theory of natural selection they saw erected a philosophy of atheism that insisted upon its own description of the method of creation but in truth denied creation "in the sense of a procession from a power higher than a blind *atom*."[19] To say that each new species was the result of myriad fortuitous combinations through immeasurable periods of time, the antimaterialists argued, was to deny both purpose and final causation.[20]

For Haeckel and others who seized upon the philosophical

implications in Darwin's thesis, man had lost his freedom of will and had become, like the rest of the animal and plant kingdoms, subject to the fixed laws of natural phenomenon. "The action of our free will," the German morphologist wrote in *Evolution of Man* (1876), "shows that the latter is never really free, but is always determined by previous causal conditions, which are eventually referrable either to heredity or adaptation."[21] It seemed to the antimaterialists that Haeckel's relegating of free will to the confines of heredity or adaptation had removed forever any accountability for human conduct. Conscience had become a fiction, and society existed only by the sufferance of the strong. Surely, the antimaterialists argued, immortality was more than a dream, God was greater than a fancy, and man's destiny was other than the void of ultimate annihilation.[22] "While we are influenced by wind and currents, and even the variation of the compass, and the tricks played by the mirage with the coast and sea-marks," physician Edward Waldo Emerson commented, "yet *we* stand at the helm, and may change our course, or even put the ship about at will." Emerson, like his father before him and the pragmatists of a later generation, refused to accept a universe in which man was not in some small way a master of his own destiny.[23]

The antimaterialists were not always anxious to salvage Christian mythology at the expense of science. There was nothing intrinsically embarrassing, some argued, in Darwin's assertion that man had evolved from a branch of catarrhine apes. What bothered them more was the popular misconception of Darwin's theory that man was a sort of *édition de luxe* of the gorilla or chimpanzee. The idea that man and anthropoid descended from a common ancestor and, over the course of time and as a result of natural and sexual selection, the branches diverged, appeared lost in the din of battle. Neither the theory nor its popular misconceptions concerned the antimaterialists as much as the willingness of scientists to accept the theory without sufficient evidence. Doctors sometimes remarked that while they discovered very attractive features in Darwin's thesis, they held their final opinion in judicious reserve, agreeing with Rudolph Virchow of Germany that the theory was too quickly becoming a "dogmatism" among modern biologists.[24] Virchow, for exam-

ple, feared that the youthful vigor with which the new generation of scientists and philosophical speculators had seized
upon Darwin's thesis would transform biology into the same
romantic philosophy that had tyrannized and retarded the
science of his own generation. Concerning Darwin's theory
Virchow remarked: "I have spoken as a friend, not as an ad-
versary of transformism, and at all times I have approached
the immortal Darwin in a friendly, not a hostile way. But I
have always differentiated between friend and partisan. I can
salute and even support a scientific hypothesis, before it is
proven by facts. But I cannot become its partisan as long as
sufficient proof is lacking."[25]

The proofs which the Darwinists had recounted in such
glowing terms had yet to be weighed in the scales of exact
observation or demonstrated from sufficient evidencial material. Already history was resplendent with hypotheses that
had been established over the objections of man's searching
questions only to vanish like a vision of the night.[26] In a
speech before the Hardin County Medical Society of Kentucky in 1894, T. B. Greenley, M.D., reflected Virchow's remarks in a recitation of several scientific claims of the day,
among them the Burgeon method of treating consumption,
Koch's remedy for tuberculosis, and the rejuvenating liquid
of Brown-Séquard, which had resulted in widespread medical acceptance without sufficient investigation of the facts.
The medical profession had erred in placing the high standing of the authors of those products apart from the careful
criticism that must necessarily accompany all new ideas. The
same was true also of the theory of evolution.[27]

For Virchow, Greenley, and others like them, the scientific
community had unwittingly exchanged the healthy attitude
of scientific skepticism for that of worshipful credulity. This,
they argued, laid modern science open to objections and
ridicule. "The progress of discovery has been so rapid of late
years, and the triumphs of scientific research so brilliant,"
one doctor observed, "that a glamour of something like 'mutual admiration' seems to have come over the minds of many
of our eminent savants, which leads them to hail each other's
theoretical speculations beforehand; and in fear or impa-
tience of being anticipated in the arrival of final truths, allows them . . . to jump to the conclusion of problems that

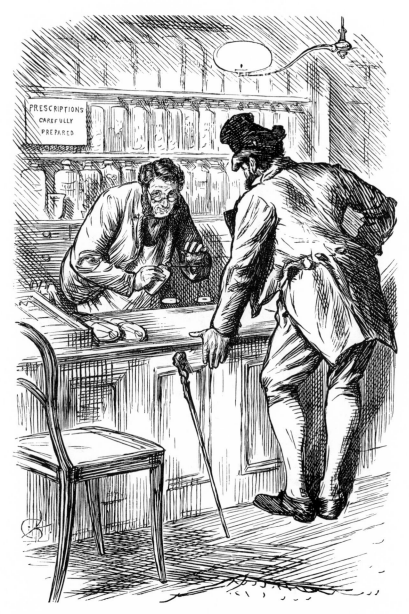

A druggist prepares a prescription for a waiting customer. *Punch, or The London Charivari*, November 28, 1874. Courtesy of Historical Pictures Service, Inc., Chicago.

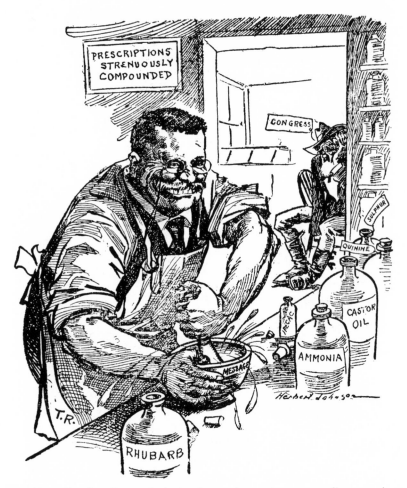

President Theodore Roosevelt depicted as a pharmacist compounding a noxious prescription (his annual message) for a hostile Congress (1903). Courtesy of Historical Pictures Service, Inc., Chicago.

have really not been half worked out." And the public had been inundated with so swift a succession of discoveries that it had lost its capacity for surprise and was prepared to accept almost any announcement without inquiring whether it was a mere theory of imagination or a truth established by the unquestionable evidence of all the facts. When science began to extend the conclusions of a partial induction over an area broader than human observation, it dressed imagination in the cloak of science and encouraged insidious dogmatism.[28]

Rather than accept criticism for deficiencies in its ratiocination, the new science had adopted a bigotry demanding complete and total acceptance. Exemplary of this attitude was the remark of Dr. John A. Rider in the *American Naturalist*. He observed that "judging by centuries of experience, as attested by unimpeachable historical records, it is safe enough for an intelligent man, even if he knows nothing about the facts, to accept promptly as truth any generalization of science which the church declares to be false, and conversely to repudiate with equal promptness as false any interpretation of the behavior of the universe which the church adjudges to be true."[29] But as one individual commented sarcastically, the scientific community had assumed in its tone and manner the very pretensions of the ministry. "Dogmatism, which for centuries droned upon the standards of the theological army, had taken flight and perched upon the banners of the scientists, where it is very noisily flapping its wings." Scientists were the new dogmatists of the age, while theologians had become faint-hearted and humble. Scientists, like the theologians before them, knew that few were competent to test their conclusions, thus causing them to make rash assertions, and "to take vast leaps over pure vacancy."[30]

Evolutionary Teleology

By the latter decades of the nineteenth century, the medical men who had accepted evolution tended to ignore the dysteleology implicit in Darwin's theory and, avoiding the warning of Charles Hodge (who perceived that Darwin had relegated God to a role of ontological nonexistence), transformed evolution into a benevolent and progressive teleology behind which worked the ever-present hand of Design. Like Asa Gray of Harvard, they were inclined to believe that evolution originated in the will and wisdom of the Creator. "If evolution be the result of foresight and contrivance," Samuel Haughton, M.D., wrote, "it becomes merely the expression of the chain of Second causes by means of which the purposes of the First Cause are harmoniously carried out."[31] As Stanford E. Chaille, M.D., professor of physiology and pathology at the University of Louisiana explained it, evolutionary theory defined God as a merciful and benevolent deity who revealed his thoughts in the progressive unfolding of creation. While man still bore in his frame the stamp of lowly origin, he had at least, in the developmental theory, demonstrated some progressive development away from his early beginnings. Now he could claim membership in a risen species rather than a fallen one, a "degradation from a perfect parent."[32]

In responding to critics who claimed that atheism, materialism, and determinism were the stepchildren of evolution, supporters of the theory argued persuasively that those "isms" were much older than the theory of natural selection and would persist as philosophical problems regardless of Darwin's thesis. The theory of biological evolution was no more atheistic or materialistic than it was idealistic or spiritualistic, since individuals holding all of those antagonistic views had embraced the theory at one time or another. Furthermore, the suggestion that determinism had removed the moral imperative from man's actions was simply untrue, particularly since the deterministic position was already imbedded in the theology of second-century Christian sects and stood on no firmer ground than the writings of Augustine, Aquinas, Calvin, and Jonathan Edwards, whose demonstrations of ontological determinism were derived wholly from theology. "If evolution, in strengthening our belief in the universality of causation and abolishing chance as an absurdity, leads to the conclusions of determinism," P. Dougherty, M.D., observed in 1896, "it does no more than follow the track of consistent and logical thinkers in theology and philosophy, before it existed, or was thought of." Surely, whoever accepted the existence of an omniscient Deity affirmed that the order of things was fixed from eternity; that foreknowledge of all that is and ever will be was fixed and fated in the mind of God. "If the belief in the uncausedness of volition is essential to mortality," Dougherty argued, "evolutionists have no more to say against that absurdity than the logical theologian or philosopher." No impartial observer in the conflict between evolution and special creation, Dougherty considered that the theory of special creation belonged to a system of belief which could no more be affirmed in light of current knowledge than the Ptolemaic notion of the universe could have been affirmed by early astronomers. Like many evolutionists in his day, he viewed the Church as an implacable foe of the Darwinian theory, just as it had been a foe of the achievements of astronomy and geology in years past.[33]

The American School of Biology

Although by the 1880s and the 1890s overwhelming evidence existed in favor of the theory of biological evolution, a growing number of American zoologists, entomologists, and paleontologists had begun to seek alternative explanations for the actual process of evolution. While Darwin had explained evolution as natural selection and Herbert Spencer as the instability of the homogeneous and the survival of the fittest, a group of American scientists advanced the law of acceleration and retardation.[34] This latter school of interpretation, which published many of its views in the *American Naturalist*, formed around the research and writings of Edward Drinker Cope (1840–97), Alpheus Spring Packard (1839–1905), and Alpheus Hyatt (1838–1902). Although this school was designated by some as the American School and by others as the Hyatt School, Packard preferred the designation Neo-Lamarckism to clarify its environmentalist position.[35]

According to the Neo-Lamarckians, there were two modes of species development: (1) the law of natural selection, and (2) the law of acceleration and retardation. Darwin's elaborate evidence accounted only for the reality of natural selection, and it made no attempt to explain the origin of variations.[36] Because natural selection was a preservative rather than originative principle, Packard argued that Darwin's natural selection and Spencer's survival of the fittest were misused to state the cause, when they simply expressed the re-

sult, of the action of a chain of causes.[37] Recognizing the dual
function of natural selection and the increments of change
impressed upon individuals during their lifetime and perpetuated in some measure through heredity, the Neo-Lamarckians attempted a reconcilation of both Darwin and
Lamarck.[38]

To this end, the American School relegated Darwin's natural selection to a secondary position in the conviction that an
animal's relation to its environment was the primary cause of
evolution.[39] Species, Cope wrote, developed from preexistent
species by an inherent tendency to variation and were preserved in given directions and repressed in others by the operations of the law of natural selection. In other words, Darwin's law of natural selection was simply part of a much
larger process of development. Natural selection operated by
the preservation of the fittest, while retardation and acceleration acted without reference to fitness at all. Instead of
being controlled by fitness, the principle of acceleration and
retardation was the controller of fitness. Once change had
begun, it would follow the laws of acceleration and retardation and would move at a pace more rapid than Darwin
allowed.[40]

Reflecting the viewpoint of this American School, Cora
Hosmer Flagg, M.D., instructor in comparative embryology
at the College of Physicians and Surgeons in Boston, observed that the work of Robert Wiedersheim, Daniel Cunningham, Henry F. Osborn, J. B. Sutton, Edward Cope, Wilson, Howes, Humphry, and Rathke had made comparative
anatomy the most progressive of the biological sciences.
Medical schools would need to present the subjects of physiology and pathology from a comparative standpoint, since
man was no longer in a separate order by himself but rather
the last link in a long chain of development. "It now remains
for physiology and pathology, based as they necessarily are
upon morphological data, to profit by the consideration of
the possibilities of comparative anatomy for elucidating
many of the pathological conditions to which man is subject."
Accordingly, Flagg thought it necessary to replace the prevailing belief that the human body was stable in its structure
and perfectly adapted to "supposed uses for definite ends"
with the evidence from comparative anatomy, embryology,

and physiology, which indicated that most organs were "combinations, rearrangements, and compromises necessitated by the accidents of growing complexities."

Moreover, the human organism was still undergoing change; and it was precisely in those areas where the body's retrogressive and progressive structures had changed to secondary uses or were "becoming more highly differentiated by the modification of their cell habits," that it offered less vigorous resistance to disease.[41] In other words, those structures which had retained their cell habits over long periods of time were less apt to succumb to disease than those which had been most affected, either in a progressive or retrogressive manner, by the forces of evolution. In *Evolution and Disease* (1890), J. Bland Sutton wrote, "It was clear that as there has been a gradual evolution of complex from simple organisms, it necessarily follows that the principles of evolution ought to apply to diseased conditions if they hold good for the normal, or healthy states of organisms: in plain words there has been an evolution of disease pari passu with evolution of animal form."[42]

In this regard Flagg noted that the details of pathology had been studied in a comparative manner that took into account not only an existing disease but also, as far as possible, "the factors in the long history of our growth that gave rise to it and from which it too has evolved." Those portions of the brain which "have developed and specialized in response to individual need rather than of species necessity" were more susceptible to disease than those deeper parts of the brain where the primal emotions and desires were to be found. Since the most complex parts of the brain were the most recently acquired, they were also the most easily disturbed, and their derangement furnished a satisfactory explanation for the study of insanity, idiocy, and kindred diseases. The comparatively rapid mental evolution of the Aryan peoples over four or five thousand years had been responsible for the high incidence of insanity in the modern civilized world, "since the stability of any form, function, or faculty in any race is dependent upon the time it has existed in that race, and therefore the more recent a faculty is in a race the more frequently will it be found absent, defective, or unstable in the individuals of the race."

Similarly, there was a greater frequency of disease due to the mechanics of man's upright position and the fact that the body with its quadrupedal ancestry had not fully adapted to its present conditions. Many pathological conditions of the viscera in the adult body had risen from the downward shifting of the pelvic organs because of the upright position. Problems included: inequality of muscular development, as individuals became either right- or left-handed; more frequent fractures of the femur as a result of the increased weight it had to assume; impaired circulation of the intercostal and lumbar veins as a result of their being maintained against gravity; congestive diseases, such as hemorrhoids or piles; frequent occurrence of varicose veins, varicocele, and anasarca; and weak spots in the abdominal walls that brought on hernia. Among the pelvic organs that were affected by evolutionary change, Flagg believed the woman's uterus probably had suffered most. The curved birth canal and changed pelvic inclination in the civilized races were modifications that brought increased danger to the life of both mother and child in delivery.[43]

Germ Theory and Evolution

Chicago physician G. Frank Lydston found it unthinkable that doctors would renounce the doctrine of evolution as unscientific, when its application bound together the natural sciences and, indeed, was basic to the correct medical understanding of infectious diseases. Although medical science owed much to the achievements of Louis Pasteur (1822–95) and Robert Koch (1843–1910) in germ theory and pathology, Lydston estimated that their contributions had "played an active part in deranging the substratum of rational philosophy upon which rested the entire superstructure of medical science." Moreover, he felt that germ theory, which shed significant light on the origin of infectious diseases, unfortunately brought an end to the search for causality. Koch's belief in the immutability of specificity in pathogenic microorganisms had given rise to great optimism in therapeutics as doctors assumed that, once having posited "a specifically constant" germ, they had only to find a specific remedy to kill the germ and cure the disease.

In effect, Lydston argued, Koch's germ theory had inadvertently retarded medical science by too parochial an approach to theories of infectious particles. Why not, he asked, apply the laws of evolutionary progression, differentiation, and development to germs in the same manner as they applied to other life forms? In other words, disease germs were no different from bodily characteristics that had become differentiated through changes in man's environment. Realizing that age, exposure, lowered resistance, and special conditions (the culture-bed or soil in which the germ was sown) were important in the proper understanding of disease, Lydston urged his fellow doctors to question the unvarying, specific entity of the germ as the prime cause of disease, for he doubted that a specific poison *always* existed.[44]

The interest of European scientists like Max von Pettenkofer of Bavaria, John Hughes Bennett of Edinburgh, Henry C. Bastion of Truro, and Lionel S. Beale of Cambridge contributed much to the stimulus for Lydston's ideas. Beale's two books, *Disease Germs: Their Real Nature* (1872) and *Disease Germs: Their Supposed Nature* (1879), as well as his earlier report on the "Microscopical Researches on the Cattle Plague" (1866) set forth the thesis that germs are in crucial ways dependent upon the *conditions* of the host. Only when scientists discovered the conditions under which an innocuous germ presented its virulent properties would they be able to place the true etiology of disease on a secure foundation. Influenced by these ideas, Lydston argued that the etiology and pathology of infectious diseases would stand not upon the germ but upon the myriad of conditions yet unknown that lie behind the germ. "The germ," he said, "bears the same relation to the true etiology of disease as the cosmogony of Moses does to the universe. It crudely attempts to explain but a small part of a great whole."[45]

Lydston was not upholding a belief in the spontaneous generation of germs, as some critics claimed, but a belief in "the spontaneous generation of new and virulent properties in hitherto innocuous germs, and a natural variation of type and pathogenic effect of germs supposed to be invariably specific"—a transformation made possible in venereal disease by the favorable environment of the female generative apparatus. In its relation to disease, evolution was thus a double-purpose law which controlled and modified not only the parasite but the host as well.

> Disease is incident to the very life of every animal. Disease is largely dependent upon living micro-organisms. As we study the evolution of the animal so should we study the evolution of the disease germs which affect it. Every phase of organic evolution is subject to adverse as well as favorable elements of various kinds. Each organism is relentlessly pursued by foes of a higher or lower order of evolutionary development and differentiation. Even the germs of disease are, in some cases, pursued by other germs which destroy them. How much of this phase of organic evolution is manifest in infectious diseases of a mixed type science has not yet determined. We know that some germs prepare a favorable field for other germs. The converse seems also to be true. . . . It is unfortunate that the human system should be the battleground of the warring micro-organic factions. Man, with his superior power born of the forbidden fruit—knowledge—has been able to contend pretty successfully against most of the elements unfavorable to him. He has not acquitted himself so brilliantly as regards those apparently insignificant little foes, the germs of disease. Evolutionary law he may not abrogate, though he may sometimes direct and modify its operation.[46]

Lydston applied the evolutionary approach to his own research in venereal disease which, he stated, was still suffering a period of etiological and pathological confusion. Too much optimism had been placed on the discovery of the gonococcus by those who believed in specificity in germs. He hoped that in time the emphasis placed upon the gonococcus would lessen and the conditions governing the evolution of the germ would draw greater concern. Wide variations existed in venereal infection, from simple urethritis to virulent chancroid. To these variations, he emphasized, environmental influences were important. "It is my firm belief," he wrote, "that gonorrhoea and chancroid develop *de novo* in the medium afforded by the secretions of the unclean and pathologically contaminated vagina. This development depends upon the adaptation changes in innocuous or comparatively non-virulent germs—a spontaneous culture modification." The virulence of the germ depended upon the nature and conditions in which it developed: decomposition of vaginal fluids, the age of the process of germ development, frequency of coitus, habits and constitution of the woman, character of discharge from the male, and uncleanliness of the woman. "If evolutionary adaptation did not control infection," he remarked, "comparatively benign infections would be malignant and fatal." The reason behind benign and malignant germ infection was the adaptative success of the germ or cell. A gonococcus, for example, might be shorn of its pathogenic properties by adaptation, while retaining its physical characteristics; yet deposited on other more suitable cells, it would evolve into a pathogenic microbe. A man with latent gonorrhea could infect his wife with typic pelvic infection, which at a later time might be imparted back to the man as a typic, virulent gonococcic urethritis. In another illustration of germ adaptation, Lydston referred to a woman with latent gonorrhea who showed no symptoms until the onset of her menstrual period when, because of environmental changes in the sexual organ, she developed acute infection.[47] On the whole, however, Lydston believed that the effect of evolution had been to decrease the virulence of syphilis on the human system. "The human race has become fairly well syphilized," he observed, "and hereditary immunity should count for something in a disease which in its active period so seldom kills as to permit the race to secure the full benefit of hereditary immunity, if such there be." As for the more virulent forms of syphilis, Lydston suspected that their occurrence resulted from "atavism of micro-organisms combined with atavism of susceptibility."[48]

Evolution and Social Reform

By the 1880s perceptible changes had occurred within American culture with respect to the developmental theory. Along with the genuinely philosophical and scientific discussion of natural selection as it affected Christian theology, anthropology, and the medical sciences, a highly speculative literature emerged, which seemed to float on an evolutionary sea, with writers from all disciplines grasping bits of evolutionary thinking and consuming them without thought or question. The unusual phenomenon resulted from the popularization of the developmental theory by the Darwinists (or, more correctly, Spencerians) who read less of Darwin than they had of the philosophical evolutionists before him.

Every discipline, from mechanics, music, and art, to science and philosophy, became enveloped in the elaborate system of evolutionary law; and doctors, no less than the rest of society, consumed large chunks of evolutionary theory with never a thought to its assimilative difficulties.

For the first time science carried popular culture out into celestial space, pointing out nebulae and showing how worlds and suns first formed. Overwhelmed by the conceptions they were asked to grasp—the eons of time and the immensity of space through which the law of development operated—society seemed unable to comprehend, let alone question all that was said to be true. The disciples of Spencer and Huxley passed through society like gigantic reapers cutting broad swaths across the sciences and suggesting that whatever gaps existed in the supraorganic chain would be reconciled in time and with faith in the evolutionary (i.e., teleological) process. At their best, evolution's zealots laid the groundwork for more serious thought and reflection; at their worst, they turned listeners into veritable rustics who, on hearing their discourses, could only gaze in wonderment that men could know so much.

For many of these new evolutionists, the developmental theory demonstrated two significant phases in its effect upon life forms: the struggle of each organism for its own life, and its struggle for the life of others. Biologists and sociologists identified these two activities of living forms as those which were directed toward the nourishment and preservation of self, known as *egoism*, and those directed toward the preservation of the race, which they termed *altruism*. Henry Maudsley in *Body and Mind* (1870) and Herbert Spencer in *Principles of Ethics* (1892–93) depicted the principle of altruism as gradually gaining ascendancy over egoistic principles as human society advanced from its more primitive organizations.[49] Thus, for those inclined to employ the theory as a touchstone for the foundation of moral government and civilization, evolution implied an advance of ethical progress or an ascent in the development of laws to guide human conduct. J. S. Foote, M.D., remarked: "The ethics of evolution is the ethics of an ever changing series; it began with katabolism and will continue through eternity; as we find it more highly developed in man than in the lower animals, more highly developed in modern man than in primitive man, and more highly developed in some modern men than in others, so we will find it more highly developed in the spiritual life than in this, and it will reach its highest type only in the universal perfection of the future. The time is come when we ought to have a better understanding of human life, and the time is also come when we ought to know better how to deal with it."[50]

Although Herbert Spencer, the pseudomoralist for the status quo, believed that evolutionary law expressed an inherent bias toward perfection, he interpreted evolution as an impersonal process in which the environment was omnipotent and man was all but helpless to either hasten or retard the sequence of events. In effect mankind must accept the slow and natural working out of age-old problems. In *Social Statics* (1850), Spencer argued against the wisdom of embarking on any cooperative work in the field of preventive medicine by the state or the medical profession. Both he and his American counterpart, William G. Sumner of Yale, had urged the maintenance of a strictly neutral government motivated simply to ensure an unhampered laissez-faire environment. By the 1880s, however, with the encouragement of second-generation evolutionists like Lester Ward (1841–1913), who looked to telic change (the ability, though limited, of the mind to impose its will over environment), the state became a positive instrument in the erection of a man-made environment. Accepting the ideas of Ward, as well as those of August Comte and the French hygienists, doctors began seeking cooperative ventures between medicine and government in areas of hygiene, contagious diseases, and epidemics. Recognizing that medical men working in their private capacities had done much to develop, systematize, and teach the principles of sanitary science, doctors were inclined to believe that much more could be accomplished with additional support from the government. If a government was willing to equip a scientist for an expedition or to make a large appropriation for an international exhibition, how much more valuable might it become in providing a department of health to act as watchman over the health of the nation. Had there been a corps of doctors ready to rush to the scene of the 1873 epidemic of cholera in Tennessee and Alabama or of the outbreak of yellow fever in Alabama in 1878, valuable information might have been obtained through medical investigation to afford future protection of human life.[51]

As a group, however, nineteenth-century physicians were more inclined to ply their patients with pills than teach them sanitary science. Indeed, the byword of medicine seemed to be: "Millions for cure, but not one cent for prevention."[52] One had only to peruse the patent-medicine shelves to understand the prevailing temper of the medical arts. Part of this problem stemmed from age-old biases that derived from the theory of constitutional pathology and the priority the theory gave to individual disposition over environmental causation. Not until the general acceptance of germ theory in the later decades of the century following Koch's demonstration of the tuberculosis bacillus (1882) did preventive medicine move from a supportive or secondary role to take a position of preeminence in medical science. Only then did medical men move firmly in the direction of preventive medicine, with the understanding that disease could not be rationally and successfully treated until its causes and nature were better understood. In a speech before the American Academy of Medicine in 1882, Nathan Allen, M.D., remarked, "Formerly *cure* was the supreme if not the leading object of the physician, but the time is fast approaching when *prevention* will be the watchword."[53] Unfortunately the preventive measures undertaken by American doctors lagged noticeably behind programs inaugurated by their European counterparts. One reason for this lag was the fact that Europe's medical profession was much older and more established than the American. More important, however, was the fact that American medical men, on the whole, were far less involved in affairs of state than were European doctors; in America social medicine emerged first from philanthropic charity rather than from state or public efforts.

Those doctors who recognized the need for preventive medicine (commonly identified as "sanitary science" in America as opposed to "state medicine" or "science for the state" in Europe) operated on the premise that the external elements of the environment (pure air, pure water, and pure soil) and the internal relations of the body (physical exercise, proper diet, and suitable clothing) affected the entire physical, intellectual, and moral education of the individual, and even extended beyond the individual to the family, school, state, and church.[54] Doctors talked of an organic relationship between the greatness of every nation and the physical health of its people. Insuring a healthy coexistence between these external and internal factors was the responsibility of each physician who studied nature's laws and their relationship to society. The duties of each physician involved "the scope of the human mind, the dignity of the human character, and the brightness of the nation's glory"; and the degree to which those virtues were encouraged or sustained depended in the last analysis on the ability of every physician to teach the laws of health among his patients.[55]

Selective Reform

While the origins of sanitary science certainly predate the zealots of evolutionary theory, the rationale for late-nineteenth-century involvement in sanitary science drew substantively from social Darwinists who chose to expand the tools of the physician so as to better serve the public in areas of preventive medicine. One of the more significant signs that evolutionary theory was influencing medicine came from physicians who expressed alarm at mankind's inability to move satisfactorily toward a higher development. The villains in this regard were the artificial mechanisms of altruism and philanthropy which had complicated the engine of natural selection by allowing for the preservation of the unfit. Indicative of their impact were census reports for the United States and England which showed that the number of insane, idiots, epileptics, deaf and dumb, chronic drunkards, and persons with constitutional tendencies toward such diseases as scrofula, phthisis, cancer, and rheumatism had increased at a faster rate than the population.[56]

Those doctors who expressed alarm at the changes affecting national health patterns and the corresponding tendencies in ameliorative legislation were quick to identify with Robert J. Dugdale's 1877 study of Margaret Jukes's progeny through six generations. Of the 709 individuals who constituted the basis of the study, the majority became thieves, prostitutes, and idiots.[57] Along similar lines, the writings of

William R. Greg (1809–81) regarding the degenerate Irish, Galton's *Hereditary Genius* (1870), Lawson Tait's essays on the laws of evolution, and Erwin Ray Lankester's *Comparative Longevity* (1870) had given Charles Darwin much of the argument he eventually employed in *Descent of Man*, when he expressed his reservations about society's inclination to prolong the capacity of the unfit for survival.

> With savages, the weak in body or mind are soon eliminated; and those that survive commonly exhibit a vigorous state of health. We civilized men, on the other hand, do our utmost to check the process of elimination; we build asylums for the imbecile, the maimed, and the sick; we institute poor-laws; and our medical men exert their utmost skill to save the life of every one to the last moment. There is reason to believe that vaccination has preserved thousands, who from a weak constitution would formerly have succumbed to small-pox. Thus the weak members of civilized societies propagate their kind. No one who has attended to the breeding of domestic animals will doubt that this must be highly injurious to the race of man. It is surprising how soon a want of care, or care wrongly directed, leads to the degeneration of a domestic race; but excepting in the case of man himself, hardly any one is so ignorant as to allow his worst animals to breed. . . . We must . . . bear the undoubtedly bad effects of the weak surviving and propagating their kind; but there appears to be at least one check in steady action, namely that the weaker and inferior members of society do not marry so freely as the sound; and this check might be indefinitely increased by the weak in body or mind refraining from marriage, though this is more to be hoped for than expected.[58]

The danger to society, as Darwin, Galton, and their disciples understood it, was that the humanitarian nature of the age (in particular, the element of altruism that emerged among the higher races) had kept alive the sick and defective classes who were as prolific as they were inefficient. Though institutions such as almshouses, reformatories, asylums, and hospitals were a necessity, doctors cautioned society not to abuse their intended purpose.[59] Recognizing that people had no wish to be guided by heredity in matters so personal as marriage, Darwin's supporters nevertheless advocated the passage of hereditarian laws that, when accompanied by proper education, would cause the public to appreciate the value of the law and the consequences of public indifference.

The hereditarian experiments of Darwin's cousin, Sir Francis Galton (1822–1911) on rabbits and basset hounds, his laws of filial regression and ancestral inheritance, and the opening of his eugenics laboratory (1904) in London, became the basis of statistical material bearing on the mental and physical condition of man and the relations of those conditions to environment and inheritance. Galton's theory of ancestral inheritance was the starting point of Karl Pearson's biometric methodology and the extension of evolutionary theory into the area of national eugenics. Pearson, in *Darwinism, Medical Progress, and Eugenics* (1912), urged a full scale study of the degenerate (i.e., insane, tubercular, epileptic, idiot, hysteric, and mental defective) in the belief that mankind "can only progress as a race, mentally and physically, by stringent selection for parenthood."[60]

Exemplary of the hereditarian legislation suggested to state governments by individual physicians or medical societies was that of E. O. Sisson, M.D., of the College of Physicians and Surgeons in Keokuk, Iowa.

1. That each state should pass laws preventing the intermarriage of all persons who would come under the following headings:

    a. All those suffering from such constitutional diseases as consumption, scrofula, syphilis, and leprosy.

    b. All those suffering from various neuroses, epilepsy, insanity, and severe cases of chorea.

    c. All criminals coming under the head of murderers, thieves, prostitutes, etc.

2. A systematic crossing of the breeds in cases of a mild character, thus aiding nature to revert to the normal.

3. That the physicians of each community constitute an examining board before which all parties contemplating marriage shall be required to appear and submit to the necessary examinations before they can be allowed a license, a record being kept showing the results of such examination, to which shall be added the births resulting from such unions, with a record of the physical and mental condition of the child.

4. That the violator or violators of the first law be liable to punishment the same as in the violation of any law.

5. That the physician or physicians who neglect to fulfill his or their duty, as mentioned above, be liable to punishment the same as in the violation of any law.

6. That there will be instituted into our educational system studies by which the masses will become more enlightened on, and have a more thorough understanding of, the great laws of nature, and the evil results arising from their abuse.[61]

"By evolution," Sisson wrote, "we are taught that the tendency of man under congenial environments is ever towards a higher plane, be that plane mental, moral or physical." But for evolution to improve the individual, the tendencies that frustrated or selfishly ignored the laws of hereditary transmission had to be stamped out.[62] As one physician remarked, "Men and women have no right to bring into the world children to either suffer and die prematurely or to drag out a miserable existence and transmit again to their children the fatal inheritance." Society had unfortunately permitted the mentally, morally, and physically degenerate to perpetuate themselves through the misguided patchwork of philanthropy and government reform.[63]

Sanitary Science and Politics

While hereditarian zealots within the medical profession wrote of the long-term evils of ameliorative legislation, others chose to disregard the warnings of Darwin, Galton, and Pearson and appealed instead for a dedicated effort to stamp out causes rather than temporize with effects. To this end they encouraged the allocation of funds to remedy overcrowded tenements, solve the problems of polluted air and foul gases, ensure the production of cheap and nutritious foods, educate the population in the principles of hygiene, close saloons, and face the evils of improper sanitation and unhealthy working conditions.[64] Partisans of sanitary science observed that, while government and medicine had long operated as independent factors in social evolution, the conditions present in the industrial age made it imperative for them to continue serving their responsible trusts through closer cooperation.[65]

National existence, the advocates of sanitary science argued, was the crystalization of such diverse elements as presidents, cabinets, legislative bodies, families, and individuals and required the expertise of the capable physician as well as the astute politician. Together they could accomplish what individually they could only aspire to achieve. From sanitary plumbing, regulation of working hours, immigration restriction, and food preparation to property condemnation, water purification, and urban planning, the responsibilities of medicine and government seemed to intersect with increasing regularity. Thus, the widely held belief that medicine should remain aloof from the rough-and-tumble world of politics fell before the needs of the public in the new industrial and urban age. "Are we merely diagnosticating and healing machines, grinding out opinions and advice as the grist from the mill?" one practitioner inquired in the 1890s. "Is our outlook upon the world only on perverted function and diseased action? Is humanity only one vast museum of pathological specimens for our contemplation and study?" More and more, medical men answered these questions with a definitive no. Concerned with the need for taking stock of themselves and considering whether the profession ought not to enlarge its responsibilities, practitioners began to lay aside older attitudes and, under the aegis of their own association, to move into the turbulent waters of American politics. In a culture that was beginning to place the doctor in an eminent position within the value structure of Victorian society, the problems of etiology, pathology, and therapeutics were becoming springboards to political involvement.[66]

Part of the incentive for this change in attitude came from the industrial culture itself, where man's inventive skills seemed unending as the era burgeoned with accomplishments of mechanical and organizational genius. It was an age of entrepreneurs, whose vast fortunes spoke not only of their financial ingenuity but of their ability to carve out and control important areas of the American economy. Doctors not only expressed admiration for these industrial barons, but assumed positions of trust and responsibility over their various philanthropic gifts to society. In doing so, medical men gave direction to programs without which the era's material prosperity might have spawned resentment, class conflict, and punitive government reform. Physicians, with their knowledge of disease, became consultants and administrators over these charitable bodies, providing them with plans of operation that promised practical results. By reinforcing in the public mind the need for the scientific management of contagious and infectious diseases, by warning against sanitary negligence, by proposing regulations designed to extinguish or control diphtheria and typhoid, and by instituting procedures for isolation during epidemics, the medical profession provided invaluable service to help solve the problems facing Victorian cities.[67]

By the latter decades of the nineteenth century, the AMA had begun to urge that doctors and their medical societies become more involved in local, state, and national issues affecting the profession: the complications of poor laws; the regulation of school boards; the question of coeducation; the licensing of doctors, druggists, dentists, and barbers; the control of quarantine, prostitution, and related social matters. Readers of its national journal were reminded that any program designed to raise the standard of medical education in the United States would require legislative enactment on a state, and perhaps even a national, level to make the goal meaningful. The successful efforts of homeopaths to control 110 hospitals, 145 dispensaries, 16 insane asylums, and numerous sanatoria and nursing homes, many of which were supported by state and community appropriations, were indicative of the problems at hand. State examinations rigid enough to exclude homeopaths and osteopaths from general practice would necessitate active lobbying by the medical profession in the halls of government. Protection from patent-medicine claims, the devastating results of opium addiction, and the evils of over-the-counter prescribing were added problems that the medical profession could successfully control only by political means.[68] "You will find that public health legislation is a matter to which you cannot remain indifferent," J. S. Billings remarked before the graduating class of Bellvue Hospital Medical College in 1882, "and if you are wise you will study the subject so that you can aid in shaping this legislation to what it should be, for in this respect knowledge is power."[69]

There were, of course, those who regarded medicine as a jealous mistress who tolerated no rival. One physician wrote in 1860, "The man who educates himself in such a way, that he is capable of wielding the vast stores of knowledge embraced in the science and art of medicine will find no time or opportunity to distract his attention with other pursuits."[70] But H. Bert Ellis, M.D., president of the California State Medical Society, reminded his sometimes reluctant colleagues that "a positive and vital relationship between medicine and the scientific principles underlying social conditions and phenomena" made it both selfish and unjustifiable for physicians to neglect political problems. Their particular educational advantages, knowledge of hygiene and sanitation, critical judgment, and understanding of human nature made them especially qualified for both participation and leadership in political affairs.[71]

Another medical writer remarked, "The physician is better acquainted with men and has a deeper knowledge of human nature than the average citizen, and therefore is in a position to understand thoroughly many of the requirements of the community."[72] In effect physicians were more able to understand the social organism; and since they were presumably more emotionally stable than the public at large, they could carry their strength into the field of politics. "We look on, amused, and perhaps with offended dignity when we see audiences swayed by some trivial matter, which so forcibly appeals to their emotions," a doctor commented in 1891. The same training in scientific observation that shaped the thinking of the studied physician could provide an excellent foundation for judgment in political matters.

In a speech before the Medical Society of the District of Columbia, Swan M. Burnett, M.D., remarked, "If all men who follow callings which are classed as respectable, and all men belonging to the learned professions and the cultured classes kept themselves away from affairs of State and took no interest in the workings of government, then indeed would the advance of civilization be in peril." If politics had become a reproachful word, it was because intelligent and informed men had failed to participate in the conduct of political parties, but had instead allowed them to fall into the hands of deceitful men. In Burnett's opinion the medical profession in the United States owed to itself and to the community a greater representation in public assemblies, legislatures, and commissions. Questions relating to public health, sanitation, and hygiene demanded the physician's advice and good counsel. "It cannot be derogatory to the dignity of the profession to thus put itself and its accumulated experiences at the service of the State," Burnett wrote; "and, by so doing, in the proper manner, it elevates itself in the opinion of the community, and by this added respect, is enabled to work a greater advantage in its own special field of activity." [73]

Advocates of greater political involvement looked to European examples, such as Albrecht von Haller (1708–77), who during the days of his practice was also a poet, litterateur, botanist, and legislator; Senator Samuel-Jean Pozzi (1846–1918) of France, who was also a skilled surgeon and specialist in gynecology; and Rudolph Virchow, whose work in cellular pathology, anthropology, ethnology, and archaeology did not prevent him from carrying on an active political career in the Prussian lower house from 1861 to 1902. [74] They also noted the participation of Greek scholars and professional men in the affairs of state. Burnett observed that "The Grecian of culture touched life on all sides, and the result was that he grew in all directions and became a symmetrical being, and intellectually the model for men of all time." [75]

In colonial America, twenty-two physicians had been members of the Provincial Congress of Massachusetts in 1774–75; and Josiah Bartlett and Matthew Thornton of New Hampshire, Oliver Wolcott of Connecticut, Lyman Hall of Georgia, and Benjamin Rush of Pennsylvania had all been noted practitioners whose responsibilities were truly civic in the broadest sense. Rush, one of the leading spirits in the political and social scene of the eighteenth century, had been a member of the Pennsylvania legislature, a signer of the Declaration of Independence and a prominent abolitionist as well as an active medical man throughout his life.

In contrast with these illustrious participants in early American government, at the turn of the century the medical profession could claim only two senators (L. H. Ball of Delaware and J. H. Gallinger of New Hampshire) and one representative (W. G. Hunter of Kentucky), all of whom had retired from practice. This contrasted sharply with the French Senate, which boasted no less than forty medical men among its three hundred members. "Think what might be accomplished in the way of needed and wholesome legislation in the United States if our medical profession were only represented in similar proportion in the two branches of Congress," one advocate of political involvement remarked.[76]

Recognition of the need for this involvement came not just from the medical profession but from national leaders like President Grover Cleveland, who, in a speech before the New York Academy of Medicine in the 1890s, criticized the notable absence of physicians in community affairs. "We cannot but think that the discoveries and improvements in medical practice which we now enjoy are dearly bought if the members of the profession in their onward march have left behind them their sense of civic obligation and their interest in the general public welfare." Although the nation required the watchful eye of the medical profession, the greed for scientific achievements had consumed excessive amounts of time, causing doctors to forget their obligations to the state— obligations manifest at all levels of government. The jurists on the county courts, for example, were continually faced with judgments on insanity; and these crucial decisions, for lack of medical cooperation, were too often left to unschooled laymen. It was obvious from all available evidence, the President added, that a permanent corps of medical examiners was needed to reduce the number of contagious diseases in the schools, to attend the sick, and to provide a watchful eye over the condition of educational facilities in general. Boston, a pioneer city in educational improvement, discovered that out of 16,780 pupils examined in its school system, 10,737 were ill. If laws were to be just and appropriate, Cleveland observed, the legislatures would need the help of medical men to formulate health laws and police their enforcement. "If laws were needed to abolish abuses which investigations have unearthed," he concluded, "your fraternity should not be strangers to the agencies which make up the laws."[77]

The most obvious need for medical expertise was in the field of hygiene, the lack of which was the major source of plagues, choleras, typhoids, and all the assorted "death-breeding customs of mankind." In order for governments to grapple with the problem, it was necessary for them to obtain accurate statistics, which meant reliable records of births and marriages and correct mortality figures based upon immediate registration of deaths. When properly plotted, statistics were especially meaningful in alerting health officers to the mortality of the population from certain diseases or environmental hazards. Knowledge of the duration of life and the mortality rates in every town invariably lightened the burden of physicians in their efforts to ascertain the influence of environment on the causes of disease. Statistics were also valuable in the matter of inheritance, the relations of guardians and wards, administration of vaccination, settlement of insurance claims and pensions, child labor, and disability problems. Although the contributions of Quételet, Louis, and the French clinicians had predated Darwin's influence, modern statistics applied to man owed much to the new attitude that Darwin lent to the study of human correlations and measurements. His *Origin of Species* and *Descent of Man*, along with the translation of J. G. Mendel's monograph in 1902, Francis Galton's anthropometric laboratory, and the School of Biometry founded by Karl Pearson at University College, gave clear indication that medical statistics, sampling, averages, and variability of observation were essential to a clear and accurate understanding of man and his diseases.[78]

In responding to American cities, which had grown at a rate that far exceeded their ability to control social problems, doctors urged the creation of state and local boards of health with power to disseminate information for the preservation of health. More than ever before physicians were called upon to write pamphlets explaining the dangers of consumption and the need for its proper care and control; the importance of nutritious foods, exercise, and recreation; the necessity for proper drainage, disinfection, and vaccination; the need for well-equipped hospitals; the necessity for study of lung diseases and their relationship to living conditions; and the dangers of improper ventilation and light in factories. "Should not physicians . . . take steps to create public opinion, to prepare newspaper articles, leaflets, pamphlets, and books that shall be at the same time scientifically accurate and to the lay mind intelligible?" the New York Medical Association asked.[79] To aid in this form of public education, the association urged the creation of a special committee on "popular sanitary science" in each state to supervise the writing of articles for the secular press and publication and distribution of pamphlets on the principles of sanitary science.[80]

Those medical men who advocated greater participation in politics carefully distinguished themselves from the proverbial "doc" who was simply part of a political machine and whose conduct was "not the function of a scientific or strictly medical man." Few such individuals could maintain the dignity of their profession, and eventually they overreached themselves to a point where they appeared unprofessional. "More results can be obtained by quiet, earnest work than by the blare of trumpets, as illustrated by the work of the successful politician," one nineteenth-century practitioner commented. The medical profession must first be respected for its medical skills; then its influence, when properly directed, would effect quiet change and honest politics.[81]

The AMA preferred not to strike a new path in politics by seeking third-party involvement; rather, the association saw its responsibility in teaching and purifying the parties that already existed. With the creation of a National Committee on Medical Legislation, the AMA sought to identify and inform its membership of the wishes and desires of the association on various political issues. Several states, following the lead of Colorado, provided the framework for the national committee by organizing medical legislation leagues. Political organization was a fact of modern society, Charles Fisher Andrew, M.D., of Colorado argued. "The essence of a free government," he wrote, "lies in the submission of will to will, sanctioned by physical force and justice." It was in the interest of each doctor that his ideas be heard and his suggestions be accepted. Too long had the public been at the mercy of patent-medicine men, quacks, and advocates of new dogmas and pathies. "The time," Andrew wrote, "is opportune for us to take the public into our confidence and for us to educate them properly in a medical way, for with the people lies the power to bring out great changes in our medical laws."

> Let us put on our armor and go before the people with a determination to be heard. Let us do it individually and collectively, and let us have the A.M.A. behind us. Let a doctor arise in our midst who, having the love of his profession at heart, will lead and point the way. Let us follow him to the primaries,

to the county, state and national conventions; let him be a man who has the wisdom of a King Solomon and the vigor of a Teddy Roosevelt. Let him be a man who places his faith in the upbuilding of our noble profession far above party politics. Let each one of the members of the A.M.A. consider himself a committee of one to educate his friends in his political party to justness and righteousness of medical politics.[82]

Yet another advocate of greater political involvement was Charles A. Reed, M.D. (1856–1928), chairman of the National Committee on Medical Legislation of the AMA, who insisted that the medical profession maintain vigilance over the constitutional and statutory laws of the states and nation. From their work in the very foundations of human existence, medical men had the advantage of analyzing individual health problems against the larger perspective of national purpose. Devotion to strictly professional labor could not be used to plead exemption from responsibilities and duties as a citizen. Reed stated that the lack of an organized profession had hampered the enactment of appropriate sanitary laws for the country and that the few successful achievements had been the result of voluntary associations which were patently limited in their influence and capability.[83]

The failure to control entomologic problems, food contamination, and purity of pharmaceutical and proprietary medicines reinforced in Reed's mind that the duty of the profession lay "in the direction of securing legislation by the Congress, whereby our medicines, like our foods, shall be subject to inspection and certification by the National Government." Reed observed that state laws regulating the practice of medicine lacked uniformity; thus, "there could be neither complete cooperation in health matters nor reciprocity in medical licensure between the different states." Only uniform health laws, consistent gathering of vital statistics, and national regulation over the practice of medicine could hope to bring order out of the chaos of state practices. It was the responsibility of the medical profession to work for the adoption of uniform laws in all states or to insist on the development of national legislation.[84]

To effect uniform laws and regulations over the health and practice of medicine, the AMA created a National Committee on Medical Legislation, a Legislative Council, the membership of which included the National Committee and one member for each state and territory and each of the public services (i.e., Army, Navy, and Public Health and Marine Hospital Service), and finally, a National Auxiliary Congressional and Legislative Committee, with its membership including one member from each county in the United States. The National Committee on Medical Legislation was to examine "the merits of all proposed legislation affecting either the efficiency, status, or personal welfare of the medical profession, as represented in the public services; and all proposed legislation in any way relating either to the science of medicine or to the correlated sciences." The result of its deliberations would be placed before the Legislative Council, where the findings would be either accepted or rejected. The National Committee would then communicate the views of the profession to the proper legislative committees, before whom specific bills were pending and when necessary communicate instructions to the National Auxiliary Congressional and Legislative Committee, whose members were to bring "such matters of pending legislation as may be thus referred to [them], to the attention of the medical profession and to the people of [their] respective counties, and by every honorable means . . . secure desired action thereon by [their] representatives in both branches of the Congress of the United States."[85]

The Darwinian Legacy

For everyone who vehemently dismissed the possibility of Darwin's evolutionary hypothesis, countless others appreciated the Englishman's observational methods and expressed a quiet confidence in the future advance of medicine along more scientific paths. Claude Bernard, in *Introduction to the Study of Experimental Medicine* (1865), noted that by "the very nature of [medicine's] evolutionary advance, it is little by little abandoning the region of systems, to assume a more and more analytic form, and thus to join in the method of investigation common to the experimental sciences."[86] Above all else, the progress of medicine depended upon the establishment of "a good experimental standard," which, freed from previous system approaches, meant "solid instruction in experimental physiology."[87] As Bernard expressed it, "systems are not found in nature, but only in the mind of man."

> The experimental method, on the other hand, is impersonal; it destroys individuality by uniting and sacrificing everyone's particular ideas, and turning them to the advantage of universal truth as established with the help of the experimental criterion. It advances slowly and laboriously and in this respect will always be less pleasing to the mind. Systems, on the contrary, are alluring because they give us a science absolutely regulated by logic alone; and that frees us from studying and makes medicine easy. Experimental medicine, then, is antisystematic and anti-doctrinal in nature, or rather, it is free and independent in its essence and does not try to attach itself to any kind of medical system.[88]

In a lecture delivered in 1876 at University College, London, Henry Maudsley, M.D., reflected on the new role of medical science in modern thought. For Maudsley no education was more relevant to man than that of students seeking to become physicians. In medical education students were brought face to face with facts of nature as they advanced through steps of observation and induction, by which they sought to order their ideas and bring them into conformity with nature. Admitting that many misconstrued the concept of induction as a sort of "mechanical process of knowledge-getting which rendered mental capacity unnecessary," Maudsley insisted that man "does not see with his eye, but through it; that seeing in the sense of observation is impossible unless there be behind the eye the intelligence to interpret what is presented to it." Like Darwin, medical students must not be students of observation alone; they must also be students with minds capable of making sense out of so-called facts. "Happy is the observer who, when he sets to work, has a good theory in his mind," Maudsley wrote. But men untrained in habits of accurate observation theorized frivolously. Thus, it was of utmost importance that the medical mind be trained not only for sound reflection but also for close observation of the facts of nature.[89]

Just as it was impossible to understand the mind without first understanding the body, so Maudsley believed one could not understand the body unless the processes and laws of nature that lay underneath (i.e., anatomy and physiology) were correctly known. While classical knowledge rounded out a medical student's education, a thorough knowledge of science was the bedrock of modern medicine. The proper training of medical men must begin by following the order of nature—by starting with the less complex and moving towards the more complex, "using the lower as a ladder by which to mount up to the higher." This implied that the training of a physician must begin with a knowledge of mathematics and physics and proceed to the study of chemistry, and from there pass on to anatomy and the study of physiology.[90] To know man, a doctor must first know nature and those relationships which constitute life. Only after he mastered the phenomena of living beings would he be competent to treat the sick. Without a thorough understanding of the properties of the human organism and of their relations to the environment, it was impossible, "except in the most lamely empirical fashion," to treat disease and restore harmony to the body. Until medicine broadened its field of vision by regarding man in his essential relationship with surrounding nature, medical science would remain empirical and defective—a world in which physicians would simply wait patiently on nature and aim to do the least harm by the drugs they employed.[91]

From Claude Bernard and Maudsley to Abraham Flexner there existed a concerted effort on the part of the educators to use observation, reflection, verification, and generalization as the touchstones of modern medicine. Flexner wrote: "Science resides in the intellect, not in the instrument. To call a careful and correct bedside observation clinical and a laboratory examination scientific, as if there were some qualitative distinction between the two, is absurd. Whether the observer be seated at the bedside or bending over his microscope, he observes, elicits data, frames an hypothesis, and tentatively pursues the course of action suggested by reflection upon all the facts of his possession, regardless of where or how obtained." The same quality of intelligence was demanded in both for the solution of the problems at hand. "Though the experienced practitioner may, by a process of apparently instinctive 'short circuiting,' achieve a diagnosis so swiftly that he seems to be guided by something called 'clinical instinct,' we may be quite sure that, as a matter of

fact, the processes actually involved are observation, elimination of the irrelevant, inference—in other words, induction—even though the pace has been so rapid that the several steps are indistinguishable." Neither in the intellectual
attitude nor in the scientific method was there a difference
between the tools of the laboratory investigator and the practicing doctor or, for that matter, between clinical medicine
and preventive legislation designed to preserve the social
organism.[92]

Although doctors did not easily throw off their age-old
habits of thinking, they were compelled by temperament to
render the future amenable to human control. In this sense,
Darwin's theory proved responsive to the needs and direction of medicine in the late nineteenth century. Its strength
in defining the perimeters of the new age was clear acknowledgment that medicine had outgrown the scholastic premises that for centuries had delineated its thought and activity.
After having wandered amid the complexities of abstruse
system formulations that had transformed therapeutics into
intellectualized busy-work dedicated to "truth," doctors now
emerged relatively free of rationalistic thinking and prepared to follow a more rigorous pragmatism. Moreover, evolutionary theory became a welcome kinsman to medicine's
expanded definition as it moved to encompass prevention as
well as cure. By the dawn of the twentieth century, sanitary
science had become a recurring theme in the shaping of pub-
lic-health legislation. Stressing unremitting observation and
thorough testing of hypotheses, the proponents of sanitary
science saw medicine impregnated with a new consciousness
of social values. The process of growth, improvement, and
progress became less the subject of theological or metaphysical discussion and more the practical obligation of human
endeavor.

All of this was perhaps distant from the original intent of
Darwin's thesis. But not really. Just as the eighteenth century
had witnessed the application of physics, government, and
the "natural" man to the Newtonian world-machine, so also
the nineteenth century undertook a step-by-step application
of the biological, social, and behavioral sciences to a Darwinian universe. Darwin's interpreters provided society with an
optimistic assurance of stability amid the uncertainties of

change by offering the promise of improved health—if not a new and better citizen—as a result of the evolutionary formula. The philosophic climate of evolution forced the intellect to accept possibilities only hinted at before and which existed for the harmony of the individual in society. So considered, Darwin's theory of natural selection demonstrated not only a new way of interpreting life, but also a new method of employing intelligence in problem solving. Although the theory began as a mechanism for explaining transformation, it soon provided the intellectual equipment in ideas necessary to articulate the needs of society during medicine's coming of age.

9

Problems and Prospects

ALTHOUGH THE MEDICAL ACHIEVEMENTS of the nineteenth century were formidable, as doctors made conspicuous departures from the orthodox positions of previous system-builders, their achievements did not bring wisdom beyond years. Medicine's coming of age brought immaturity along with strength, and together these characteristics helped plot a course between old ways and new ideals. It is important, therefore, not to judge medicine's emergence into the modern world as simply a reflection of the scientific and philosophical triumphs that labeled the century; one must also consider the reinforcements, associations, and deviations that were common to the age and its doctors. From this perspective, nineteenth-century medicine was as much a record of experiences that deviated from the spirit and texture of the age as a paean to the creative activities of its intellectuals. Both tendencies grew side by side and occasionally intersected to obscure careful delineation. Medical practices formed an aggregation of particular ways in which physicians answered practical needs—practices that were borrowed from the past, modified, and combined with new techniques or were abandoned altogether according to chance or circumstance.

The period from 1840 to 1910 provided a rich inheritance for the twentieth century by leaving a wealth of information from which opinions could be checked against experience and doctrinal pretenses. The search for "systems" continued to tempt a few, but more and more doctors seemed content to replace them with case studies, using the inductive procedures of laboratory research. Contributors to the art and science of medicine worked to fit the pieces of the human organism into a coherent relationship and in doing so brought new standards of rigor to medical discourse. Though doctors failed to speak with one voice, they nevertheless agreed that while logic and theory were essential parts of the scientific method, their reliability rested utimately on relevant methods of observation. The strength of this position, though often subject to bitter debate, provided the impetus that took the "art" of medicine to the frontiers of "science."

One unpredicted by-product crept in upon the twentieth century unheralded. The scientific method Darwin, Bernard, Maudsley, and Flexner had encouraged as the basis of intellectual thinking burst forth upon a nonscientific culture unable to accommodate to change in the same spirit as the scientific community. Moreover, the nonscientific culture became increasingly mystified by the tools and techniques of the new medical sciences; and doctors, for their part, did little to enlighten their patients. Clearly the power of the medical profession was in no small way related to the aura of truth with which doctors surrounded themselves. Though surely not an objective of Darwin's methodology, some of the temper of classic philosophy clung to the coattails of twentieth-century medicine. Rather than freeing men from bias and enlarging their perceptions, medicine and its purveyors became overly pretentious and, worse, arrogant in authority and demanding in privilege. The professionalization of medicine that absorbed the energies of nineteenth-century doctors succeeded in transforming the profession into an unprogressive caste tied to a technological revolution.

Unlike the ages that had preceded it, the twentieth century gave doctors and their patients one technological breakthrough after another—all of which created a somewhat deceptive picture of what medicine could and could not accomplish. On the positive side, it demonstrated a remarkable ability to purchase health advantages that previous generations could only imagine. But while enriching the age with its materialistic capabilities, it often blinded scientists to the humanity before them. This was especially evident as doctors assumed added importance in society at the same time as the tools of their profession were removing them farther from the patient. The age became one of progressive specialization in particulars that added to the total sum of knowledge but produced minds reluctant to stray beyond narrow corridors of vision. Discussion, let alone contemplation of the whole, received only the most superficial treatment, a symptom of the age's fear of abstractions. As a result, medical breakthroughs that touched human hopes and resignations at critical junctures seemed often to misconnect for lack of a human touch.

So rapid has been the pace of medical innovation in the twentieth century that larger issues have appeared only as coincidental happenings bearing an unfortunate likeness to fads that burn quickly and are forgotten until another generation. It is questionable whether ethical or aesthetic issues will ever bring medicine into meaningful dialogue with itself and the nonscientific culture. The assumption by the federal government of these responsibilities has thus far only substituted inanimate forms and impersonal committee action for what should be acts of individual conscience. The fear is that medicine will proceed on a course that, with few lapses of self-doubt, will carry society into an unquestioning but highly productive era of medical technology void of ethical and aesthetic discussion. The extent to which medicine has been devoid of these issues speaks to the strife that already abounds. The growth of positive knowledge and of the spirit of inquiry has brought untold advantages to medicine by developing a method of rational investigation that placed verifiability on the side of new knowledge. But knowledge in and of itself is no substitute for the human side of medical care. As Maudsley observed, "science has not rendered the philosopher, the poet, and the moral teacher superfluous, nor will it ever supersede them; on the contrary, it will have need of them to attain . . . the bettering of man's estate . . . which the labored acquisitions of science will ever fail to satisfy."[1] Questions of ethics and aesthetics extend backward through time as footnotes to Plato and will exist into the future—if society is willing to accept questions without answers and ideals never to be realized.

The question of new directions, of change, and of leadership need also to be addressed. For better or worse, governments have become steadily more important forces in health care. They have had enormous influence over the size, education, research, and services of the profession; and their regulatory powers will continue to exercise a wide discretionary role. At question in the United States is whether the profession will be permitted to implement change (i.e., choose when and how to achieve its stated goals) as it did at the time of Flexner or will relinquish both direction and process of health-care issues to federal prerogative.

As federal support of education, services, and research replace philanthropic spending, both the function and role of private funding have taken a back seat to "planning" operations within the federal bureaucracy. While such planning is justified on the basis of goals that are national and social in scope, at question is whether there is true "vision" in government planning, since public servants, whose activities are caught up in a plethora of detail, fail miserably in the larger comprehension of human life. Nevertheless, governmental authority is bound to be more widespread than before—the magnitude can only be guessed. The future direction of American medicine can be found in a review of present and past politics and the profusion of social planning that has become the byword of federal involvement in the nation's health care.

Appendix A

Table of States and Territories Showing the Relation between Population and the Number of Physicians.

(From J. Howe Adams, "The Physicians of the United States," *Medical Times*, XXV [1907], 107.)

	POPULATION	PHYSICIANS	RATIO 1 TO
Dist. of Columbia	278,718	1,086	255
Colorado	539,700	1,670	323
California	1,485,053	4,369	340
Indian Territory	391,960	1,049	373
Oklahoma	398,331	1,003	397
Arkansas	1,310,564	2,780	471
Vermont	343,641	724	477
Missouri	3,106,665	6,439	481
Indiana	2,516,462	5,203	483
Ohio	4,157,545	8,582	486
Illinois	4,821,550	9,609	502
Tennessee	2,020,616	3,802	505
Arizona	122,212	339	511
Oregon	413,536	807	512
Massachusetts	2,805,346	5,434	514
West Virginia	958,800	1,845	519
Maryland	1,190,050	2,258	531
Texas	3,048,710	5,694	533
Maine	694,466	1,295	537
Michigan	2,530,016	4,651	544
New Hampshire	411,588	735	559
Kansas	1,544,968	2,732	565
New York	8,067,308	14,238	566
Pennsylvania	6,302,115	10,954	575
Kentucky	2,147,174	3,628	578
Iowa	2,231,853	3,835	582
Rhode Island	428,556	715	596
Connecticut	908,355	1,494	607
Florida	528,542	786	672
Delaware	184,735	267	691

	POPULATION	PHYSICIANS	RATIO 1 TO
New Mexico	195,310	281	695
Wyoming	101,816	147	719
Washington	874,310	1,158	755
Georgia	2,216,331	2,855	776
Utah	276,749	351	788
Virginia	1,854,184	2,293	808
New Jersey	2,144,143	2,634	814
Louisiana	1,381,625	1,664	820
Wisconsin	2,228,949	2,660	838
South Dakota	455,185	536	849
Alabama	1,828,697	2,261	852
Idaho	250,000	284	880
Mississippi	1,551,270	1,749	889
Minnesota	1,979,912	2,141	924
North Dakota	437,070	446	980
North Carolina	1,893,810	1,812	1,045
South Carolina	1,340,316	1,255	1,067
Alaska	63,592	57	1,106
Hawaii	154,000	106	1,452
Puerto Rico	953,243	172	5,540
Philippines	7,635,426	578	13,210

Appendix B

Table Showing Numerical Strength of Theology, Law, and Medicine in the United States, 1850–70; the Proportion Each Bears to the Whole Population; and the Mortality of Each for the Year 1970.

(From J. M. Toner, "Statistical Sketch of the Medical Profession of the United States," *Indiana Journal of Medicine*, IV [1873], 14–17.)

STATES AND TERRITORIES	PROFESSION (C = CLERGY; L = LAWYERS; P = PHYSICIANS)	1850	1860	1870	RATIO TO 1870 POPULA- TION	DEATHS IN 1870
Alabama	C	702	877	821	1,204	19
	L	570	763	758	1,305	14
	P	1,264	1,760	1,418	703	30
Arizona	C	0	0	7	1,399.7	0
	L	0	0	21	459.9	0
	P	0	0	22	439	0
Arkansas	C	233	494	397	1,220	2
	L	224	467	413	1,173	9
	P	419	1,222	1,026	481.8	11
California	C	36	348	569	984.6	17
	L	191	894	1,115	502.4	29
	P	626	1,138	1,257	445.7	28
Colorado	C	0	11	54	737	0
	L	0	89	99	402.6	3
	P	0	116	70	569.5	4
Connecticut	C	705	878	908	591.9	10
	L	289	468	391	1,374.5	9
	P	560	716	680	790.3	14
Dakota	C	0	4	16	886	0
	L	0	8	23	616	5
	P	0	0	20	709	0

STATES AND TERRITORIES	PROFESSION (C = CLERGY; L = LAWYERS; P = PHYSICIANS)	1850	1860	1870	RATIO TO 1870 POPULA- TION	DEATHS IN 1870
Delaware	C	79	110	150	833	4
	L	46	87	84	488	1
	P	114	154	170	735	0
Dist.	C	94	71	174	756.9	0
Columbia	L	99	189	411	320.4	6
	P	104	148	326	404	1
Florida	C	83	159	197	953	7
	L	131	173	149	1,260	5
	P	135	268	248	757	4
Georgia	C	715	1,015	953	1,242	15
	L	711	1,168	851	1,390	12
	P	1,295	2,004	1,537	770	30
[Idaho]	C	0	0	6	2,499.9	0
	L	0	0	42	357	3
	P	0	0	33	454	0
Illinois	C	1,023	1,880	3,192	795	33
	L	817	1,602	2,683	946	31
	L	1,402	2,867	4,862	522	45
Indiana	C	1,063	1,459	1,787	940	27
	L	924	1,219	1,685	997	17
	P	2,170	2,540	3,613	465	35
Iowa	C	248	1,208	1,596	746	19
	L	272	1,161	1,456	818	8
	P	542	2,552	1,865	639	29
Kansas	C	0	207	538	677	9
	L	0	361	682	534	6
	P	0	376	906	402	10
Kentucky	C	931	1,150	1,080	1,223	10
	L	995	1,190	1,552	850	20
	P	1,818	2,198	2,414	547	32
Louisiana	C	229	333	404	1,799	8
	L	622	689	663	1,096	13
	P	912	1,149	939	774	20

STATES AND TERRITORIES	PROFESSION (C = CLERGY; L = LAWYERS; P = PHYSICIANS)	1850	1860	1870	RATIO TO 1870 POPULA- TION	DEATHS IN 1870
Maine	C	928	1,059	890	715	12
	L	560	646	558	1,121	12
	P	659	798	818	766	13
Maryland	C	453	731	938	831	13
	L	535	599	772	1,011	16
	P	990	1,108	1,257	621	23
Massachusetts	C	1,662	1,913	2,040	714	41
	L	1,111	1,186	1,270	1,147	30
	P	1,643	1,821	2,047	711	42
Michigan	C	557	1,046	1,430	828	17
	L	560	791	1,167	1,014	23
	P	854	1,285	2,034	582	23
Minnesota	C	32	311	620	709	10
	L	23	407	449	979	2
	P	13	252	402	1,093	2
Mississippi	C	471	693	749	1,105	7
	L	590	620	632	1,310	14
	P	1,217	1,708	1,511	547	20
Missouri	C	814	1,280	1,739	989	30
	L	687	1,187	3,452	498	13
	P	1,351	2,543	3,560	483	40
Montana	C	0	0	19	1,084	0
	L	0	0	23	895	1
	P	0	0	42	490	1
Nebraska	C	0	57	183	672	2
	L	0	130	204	602	2
	P	0	127	247	498	1
Nevada	C	0	0	35	1,214	0
	L	0	18	166	262	2
	P	0	21	110	386	1
New Hampshire	C	649	641	664	479	10
	L	326	375	349	820	10
	P	623	591	565	563	20

STATES AND TERRITORIES	PROFESSION (C = CLERGY; L = LAWYERS; P = PHYSICIANS)	1850	1860	1870	RATIO TO 1870 POPULA- TION	DEATHS IN 1870
New Jersey	C	650	856	1,236	733	15
	L	412	537	888	1,020	13
	P	608	865	1,208	750	20
New Mexico	C	24	37	51	1,801	0
	L	11	23	48	1,914	1
	P	9	14	27	3,402	0
New York	C	4,290	5,235	5,678	722	72
	L	4,263	5,592	5,913	743	114
	P	5,060	6,390	6,810	642	136
North Carolina	C	747	907	861	1,244	16
	L	399	500	574	1,866	10
	P	1,083	1,266	1,143	937	15
Ohio	C	2,440	2,927	3,572	746	46
	L	2,028	2,537	2,563	1,039	31
	P	4,263	4,238	4,638	574	66
Oregon	C	29	125	162	561	3
	L	22	104	194	468	0
	P	45	115	206	441	5
Pennsylvania	C	2,789	3,396	3,841	916	57
	L	2,503	2,414	3,253	1,082	50
	P	4,071	4,399	4,843	727	94
Rhode Island	C	193	231	250	869	2
	L	114	96	163	1,332	1
	P	217	225	260	836	5
South Carolina	C	474	586	553	1,458	13
	L	397	457	387	1,823	7
	P	905	1,116	789	894	10
Tennessee	C	1,081	1,186	1,256	1,002	13
	L	725	1,037	1,126	1,117	17
	P	1,523	2,240	2,220	566	23
Texas	C	308	758	831	985	9
	L	429	904	1,027	797	9
	P	616	1,476	1,906	429	33

STATES AND TERRITORIES	PROFESSION (C = CLERGY; L = LAWYERS; P = PHYSICIANS)	1850	1860	1870	RATIO TO 1870 POPULATION	DEATHS IN 1870
Utah	C	3	12	47	1,846	1
	L	5	8	23	3,904	0
	P	16	14	46	1,886	0
Vermont	C	619	631	591	559	9
	L	494	0	72	4,591	4
	P	663	594	569	580	9
Virginia	C	1,087	1,437	1,073	1,141	23
	L	1,384	1,341	1,075	1,139	15
	P	2,163	2,607	2,126	576	35
Washington	C	0	26	50	478	0
	L	0	22	56	428	0
	P	0	22	43	557	1
West Virginia	C	0	0	466	948	7
	L	0	0	400	1,105	3
	P	0	0	612	722	4
Wisconsin	C	401	1,243	1,189	887	18
	L	471	1,133	785	1,345	12
	P	581	1,110	915	1,043	22
Wyoming	C	0	0	11	829	1
	L	0	0	25	365	0
	P	0	0	24	380	0
Total No. of each	C			43,874	878	571
	L			40,736	946	552
	P			62,383	618	947

Notes

CHAPTER ONE

Every Man in His Humor

1. Background information on the humors can be found in William B. Tucker and William A. Lessa, "Man: A Constitutional Investigation," *Quarterly Review of Biology*, III (1940), 265–89; 411–55; Ralph H. Major, *A History of Medicine* (2 vols.; Springfield, Ill., 1954), I, 111–12, 123, 192; Fielding H. Garrison, *An Introduction to the History of Medicine* (Philadelphia, 1929), 88–89, 114, 270; Esmond R. Long, *A History of Pathology* (New York, 1965), 6–7; Lester S. King, *The Growth of Medical Thought* (Chicago, 1963), 27–31, 82–83; Logan Clendening, *Source Book of Medical History* (New York, 1942), 39; Brian Inglis, *A History of Medicine* (Cleveland, 1965), 29–30; Sir William Osler, *The Evolution of Modern Medicine: A Series of Lectures* (New Haven, 1921), 67; P. M. Mehta, "Origin, Growth, Decline and Re-emergence of the Humoral Tridosha Concept," *Nagarjun*, XIX (1975), 1–5; A. Hameed (ed.), *Theories and Philosophies of Medicine* (New Delhi, 1973), 64–65, 84, 179–83.

2. Quoted in Thomas W. Blatchford, "The History of the Temperaments," *Transactions*, Medical Society of the State of New York, VII (1847–49), 49–50; Arturo Castiglioni, *A History of Medicine* (New York, 1958), 134, 160, 162; W. F. Hardie, "Aristotle's Treatment of the Relation Between the Soul and the Body," *Philosophical Quarterly*, XIV (1964), 53–74.

3. Osler, *The Evolution of Modern Medicine: A Series of Lectures*, 67–68; George Sarton, *Galen of Pergamon* (Lawrence, Kans., 1954), 52–53; William H. S. Jones (trans.), *Hippocrates*, 4 vols. (Cambridge, Mass., 1939–45), I, 1–41; Richard H. Shryock, "The Interplay of Social and Internal Factors in Modern Medicine," *Centaurus*, III (1953), 113–18; Jerry Stannard, "Materia Medica and Philosophic Theory in Aretaeus," *Sudhoffs Archiv für Geschichte der Medizin und der Naturwissenschaften*, XLVIII (1964), 27–53; Owsei Temkin, "Fer-

nel, Joubert, and Erastus on the Specificity of Cathartic Drugs," in Allen G. Debus (ed.), *Science, Medicine and Society in the Renaissance: Essays to Honor Walter Pagel*, 2 vols. (New York, 1972), I, 61–67.

4. Blatchford, "History of the Temperaments," 49.

5. D. W. Yandell, "Temperament," *American Practitioner and News*, n.s. XIII (1892), 194; R. Cream, "Temperament in Relation to Disease," *Health Lectures for the People* (1887), 34.

6. Yandell, "Temperament," 195; Rosaleen Love, "Herman Boerhaave and the Element-Instrument Concept of Fire," *Annals of Science*, XXXI (1974), 547–59.

7. John W. Draper, "The Humors: Some Psychological Aspects of Shakespeare's Tragedies," *JAMA*, CLXXXVIII (1964), 259–62; id., *Humors and Shakespeare's Characters* (Durham, N.C., 1945); Nellie B. Eales, "The History of the Lymphatic System, with Special Reference to the Hunter-Monro Controversy," *Journal of the History of Medicine and Allied Sciences*, XXIX (1974), 280–94; Reginald S. A. Lord, "The White Veins: Conceptual Difficulties in the History of the Lymphatics," *Medical History*, XII (1968), 174–84.

8. Quoted in Varnum Collins, "Temperaments," *Dental Cosmos*, XI (1869), 229; William B. Powell, *The Natural History of the Temperaments; Their Laws in Relation to Marriage, and the Fatal Consequences of their Violation to Progeny, With Indications of Vigorous Life and Longevity: Followed by a Fugitive Essay on the Protection of Society Against Crime* (Cincinnati, 1856); J. S. Madden, "Melancholy in Medicine and Literature: Some Historical Considerations," *British Journal of Medical Psychology*, XXXIX (1966), 125–30.

9. Quoted in Madden, "Melancholy in Medicine and Literature," 127; George Rosen, "Nostalgia: A Forgotten Psychological Disorder," *Psychological Medicine*, V (1975), 340–54; John F. Sena, "Melancholic Madness and the Puritans," *Harvard Theological Review*, LXVI (1973), 293–309.

10. James Worrell, "Treatise on the Temperaments," *American Medical Recorder*, X (1826), 285–86; R. F. Timken-Zinkann, "Black Bile. A Review of Recent Attempts to Trace the Origin of the Teachings on Melancholy to Medical Observations," *Medical History*, XII (1968), 288–92; R. E. Siegel, "Melancholy and Black Bile in Galen and Later Writers," *Bulletin*, Cleveland Medical Library, XVIII (1971), 10–20; Lawrence Babb, *The Elizabethan Malady: A Study of Melancholia in English Literature from 1580 to 1642* (East Lansing, Mich., 1951); Raymond Klibansky, Erwin Panofsky, and Fritz Saxl, *Saturn and Melancholy: Studies in the History of Natural Philosophy, Religion and Art* (New York, 1964); T. J. Jobe, "Medical Theories of Melancholia in the 17th and early 18th Centuries," *Clio Medica*, XI (1976), 217–31.

11. Charles Heventhal, Jr., "Robert Burton's *Anatomy of Melan-*

choly in Early America," *Papers*, Bibliographical Society of America, LXIII (1969), 157–75; George Rosen, *Madness in Society: Chapters in the Historical Sociology of Mental Illness* (Chicago, 1968), 132–33, 236–37, 282.

12. Madeleine B. Stern, "Poe: 'The Mental Temperament' for Phrenologists," *American Literature*, XL (1968), 155–63; Robert Jones, "Temperaments: Is There a Neurotic One?" *Lancet*, XI (1911), 4.

13. A. P. Dutcher, "Lecture on the Temperaments: Their Influence Upon Mentality and Disease in General," *Medical and Surgical Reporter*, XV (1866), 451–52; Yandell, "Temperament," 195.

14. George M. Beard, "Neurasthenia, or Nervous Exhaustion," *Boston Medical and Surgical Journal*, III (1869), 217; George M. Beard, *American Nervousness, Its Causes and Consequences, a Supplement to Nervous Exhaustion (Neurasthenia)* (New York, 1881); John S. Haller, Jr., "Neurasthenia: Medical Profession and Urban 'Blahs,'" *New York State Journal of Medicine*, LXX (1970), 2489–97; Eric T. Carlson, "The Nerve Weakness of the 19th Century," *International Journal of Psychiatry*, IX (1970–71), 50–54; Charles Rosenberg, "The Place of George M. Beard in 19th Century Psychiatry," *Bulletin of the History of Medicine*, XXXVI (1962), 245–59.

15. F. Robinson, "On the Utility of a Knowledge of the Temperaments in Connexion with the Diagnosis and Treatment of Disease," *Lancet*, I (1846), 360–61; William Hamilton, *The History of Medicine, Surgery, and Anatomy, from the Creation of the World, to the Commencement of the Nineteenth Century*, 2 vols. (London, 1831), I, 146–50; Walter Riese, "The Structure of Galen's Diagnostic Reasoning," *Bulletin*, New York Academy of Medicine, XLIV (1968), 778–91; Owsei Temkin, *Galenism: Rise and Decline of a Medical Philosophy* (Ithaca, N.Y., 1973).

16. Walter Pagel, *Paracelsus: An Introduction to Philosophical Medicine in the Era of the Renaissance* (New York, 1958), 129; Edward G. Browne, *Arabian Medicine* (Cambridge, 1962), 44, 116–17, 120–22; Henry E. Sigerist, *The Great Doctors: A Biographical History of Medicine* (New York, 1933), 116; Walter Pagel, "Van Helmont's Concept of Disease—To Be or Not to Be? The Influence of Paracelsus," *Bulletin of the History of Medicine*, XLVI (1972), 419–54.

17. Long, *A History of Pathology*, 73–74; Lester S. King, *The Medical World of the Eighteenth Century* (New York, 1958), 59–93; Gerrit A. Lindeboom, *Herman Boerhaave: The Man and His Work* (London, 1968), 264–81; Donald E. H. Campbell, *Arabian Medicine and Its Influence on the Middle Ages*, 2 vols. (London, 1926), I, 1–13, 114–15, 152–53; Lester S. King, "Medical Theory and Practice at the Beginning of the Eighteenth Century," *Bulletin of the History of Medicine*, XLVI (1972), 1–15; Saul Jarcho, "Boerhaave on Inflamma-

tion," *American Journal of Cardiology*, XXV (1970), 244–46, 480–82; Lester S. King, "Attitudes Toward 'Scientific' Medicine Around 1700," *Bulletin of the History of Medicine*, XXXIX (1965), 124–33; Lester S. King, "Changing Concept of Scientific Medicine," *Bulletin*, Harvard Medical School Alumni Association, XLII (1968), 8–11; G. A. Lindeboom, "Boerhaave's Concept of Basic Structure of the Body," *Clio Medica*, V (1970), 203–8.

18. Blatchford, "History of the Temperaments," 53–54; George E. Stahl, *Neu-verbesserte Lehre von den Temperamenten* (Leipzig, 1723); Alexander Wilder, *History of Medicine* (Augusta, Me., 1901), 228; Sigerist, *The Great Doctors*, 199–201; Lelland J. Rather, *Mind and Body in Eighteenth Century Medicine: A Study Based on Jerome Gaub's* De Regimine Mentis (Berkeley, 1965), 85–97; Castiglioni, *History of Medicine*, 583; Theodore M. Brown, "From Mechanism to Vitalism in 18th Century English Physiology," *Journal of the History of Biology*, VII (1974), 179–216; Elizabeth L. Haigh, "Vitalism, the Soul, and Sensibility: The Physiology of Théophile Bordeu," *Journal of the History of Medicine and Allied Sciences*, XXXI (1976), 30–34; Lester S. King, "Stahl and Hoffman: A Study in 18th Century Animism," ibid., XIX (1964), 118–30.

19. Quoted in Blatchford, "History of the Temperaments," 54; Castiglioni, *History of Medicine*, 673; Lester S. King, "Basic Concepts of Early 18th Century Animism," *American Journal of Psychiatry*, CXXIV (1967), 797–802; Saul Jarcho, "Albrecht von Haller on Inflammation," *American Journal of Cardiology*, XXV (1970), 707–9.

20. Quoted in Inglis, *History of Medicine*, 129; G. M. Daniels, "Finalism and Positivism in 19th Century Physiological Thought," *Bulletin of the History of Medicine*, XXXVIII (1964), 343–63; Elizabeth Haigh, "The Roots of the Vitalism of Xavier Bichat," ibid., XLIX (1975), 72–86; Walter Pagel, "The Speculative Basis of Modern Pathology: Jahn, Virchow, and the Philosophy of Pathology," ibid., XVIII (1945), 3–40; Sigerist, *Great Doctors*, 337; George Rosen, "The Philosophy of Ideology and the Emergence of Modern Medicine in France," *Bulletin of the History of Medicine*, XIX (1946), 328–39; Owsei Temkin, "Basic Science, Medicine, and the Romantic Era," ibid., XXXVII (1963), 97–128; Erwin H. Ackerknecht, "Broussais, or a Forgotten Medical Revolution," ibid., XXVII (1953), 320–43; E. Benton, "Vitalism in 19th Century Scientific Thought: A Typology and Reassessment," *Studies in the History and Philosophy of Science*, V (1974), 17–48; J. J. Nierstrasz, "General Pathology and Therapy of Inflammations in the 1860's," *Janus*, LIV (1967), 168–82.

21. John D. Davies, *Phrenology: Fad and Science; A Nineteenth Century American Crusade* (New Haven, 1955), 4; Owsei Temkin, "Gall and the Phrenological Movement," *Bulletin of the History of Medi-*

cine, XXI (1947), 275–321; Robert E. Riegel, "Early Phrenology in the United States," *Medical Life*, XXXVII (1930), 361–76; Erwin H. Ackerknecht and Henri V. Vallois, *Franz Joseph Gall, Inventor of Phrenology and His Collection* (Madison, Wis., 1956), 8, 10, 32, 83–84; Frances Hedderly, *Phrenology: A Study of the Mind* (London, 1970); Nahum Capen, *Reminiscences of Dr. Spurzheim and George Combe; And a Review of the Science of Phrenology, From the Period of its Discovery by Dr. Gall, to the Time of the Visit of George Combe to the United States, 1838, 1840* (London, n.d.); John G. Spurzheim, *Outlines of Phrenology* (Boston, 1834); T. M. Parssinen, "Popular Science and Society: The Phrenology Movement in Early Victorian Britain," *Journal of Social History*, VIII (1974), 1–20; Anthony A. Walsh, "The 'New Science of the Mind' and the Philadelphia Physicians in the Early 1800s," *Transactions and Studies*, College of Physicians of Philadelphia, XLIII (1976), 397–415; R. J. Cooter, "Phrenology: The Provocation of Progress," *History of Science*, XIV (1976), 211–34.

22. A. Gribben, "Mark Twain, Phrenology and the Temperaments: A Study of Pseudo-Scientific Influence," *American Quarterly*, XXIV (1972), 45–68; Brian Inglis, *Fringe Medicine* (London, 1964); Alastair C. Grant, "Combe on Phrenology and Free Will: A Notion on Nineteenth Century Secularism," *Journal of the History of Ideas*, XXVI (1965), 141–47; Davies, *Phrenology: Fad and Science*, 34–38, 118–25, 135–48; Robert E. Riegel, "The Introduction of Phrenology to the United States," *American Historical Review*, XXXIX (1933–34), 73–78; Charles Caldwell, *Elements of Phrenology* (Lexington, Ky., 1824); George Combe, *The Constitution of Man Considered in Relation to External Objects* (Boston, 1833); George Combe, *Elements of Phrenology* (Boston, 1834); Ackerknecht and Vallois, *Franz Joseph Gall*, 33, 36; Graeme D. C. Tytler, *Character Description and Physiognomy in the European Novel (1800–1860) in Relation to J. C. Lavater's Physiognomische Fragmente* (Ph.D. diss., Urbana, 1970).

23. David de Guistino, *Conquest of Mind: Phrenology and Victorian Social Thought* (London, 1975), 47–48, 91–93; Davies, *Phrenology: Fad and Science*, 30–65; Madeleine Stern, *Heads and Headlines: The Phrenological Fowlers* (Norman, Okla., 1971); Orson Fowler, *Phrenology Proved, Illustrated and Applied, Accompanied by a Chart* (New York, 1851); Orson Fowler, *The Practical Phrenologist: A Recorder and Delineator of the Character and Talents . . . A Compendium of Phreno-Organic Science* (Boston, 1869); Lyman Allen, "Some Remarks on Prof. A. P. Dutcher's Lecture on Temperaments," *Medical and Surgical Reporter*, XVI (1867), 38; Collins, "Temperaments," 308–9; Lorenzo N. Fowler, *Temperaments: Their Classification and Importance* (London, 1864).

24. Webb Haymaker and Francis Schiller (eds.), *The Founders of Neurology: One Hundred and Forty-Six Biographical Sketches by Eighty-Eight Authors* (Springfield, Ill., 1970), 31; H. Tristram Engelhardt, Jr., "John Hughlings Jackson and the Mind-Body Relation," *Bulletin of the History of Medicine*, XLIV (1975), 137–51.

25. Carl von Linnaeus, *A General System of Nature, Through the Three Grand Kingdoms of Animals, Vegetables, and Minerals*, 7 vols., (London, 1806), I, 9.

26. Daniel H. Jacques, *The Temperaments; Or, the Varieties of Physical Constitution in Man, Considered in Their Relations to Mental Character and the Practical Affairs of Life* (New York, 1884), 199–202; Guistino, *Conquest of Mind*, 68–72.

27. John S. Haller, *Outcasts from Evolution: Scientific Attitudes of Racial Inferiority, 1859–1900* (Urbana, 1971), v–ix.

28. Robert Jones, "Temperaments: Is There a Neurotic One?" *Lancet*, XI (1911), 1.

29. F. H. Garrison, "Constitution and Characterology," *Bulletin*, New York Academy of Medicine, III (1927), 489; Ernst Kretschmer, *Physique and Character: An Investigation of the Nature of Constitution and of the Theory of Temperament* (New York, 1925); Charles Rosenberg, "The Practice of Medicine in New York a Century Ago," *Bulletin of the History of Medicine*, XLI (1967), 231–34.

30. A.M.A., *Code of Medical Ethics*, ch. 1, art. 2, par. 3. The homeopathic profession was likewise interested in this phenomenon and taught that correct delineation of temperament significantly modified the pathogenetic and therapeutic action of their triturated medicinal agents. Accordingly, homeopathic doctors urged their colleagues to thoroughly question patients for signs of temperament before prescribing medicine. See Rollin R. Gregg, "An Essay on Temperaments," *Philadelphia Journal of Homeopathy*, II (1853), 218–19.

31. J. E. Moses, "Recognition of Temperament: A Factor to the Selection of Remedies and Their Dosage in Disease," *JAMA*, XXI (1898), 763–65; Siegel, "Melancholy and Black Bile in Galen and Later Writers," 14–16.

32. Collins, "Temperaments," 231; Michael O. Jones, "Climate and Disease: The Traveller Describes America," *Bulletin of the History of Medicine*, XLI (1967), 254–66.

33. Beddoe, "On the Relation of Temperament and Complexion to Disease," 434; Kenneth M. Flegel, "Changing Concepts of the Nosology of Gonorrhea and Syphilis," *Bulletin of the History of Medicine*, XLVIII (1974), 571–88; Rosenberg, "The Practice of Medicine in New York a Century Ago," 235–40.

34. Dutcher, "Lecture on the Temperaments," 450–51; Worrell,

"Treatise on the Temperaments," 284–85; Collins, "Temperaments," 228; Moses, "Recognition of Temperament," 765.

35. Dutcher, "Lecture on the Temperaments," 452; Worrell, "Treatise on the Temperaments," 285; Moses, "Recognition of Temperament," 765; Collins, "Temperaments," 226.

36. Jonathan Hutchinson, "Temperament, Idiosyncracy, and Diathesis in Relation to Surgical Disease," *Medical Press and Circular*, XXX (1882), 523.

37. Worrell, "Treatise on Temperaments," 285; Cream, "Temperament in Relation to Disease," 37; Yandell, "Temperament," 195; Collins, "Temperaments," 226–27; Moses, "Recognition of Temperament," 765; Dutcher, "Lecture on the Temperaments," 450.

38. W. H. Sheldon, "The Lymphatic Constitution," *Wisconsin Medical Journal*, II (1904), 472; J. R. Bryan and J. Walsh, "Lymphatic Constitution," *Proceedings*, Pathological Society of Philadelphia, n.s. II (1898–99), 216–17; J. Hogarth Pringle, "Notes on the Lymphatic Constitution," *Glasgow Medical Journal*, LI (1899), 351–56.

39. Dutcher, "Lecture on the Temperaments," 452; Moses, "Recognition of Temperament," 765.

40. Alexander Stewart, *Our Temperaments: Their Study and Their Teaching* (London, 1887), 387; A. R. Mitchell, "Temperaments," *Western Medical Review*, I (1896), 201; Mutual Life Insurance Co. of New York, *Instructions to the Medical Examiners of the Medical Insurance Company of New York* (New York, 1866).

41. Charles J. Stillé, *History of the United States Sanitary Commission, Being a General Report of Its Work during the War of the Rebellion* (Phila., 1866), 84; Haller, *Outcasts From Evolution*, 20–32.

42. Charles Darwin, *The Descent of Man and Selection in Relation to Sex* (London, 1871), 553.

43. Ely Van de Warker, "Temperaments," *Popular Science Monthly*, XII (1877–78), 307–11; Jedediah H. Baxter, *Statistics, Medical and Anthropological of the Provost-Marshall-General's Bureau*, 2 vols. (Washington, D.C., 1875); Francis Galton, *A Descriptive List of Anthropometric Apparatus, Consisting of Instruments for Measuring and Testing the Chief Physical Characteristics of the Human Body* (Cambridge, 1887), 3.

44. Van de Warker, "Temperaments," 310; George Owen Rees, *On the Analysis of the Blood and Urine, in Health and Disease; With Directions for the Analysis of Urinary Calculi* (London, 1836); Louis-René LeCanu, *Études chimiques sur le sang humain* (Paris, 1837).

45. Long, *History of Pathology*, 107–8; Karl von Rokitansky, *Manual of Pathological Anatomy* (London, 1849–54); Rudolph L. K. Vir-

chow, *Cellular Pathology as Based upon Physiological and Pathological Histology* (New York, 1860); Jerome Tarshis, *Claude Bernard: Father of Experimental Medicine* (New York, 1968), 94–95; Artur Biedl, *The Internal Secretory Organs: Their Physiology and Pathology* (London, 1912); Wilhelm Falta, *Endocrine Diseases: Including Their Diagnosis and Treatment* (Phila., 1923); Robert J. Miciotto, "Carl Rokitansky: A Reassessment of the Hematohumoral Theory of Disease," *Bulletin of the History of Medicine*, LII (1978), 183–99.

46. Reino Virtanen, "Claude Bernard and the History of Ideas," in Francisco Grande and Maurice B. Visscher (eds.), *Claude Bernard and Experimental Medicine: Collected Papers from a Symposium Commemorating the Centenary of the Publication of* An Introduction to the Study of Experimental Medicine (Cambridge, Mass., 1967), 21. See also James Pi-Sunyer, "De la Physiologie Genérale," ibid., 171–78; Frederick L. Holmes, "Origins of the Concept of Milieu Intérieur," ibid., 179–91; Hans Selye, *The Stress of Life* (New York, 1956), 205; Iago Galdston, "The Concept of the Specific in Medicine," *Transactions and Studies*, College of Physicians of Philadelphia, IX (1941), 25–34.

47. Hutchinson, "Temperament, Idiosyncracy, and Diathesis in Relation to Surgical Disease," 503; French E. Chadwick, *Temperament, Disease and Health* (New York, 1892).

48. F. B. Stephenson, "Temperament and Diathesis in Disease," *Medical Record*, XXXIV (1888), 615.

49. Quoted in Fielding H. Garrison, *Contributions to the History of Medicine* (New York, 1966), 362.

50. Quoted in Homer Wakefield, "A Dissertation on Temperament," *American Medicine*, IX (1905), 434.

51. Hutchinson, "Temperament, Idiosyncracy, and Diathesis in Relation to Surgical Disease," 44, 170; G. V. Mann, "The Concept of Predisposition," *Archives of Environmental Health*, VIII (1964), 840–45; K. W. Starr, "Diathesis in Human Disease," *Postgraduate Medicine*, XXXV (1964), 115–16; Oliver W. Holmes, "The Young Practitioner," *The Writings of Oliver Wendell Holmes*, 14 vols. (Boston, 1911), IX, 377.

52. Quoted in Collins, "Temperaments," 226.

53. Knud H. Faber, *Nosography in Modern Internal Medicine* (New York, 1923), 194.

54. Quoted in ibid., 183; Max H. Lewandowsky, *Praktische neurologie, für ärzte* (Berlin, 1912).

55. Blatchford, "The History of the Temperaments," 57–58; F. Thomas de Troisvèvre, *Division naturelle des tempéramens, tirée de la fonctinomie* (Paris, 1821); F. Thomas de Troisvèvre, *Physiologie des tempéramens ou constitutions; nouvelle doctrine applicable à la médicine—practique, à l'hygiène, à l'histoire naturelle et à la philosophie; pré-*

cédée d 'un examen des diverses théories des tempéramens (Paris, 1826); Arturo Castiglioni, "Neo-Hippocratic Tendency of Contemporary Medical Thought," *Medical Life*, XLI (1934), 115–46.

56. George Draper, *Acute Anterior Poliomyelitis* (Phila., 1917).

57. George Draper, *Human Constitution: A Consideration of Its Relationship to Disease* (Phila., 1924), 19. See Aleš Hrdlička, *Anthropometry* (Phila., 1920); Harris H. Wilder, *A Laboratory Manual of Anthropometry* (Phila., 1920); Lambert A. J. Quételet, *Anthropométrie ou Mesure des différentes facultés de l'homme* (Brussels, 1871); Paul Broca, *Mémoires d'Anthropologie de Paul Broca* (Paris, 1871); Giuseppe Sergi, *L'Uomo secondo le origini, l'antichita, le variazioni e la distribuzione geografica* (Turin, 1911); Paul Topinard, *L'Anthropologie* (Paris, 1877); Sir Arthur Keith, "The Evolution of Human Races in the Light of the Hormone Theory," *Bulletin*, Johns Hopkins Hospital, XXXIII (1922), 155.

58. Draper, *Human Constitution*, 28; Thomas Laycock, "Physiognomical Diagnosis," *Medical Times and Gazette*, I (1862), 1; Thomas Addison, *Collection of the Published Writings of the Late Thomas Addison, M.D., Physician to Guy's Hospital* (London, 1868); Sir Jonathan Hutchinson, *The Pedigree of Disease: Being Six Lectures on Temperament, Idiosyncracy and Diathesis* (London, 1884).

59. Draper, *Human Constitution*, 25. See also Achille deGiovanni, *Clinical Commentaries Deduced from the Morphology of the Human Body* (London, 1909).

60. Julius Bauer, *Constitutional Principles in Clinical Medicine* (New York, 1934); Julius Bauer, *Genetics in Cancer* (Lancaster, Pa., 1934); Karl Pearson, "Report on Certain Cancer Statistics," *Archives of the Middlesex Hospital*, II (1904), 127–37; Karl Pearson, *A First Study of the Statistics of Pulmonary Tuberculosis* (London, 1907); Karl Pearson, *On the Relationship of Health to the Psychical and Physical Characters in School Children* (Cambridge, 1923).

61. Guistino, *Conquest of Mind*, 145–52; Cesare Lombroso, *The Female Offender* (London, 1895); Blake McKelvey, *American Prisons: A Study in American Social History Prior to 1915* (Chicago, 1936), 27; Cesare Lombroso, *Crime, Its Causes and Remedies* (Boston, 1911); Davies, *Phrenology*, 98–115; Ackerknecht and Vallois, *Franz Joseph Gall*, 30; W. A. Lessa, "Somatomaney, Precursor of the Science of Human Constitution," *Scientific Monthly*, LXXV (1952), 355–65.

62. Robert A. Nye, "Heredity or Milieu: The Foundations of Modern European Theory," *Isis*, LXVII (1976), 335–55; Charles B. Goring, *The English Convict: A Statistical Study* (London, 1913); W. R. McDonell, "On Criminal Anthropometry and the Identification of Criminals," *Biometrika*, I (1901–2), 190; Edward Hitchcock, *The Need for Anthropometry. A Paper Read Before the American Association for the Advancement of Physical Education at its Second Annual*

Meeting in Brooklyn, New York, November 26, 1886 (n.p., 1887), 6–7;
T. S. Cloudston, "The Developmental Aspects of Criminal Anthropology," *Journal of the Anthropological Institute of Great Britain
and Ireland*, XXXIII (1893), 214–25.

63. See appendix of Francis Galton, *Inquiries into Human Faculty
and Its Development* (London, 1883); Derek W. Forrest, *Francis
Galton: The Life and Work of a Victorian Genius* (London, 1974),
133–48, 251–52.

64. Galton quoted in *Biometrika*, I (1901–2), 8, 9; Lindsay A. Far-
rall, "Controversy and Conflict in Science: A Case Study—the English Biometric School and Mendel's Laws," *Social Studies of Science*,
V (1975), 269–301.

65. See Karl Pearson, *National Life from the Standpoint of Science*
(London, 1905); id., *Darwinism, Medical Progress, and Eugenics*
(London, 1912).

66. Earnest A. Hooton, *Crime and the Man* (Cambridge, Mass.,
1939), 7.

67. Earnest A. Hooton, *The American Criminal: An Anthropological Study* (Cambridge, Mass., 1939), 3, 7.

68. Earnest A. Hooton, *Why Men Behave Like Apes and Vice Versa;
Or, Body and Behavior* (Princeton, 1940), 205; Sheldon and Eleanor
Glueck, *Juvenile Delinquents Grown Up* (New York, 1940), 272.

69. Eric T. Carlson, "The Influence of Phrenology on Early
American Psychiatric Thought," *American Journal of Psychiatry*,
CXV (1958), 535–38; David Bakan, "The Influence of Phrenology
on American Psychology," *Journal of the History of the Behavioral Sciences*, II (1966), 200–220; Benjamin Rush, *Medical Inquiries and Observations*, 4 vols. (Phila., 1794–98), IV, 54; Merle Curti, *The Growth
of American Thought* (New York, 1951), 361–62; George H. Daniels,
"Finalism and Positivism in Nineteenth Century American Psychological Thought," *Bulletin of the History of Medicine*, XXXVIII
(1964), 343–63; William James, *The Principles of Psychology*, 2 vols.
(New York, 1890), I, 27.

70. J. McK. Cattell and L. Farrand, "Physical and Mental Measurements of the Students of Columbia University," *Psychological
Review*, III (1896), 628. See also Edward Hitchcock and H. H.
Seeyle, *An Anthropometric Manual Giving the Average and Mean Mea-
surements and Tests of Male College Students and Methods of Securing
Them: Prepared from the Records of the Department of Physical Education
and Hygiene in Amherst College during the Years 1861–1862 and 1887–
1888 Inclusive* (Amherst, 1889), 4; Garrison, "Constitution and
Characterology," 489–95; Léon MacAuliffe, *Morphologie medicale:
Études des quatre types humains* (Paris, 1912); James A. Young, "Men-
tal Testing and Anthropometry in Early American Experimental
Psychology," *Synthesis* (1974), 35–48.

71. Ernst Kretschmer, *Physique and Character: An Investigation of the Nature of Constitution and of the Theory of Temperament*, 37.

72. Ibid., 103.

73. Ibid., 255.

74. Sigmund Freud, *New Introductory Lectures on Psychoanalysis* (New York, 1933), 210–11.

75. Henry W. Brosin, "Evolution and Understanding Diseases of the Mind," in Sol Tax (ed.), *The Evolution of Man* (Chicago, 1960), 373–422.

76. William H. Sheldon, *The Varieties of Human Physique: An Introduction to Constitutional Psychology* (New York, 1940), 28.

77. Ibid., 12–14, 58; Giacinto Viola, *Le Legge de Correlazione Morfologica dei Tippi Individuali* (Padua, 1909); Friedrich W. Beneke, *Die anatomische Grundlagen der Constitution-sanomalieen des Menschen* (Marburg, 1878).

78. Sheldon, *Varieties of Human Physique*, 238–43, 245–48; William H. Sheldon, *The Varieties of Temperament; A Psychology of Constitutional Differences* (New York, 1942), ix.

79. Garrison, "Constitution and Characterology," 489.

CHAPTER TWO

When Lancet Was King

1. G. W. Balfour, "An Episode in Medical History," *Edinburgh Medical Journal*, XL (1894–95), 578; William B. Fletcher, "A Glance at the History of Bloodletting," *Cincinnati Lancet and Observer*, VII (1864), 73–78.

2. John B. Huber, "Venesection," *Medical Times*, XXVIII (1910), 234; Mr. Wardrop, "The Diseases of the Sanguineous System," *Lancet*, I (1833–34), 236–37.

3. Balfour, "An Episode in Medical History," 578.

4. G. R. Hall, "Bloodletting: Its Past and Present Status," *Brooklyn Medical Journal*, XVI (1902), 312; Jerry Stannard, "Materia Medica and Philosophic Theory of Aretaeus," *Sudhoffs Archiv für Geschicte der Medizin und der Naturwissenschaften*, LXVIII (1964), 27–53.

5. T. K. Chambers, "The Bloodletting Question in Olden Times," *British and Foreign Medical-Chirurgical Review*, XXII (1858), 481; Huber, "Venesection," 235; Rudolph E. Siegel, "Galen's Concept of Bloodletting in Relation to His Ideas on Pulmonary and Peripheral Blood Flow and Blood Formation," in Allen G. Debus (ed.), *Science, Medicine and Society in the Renaissance: Essays to Honor Walter Pagel*, 2 vols. (New York, 1972), I, 243–75.

6. Huber, "Venesection," 235; W. Mitchell Clarke, "On the History of Bleeding and Its Disuse in Modern Practice," *British Medical Journal*, II (1875), 68; F. H. Garrison, "The History of Bloodletting," *New York Medical Journal*, XCVII (1913), 437.

7. Quoted in Joseph A. Eve,"Essay on Revulsion," *Southern Medical and Surgical Journal*, I (1837), 389.

8. Quoted in Garrison, "The History of Bloodletting," 435–36, 498–99.

9. Frederick A. Packard, "The Uses of Venesection," *University Medical Magazine*, VI (1893–94), 511; Carey P. McCord, "Bloodletting and Bandaging; Barber Surgery as an Occupation," *Archives of Environmental Health*, XX (1970), 555–58.

10. J. A. Hingeston, "The Neglect of the Use of Bleeding in the Treatment of Some of the Milder Ailments," *Association Medical Journal*, I (1854), 266.

11. John Wylie, "On Venesection," *Glasgow Medical Journal*, XIX (1883), 259; A. J. Campbell, "Venesection, or the Use of the Lancet," *Atlantic Medical Weekly*, VI (1896), 325; Hingeston, "The Neglect of the Use of Bleeding in the Treatment of some of the Milder Ailments," 267; E. Copeman, "On Bloodletting," *British Medical Journal*, II (1879), 933; James A. Leet, "Phlebotomy," *Transactions*, New Hampshire Medical Society (1897), 214–16.

12. Quoted in W. B. Giekie, "A Few Observations on the Past and Present Employment of Bleeding in the Treatment of Feeble and Inflammatory Diseases," *Canada Medical Journal and Monthly Record of Medical and Surgical Science*, VI (1870), 396.

13. Packard," The Uses of Venesection," 511; A. Lawrence Abel, "Bleeding Through the Ages," *Transactions*, Hunterian Society, XXVII (1968–69), 79–96.

14. Balfour, "An Episode in Medical History," 578.

15. C. C. Abernathy, "Blood-letting," *Nashville Journal of Medicine and Surgery*, VII (1871), 204.

16. Isaac Levene, "On the Therapeutic Value of Bloodletting—an Experimental Study," *Psychiatric Bulletin of the New York State Hospitals*, II (1897), 385–86; A. B. Davis, "Some Implications of the Circulation Theory for Disease Theory and Treatment in the Seventeenth Century," *Journal of the History of Medicine and Allied Sciences*, XXVI (1971), 28–39; Walter Pagel, "William Harvey Revisited," *History of Science*, VIII (1970), 1–31; Walter Pagel and Marianne Winder, "Harvey and the 'Modern' Concept of Disease," *Bulletin of the History of Medicine*, XLII (1968), 496–509.

17. Balfour, "An Episode in Medical History," 579; Levene, "On the Therapeutic Value of Bloodletting," 385–86.

18. Eve, "Essay on Revulsion," 395.

19. "Surgery," in *Encyclopaedia Britannica; Or, a Dictionary of Arts*

and Sciences Compiled Upon a New Plan, 3 vols. (Edinburgh, 1771), III, 643; John Reed, "On the Effects of Venesection in Renewing and Increasing the Heart's Action," *Edinburgh Medical and Surgical Journal*, XL (1836), 387–93; Wardrop, "The Diseases of the Sanguineous System," 237.

20. W. F. Barlow, "On the Value of Bloodletting as a Diagnostic," *Monthly Journal of Medicine*, III (1843), 762–83; B. M. Randolph, "The Blood-letting Controversy in the Nineteenth Century," *Annals of Medical History*, VII (1935), 178–79.

21. Wardrop, "The Diseases of the Sanguineous System," 242; John C. Hartnett, "The Care and Use of Medicinal Leeches in Nineteenth Century Pharmacy and Therapeutics," *Pharmacy in History*, XIV (1972), 127–38; John B. Beck, "On the Effects of Bloodletting on the Young Subject," *Analist*, II (1847), 105; George T. Elliot, "Remarks on Bloodletting," *New York Medical Journal*, XIII (1871), 283.

22. G. F. Knox, *The Art of Cupping; Being a Brief History of the Operation, From Its Origin to the Present Time; Its Utility, Minute Rules for Its Performance; A List of the Diseases in Which it is Most Beneficial; and a Description of the Various Instruments Employed* (London, 1836), 35.

23. S. Bayfield, *A Treatise of Practical Cupping: Comprising an Historical Relation of the Operation through Ancient and Modern Times; With a Copious and Minute Description of the Several Methods of Performing it: Intended for the Instruction of the Medical Student and of Practitioners in General* (London, 1823), 167; T. Mapleson, *A Treatise of the Art of Cupping in Which the History of That Operation is Traced; the Various Diseases in Which It is Useful Indicated; and the Most Approved Method of Performing It Described* (London, 1813), 24.

24. Knox, *The Art of Cupping*, 35.

25. M. Hills, "A Treatise on the Operation of Cupping," *Boston Medical and Surgical Journal*, IX (1833), 265.

26. Mapleson, *A Treatise of the Art of Cupping*, 1; H. A. Hare (ed.), *A System of Practical Therapeutics*, 2 vols. (Phila., 1892), II, 547, 583, 601, 623, 730, 816; Hills, "A Treatise on the Operation of Cupping," 273; W. A. Gillespie, "Remarks on the Operation of Cupping and the Instruments Best Adapted to Country Practice," *Boston Medical and Surgical Journal*, X (1834), 27.

27. Quoted in Huber, "Venesection," 297; Peter H. Niebyl, "Galen, Van Helmont, and Bloodletting," in Debus (ed.), *Science, Medicine and Society in the Renaissance*, II, 13–21; R. R. Trail, "Sydenham's Impact on English Medicine," *Medical History*, IX (1965), 356–64.

28. Quoted in "The Bloodletting Controversy," *British and Foreign Medico-Chirurgical Review*, XXII (1858), 4–5.

29. Quoted in C. D., "Remarks on Bloodletting," *New England*

Journal of Medicine, VII (1818), 155; Joseph Agassi, "The Concept of Scientific Theory as Illustrated by the Practice of Bloodletting," *Medical Opinion and Review*, V (1969), 156–69; Benjamin Rush, *Medical Inquiries and Observations*, 4 vols. (Phila., 1794–98), IV, 244–55.

30. J. B. Murfree, "Bloodletting as a Therapeutic Agent," *Nashville Journal of Medicine and Surgery*, XX (1861), 27; William P. Dewees, *A Practice of Physic* (Phila., 1833); R. H. Shryock, "Benjamin Rush from the Perspective of the Twentieth Century," *Transactions and Studies*, College of Physicians of Philadelphia, XIV (1946), 113–20; R. H. Shryock, "Empiricism versus Rationalism in American Medicine, 1650–1950," *Proceedings*, American Antiquarian Society, LXXIX (1969), 99–150; Truman Abbe, "The Surgery of the Revolutionary War," *Medical Record*, LXXXIV (1913), 277–83.

31. Samuel Jackson, "Bloodletting," *Transactions and Studies*, College of Physicians of Philadelphia, V (1853–56), 152–53; Rush, *Medical Inquiries and Observations*, IV, 253; C. D., "Remarks on Bloodletting," 156; Joseph I. Waring, "The Influence of Benjamin Rush on the Practice of Bleeding in South Carolina," *Bulletin of the History of Medicine*, XXXV (1961), 230–37.

32. W. Cobbett (ed.), *The Rush Light* (New York, 1800), 49.

33. T. L. Papin, "Venesection, Its Use and Abuse," *St. Louis Medical and Surgical Journal*, XVII (1859), 230.

34. Wardrop, "The Diseases of the Sanguineous System," 242; Elliott, "Remarks on Bloodletting," 281; B. W. Richardson, "On the Conditions of Disease Demanding Abstraction of Blood," *Gaillard's Medical Journal*, XXXVIII (1884), 603; Ernst G. Pupikofer, "Local Bloodletting in Surgery," *Buffalo Medical Journal*, VII (1852), 641–56.

35. C. D., "Remarks on Bloodletting," 153.

36. Quoted in Giekie, "A Few Observations on the Past and Present Employment of Bleeding," 399; R. H. Semple, "On the Utility of Early and Copious Blood-letting in Some Congestive and Inflammatory Diseases," *Lancet*, II (1841), 218–22.

37. George W. Campbell, "On the Utility of Blood-letting in Advanced Stages of Fever," *Transylvania Journal of Medicine and the Associate Sciences*, II (1829), 334–35.

38. Giekie, "A Few Observations on the Past and Present Employment of Bleeding," 399; John W. Ogle, "Concerning Bloodletting," *Lancet*, I (1891), 1030; "Blood-letting to the Amount of Fifty-Seven Pounds Troy," *Medical Repository*, II (1811), 295–96; Peter H. Niebyl, "The English Bloodletting Revolution, or Modern Medicine Before 1850," *Bulletin of the History of Medicine*, LI (1977), 464–83.

39. Rush, *Medical Inquiries and Observations*, IV, 300.

40. C. C. Hildreth, "On Letting Blood from the Jugular in Diseases of Children," *American Journal of the Medical Sciences*, n.s. XIII (1847), 369–74; Beck, "On the Effects of Bloodletting on the Young Subject," 103.

41. Hiram Corson, "Bloodletting in the Young," *Medical and Surgical Reporter*, L (1884), 129–30; Hingeston, "The Neglect of the Use of Bleeding in the Treatment of Some of the Milder Ailments," 267.

42. John Vaughan, "An Inquiry Into the Utility of Occasional Blood-letting in the Pregnant State of Disease," *Medical Repository*, VI (1803), 33; C. A. Murray, "Bloodletting as a Therapeutic Measure," *Buffalo Medical Journal*, XXXVII (1897–98), 194; W. C. Chapman, "Bloodletting as a Therapeutical Agency," *Toledo Medical and Surgical Journal*, II (1878), 173; Fordyce Barker, "Bloodletting as a Therapeutic Resource in Obstetric Medicine," *New York Medical Journal*, XIII (1871), 1–12; John Langley, "On the Treatment of Disease by Bloodletting," *Lancet*, II (1854), 207; Samuel D. Gross, "A Lost Art of Medicine," *Philadelphia Medical Times*, V (1875), 533; Papin, "Venesection, Its Use and Abuse," 228–31; A. W. Tupper, "Venesection," *Transactions*, Medical Society of the State of New York (1872), 218.

43. Hingeston, "The Neglect of the Use of Bleeding in the Treatment of Some of the Milder Ailments," 266; R. Hardey, "On the General Disuse of Venesection in the Treatment of Acute Diseases," *British Medical Journal*, II (1862), 463.

44. Quoted in James A. Leet, "Phlebotomy," *Transactions*, New Hampshire Medical Society, (1897), 206.

45. Balfour, "An Episode in Medical History," 583–84; Peter H. Niebyl, "Galen, Van Helmont, and Bloodletting," in Debus (ed.), *Science, Medicine and Society in the Renaissance*, II, 14; Walter Pagel, "Van Helmont's Concept of Disease—To Be or Not to Be? The Influence of Paracelsus," *Bulletin of the History of Medicine*, XLVI (1972), 419–52.

46. C. H. Spillman, "Bloodletting as a Therapeutic Agent," *Richmond and Louisville Medical Journal*, VIII (1869), 481–82; B. B. Wilson, "A Plea for the Lancet," *Medical and Surgical Reporter*, XV (1866), 482, 489; Balfour, "An Episode in Medical History," 583–84.

47. F. F. Cartwright, "Robert Bentley Todd's Contributions to Medicine," *Proceedings*, Royal Society of London, LVII (1974), 893–97; Bela Cogshall, "Bloodletting a Therapeutic Agent," *Medical Age*, XVI (1898), 326; John H. James, "Result of Experience in Bleeding, not Limited by Particular Organs, Diseases, Classes of Persons, or Seasons," *British Medical Journal*, I (1866), 200; Jackson, "Bloodletting," 148.

48. "Discussion on the Subject of Bloodletting," 500.

49. Theodore A. McGraw, "The Treatment of Inflammatory Diseases of Children by Bleeding," *Detroit Review of Medicine and Pharmacy*, I (1866), 342.

50. Quoted in D'Arcy Power, "Dr. Marshall Hall and the Decay of Bloodletting," *Practitioner*, LXXXII (1909), 323; J. Morehead, "Observations on the Abuse of Bloodletting," *Western Quarterly Journal of Practical Medicine*, I (1837), 24–36; Marshall Hall, *Researches Principally Relative to the Morbid and Curative Effects of Loss of Blood* (Phila., 1830); Marshall Hall, *Principles of the Theory and Practice of Medicine* (Boston, 1839); "The Bloodletting Controversy," 4–7; Leon S. Bryan, Jr., "Bloodletting in American Medicine, 1830–1892," *Bulletin of the History of Medicine*, XXXVIII (1964), 516–29; Erwin H. Ackerknecht, "Elisha Bartlett and the Philosophy of the Paris Clinical School," *Bulletin of the History of Medicine*, XXIV (1950), 55–60; Augustin Grisolle, *Traité Pratique de la Pneumonie aux différents âges, et dans ses rapports . . . maladies aigues et chroniques* (Paris, 1841); W. T. Gairdner, "Remarks on Dr. Bennett's Paper on Bloodletting and Antiphlogistic Treatment," *Edinburgh Medical Journal*, III (1857), 197–229; James F. Hibberd, "General Blood-letting in the Treatment of Inflammation," *Cincinnati Lancet and Observer*, III (1860), 201–31; James Jackson, *Letters to a Young Physician Just Entering Practice* (Boston, 1855), 165–66.

51. J. Hughes Bennett, "Observations on the Results of an Advanced Diagnosis and Pathology Applied to the Management of Internal Inflammations, Compared With the Effects of a Former Antiphlogistic Treatment, and Especially Bloodletting," *Edinburgh Medical Journal*, II (1857), 770–71; B. M. Randolph, "The Bloodletting Controversy in the Nineteenth Century," *Annals of Medical History*, VII (1935), 180–81.

52. Bennett, "Observations on the Results of an Advanced Diagnosis and Pathology Applied to the Management of Internal Inflammations," 771, 773, 776.

53. Ibid., 788, 791–92; James Sawyer, "The Value of Venesection in the Treatment of Disease," *Birmingham Medical Review*, VI (1877), 173–77.

54. "The Bloodletting Controversy," 9; William H. Cumming, "On the Disuse of the Lancet in Later Times," *Canada Medical Journal and Monthly Record of Medical and Surgical Science*, VI (1870), 486–87; T. H. Buckler, "A Plea for the Lancet," *New England Journal of Medicine*, CI (1879), 433–36.

55. W. T. Gairdner, "Remarks on Dr. Bennett's Paper on Blood-Letting, and Antiphlogistic Treatment," 208–9; "Discussion on the Subject of Bloodletting," 36; W. P. Alison, "Reflections on the Results of Experience as to the Symptoms of Internal Inflammations,

and the Effects of Bloodletting, during the Last Forty Years," *Edinburgh Medical Journal*, I (1855–56), 170–71; "Review of the Bloodletting Controversy," 14; C. H. Spillman, "Bloodletting Then and Now," *Medical and Surgical Reporter*, XVI (1867), 231–33.

56. T. A. Snider, "Blood-Letting," *Pacific Medical and Surgical Journal*, VII (1873–74), 160–61.

57. Cumming, "On the Disuse of the Lancet in Later Times," 481–87.

58. Hingeston, "The Neglect of the Use of Bleeding in the Treatment of Some of the Milder Ailments," 266.

59. Thomas R. Manley, "Should Blood-Letting Be More Frequently Employed?," *Medical and Surgical Reporter*, XLVI (1882), 172; Gairdner, "Remarks on Dr. Bennett's Paper on Bloodletting and Antiphlogistic Treatment," 209; Giekie, "A Few Observations on the Past and Present Employment of Bleeding," 399–400; Lester King, "The Blood-Letting Controversy: A Study in the Scientific Method," *Bulletin of the History of Medicine*, XXXV (1961), 1–13; Thomas Watson, "Note to the Lecture on Blood-Letting," *Edinburgh Medical Journal*, II (1857), 1084–88.

60. A. C. Post, "The Question of Blood-Letting," *Medical Record*, II (1867), 472–74; "Curative Effects on Bloodletting," *Bulletin*, New York Academy of Medicine, III (1868), 266–67, 284–87.

61. Thomas Kennard, "Use and Abuse of the Lancet," *St. Louis Medical and Surgical Journal*, XVII (1859), 308; James F. Hibberd, "General Blood-Letting in the Treatment of Inflammation," *Cincinnati Lancet and Observer*, III (1860), 223–25.

62. David L. Cowen, *Medicine and Health in New Jersey: A History* (Princeton, 1964), 36.

63. Campbell, "Venesection or the Use of the Lancet," 326; G. T. Elliott, "Remarks on Bloodletting," *New York Medical Journal*, XIII (1871), 283; D. B. Trimble, "Practical Remarks on Bloodletting," *Chicago Medical Examiner*, VII (1866), 129–41, 262–69, 385–97, 513–27.

64. Harvey L. Byrd, "Blood-Letting in Disease," *Medical and Surgical Reporter*, XXVI (1872), 25–26.

65. Harvey L. Byrd, "Blood-Letting in Disease," *International Dental Journal*, I (1880), 479; Benjamin W. Richardson, "On Blood-Letting as a Point of Scientific Practice," *Practitioner*, I (1868), 275.

66. Gross, "A Lost Art of Medicine," 531–32; William H. Decamp, "Report of the Committee on Remedial Substitutes for Bloodletting," *Transactions*, Michigan State Medical Society, IV (1871), 68–82.

67. W. Mitchell Clarke, "On the History of Bleeding and Its Disuse in Modern Practice," *British Medical Journal*, II (1875), 68; Henry I. Bowditch, "Venesection; Its Abuse Formerly, Its Neglect

in the Present Day," *Publications*, Massachusetts Medical Society, III (1872), 225; Elliot, "Remarks on Bloodletting," 281.

68. Gross, "A Lost Art of Medicine," 532; "Transactions of the Medical Society of the State of North Carolina," *Richmond and Louisville Medical Journal*, XI (1871), 112–13; Henry Moon, "When We May Bleed, and When We May Not Bleed," *British Medical Journal*, I (1876), 68–69; W. F. M'Clelland, "Bloodletting," *Transactions*, Colorado State Medical Society, III–IV (1874–75), 43–47; T. R. Glynn, "Remarks on Venesection with Cases Illustrating Its Value," *Liverpool and Manchester Medical and Surgical Reports*, V (1878), 126–40; N. E. Jones, "Bloodletting as a Therapeutic Agent," *Ohio Medical Recorder*, III (1878), 193–206; J. C. Thompson, "Bloodletting as a Therapeutic Agent," ibid., III (1878), 97–108.

69. J. H. Schrup, "A Plea for the Revival of Venesection," *Iowa Medical Journal*, XVI (1909–10), 528–32; Samuel Coates, "The Lancet and Bloodletting, Considered in the Light of Fifty Years Experience," *Virginia Medical Monthly*, XI (1884–85), 6–9.

70. R. Reyburn, "The Abuses and Uses of Venesection in the Practice of Medicine," *JAMA*, XL (1903), 1564–66; J. A. MacDougall, "On the Remedial Value of Bloodletting," *American Journal of the Medical Sciences*, XCIV (1887), 37–52; W. T. Hayward, "A Plea for Venesection," *Australasian Medical Gazette*, XVI (1897), 225–29.

71. Packard, "The Uses of Venesection," 511–19; Levene, "On the Therapeutic Value of Bloodletting," 386; Laws, "A Plea for Venesection," 806–10; R. L. Payne, "Remarks on Blood-Letting," *North Carolina Medical Journal*, XXIII (1889), 243–50; W. F. Mitchell, "When to Use and When Not to Use the Lancet," *Medical and Surgical Reporter*, LI (1884), 54–55; J. Clark, "On Venesection. Facts? That Are Facts, If You Please, when Theories Chose to Ignore Them," *Canada Lancet*, XIV (1881–82), 35; M. Schuppert, "Bloodletting and Kindred Questions," *New Orleans Medical and Surgical Journal*, IX (1881), 247–56; P. A. Stackpole, "Venesection, Its Necessity and Neglect," *Transactions*, New Hampshire Medical Society (1883), 141–50; R. W. Griswold, "Something about Why We Do Not Use the Lancet as of Yore," *New England Medical Monthly*, III (1883–84), 303–8; B. H. Detwiler, "Venesection: Its Remedial Properties," *Medical Times and Register*, XXIV (1892), 71–73.

72. W. Forest Dutton, "Venesection: Its Therapeutic Value," *Clinical Medicine and Surgery*, XIV (1907), 42; William Osler, *The Principles and Practice of Medicine Designed for the Use of Practitioners and Students of Medicine* (New York, 1892); Louis Jacobs, "An Improved Method of Performing Phlebotomy," *American Journal of Surgery*, XXI (1907), 117.

73. James Rodgers, "Bloodletting, a Valuable Curative Means,

Too Much Disregarded," *Atlanta Medical and Surgical Journal*, XI (1873), 223; P. S. Fulkerson, "Venesection in the Treatment of Disease," *Transactions*, Missouri State Medical Association (1898), 74–82.

74. Quoted in Cogshall, "Bloodletting a Therapeutic Agent," 329.

75. Levene, "On the Therapeutic Value of Bloodletting," 395–96; G. R. Hall, "Bloodletting: Its Past and Present Status," *Brooklyn Medical Journal*, XVI (1902), 314; J. H. Hatchett, "A Plea for Bloodletting from a Practical Standpoint," *Virginia Medical Monthly*, XIV (1887–88), 514–21.

76. Homer O. Jewett, "The Use and Neglect of Bloodletting," *Transactions*, New York State Medical Association, VII (1890), 381, 383; C. C. P. Clark, "The Lost Art of Venesection," *Medical Record*, XLII (1892), 33; Francis Warner, "On the Value of Venesection in the Treatment of Disease," *Birmingham Medical Review*, VI (1877), 18–40.

77. Bedford Fenwick, "On the Use of Bloodletting in Gynecological Cases," *Medical Times and Hospital Gazette*, XXVII (1902), 529–32.

78. G. Harley, "Visceral Phlebotomy," *Clinical Journal*, II (1893), 215.

79. Levene, "On the Therapeutic Value of Bloodletting," 395.

80. E. J. C. Beardsley, "The Indications for Venesection," *New International Clinics*, II (1916), 1.

CHAPTER THREE

The Aging Materia Medica

1. William Hooker, *Physician and Patient; Or, a Practical View of the Mutual Duties, Relations and Interests of the Medical Profession and the Community* (London, 1850), 100.

2. Robert G. Latham (trans.), *The Works of Thomas Sydenham* (London, 1848–50), c–ci, cv–cvi. The formula of mithridate (*Pharmacopoeia Londinensis*, 1782) included the following ingredients: Arabian myrrh, saffron, agaric, ginger, cinnamon, spikenard, frankincense, seeds of penny-cress, cicely, opobalsamum, sweet rush, French lavender, costum, galbanum, Cyprian turpentine, long pepper, castor, juice of hypocistis, storax, opoponax, Indian leaf, true cassia-wood, poly of the mountain, white pepper, scordium, seeds of the Cretan carrot, carpobalsamum, lozenges of cyphus, bdellium, Celtic nard, gum arabic, seeds of the Macedonian stone-parsley, opium, lesser cardamoms, fennel-seeds, gen-

tian, flowers of the red rose, dittany of Crete, seeds of anise, asarum, sweet-flag, orris-root, phu, sagapenum, meu, acacia, skunk-bellies, St. John's wort tops, Canary wine, and clarified honey. See also Dr. Holyoke, *A Collection of Choice and Safe Remedies* (London, 1712).

3. Oliver W. Holmes, *Currents and Counter-Currents in Medical Science with Other Addresses and Essays* (Boston, 1861), 27.

4. One version of the monk derivation related that Basil Valentine had thrown an antimonial preparation out a window where it was then eaten by pigs. The purgative effect on the pigs caused them to later fatten, a circumstance which led Valentine to administer the antimonial to monks emaciated by long fasts for the purpose of increasing their weight. Unfortunately, the monks died from the experiment. "The modern philological theory," A. C. Wooton wrote, "is that the early Latin *stibium* and the late Latin *antimonium* have the same etymological origin. *Stibium* was the Latinised form of the Greek *stimmi*. *Stimmi* declined as *stimmid*—and this may have found its way into the Arabic through a conjectural *isthimmid* to the known Arabic name *uthmud*, which via *athmud* and *athmoad* became Latinised again into *antimonium*." See A. C. Wooton, *Chronicles of Pharmacy*, 2 vols. (Boston, 1910), I, 377. See also Pascal Pilpoul, *La Querelle de L'Antimonie* (Paris, 1928), 15–24, 32–33, 88–89; "Bleeding and Antimony in the Seventeenth Century," *Boston Medical and Surgical Journal*, XXXVII (1847), 209–11; Alfred S. Taylor, "On Poisoning by Tartarized Antimony," *Guy's Hospital Reports*, London, III (1857), 376; Jonathan Pereira, *Elements of the Materia Medica and Therapeutics*, 2 vols. (London, 1854–55), II, 858; Homer W. Smith, "Arsenic Therapy," *Journal, American Pharmaceutical Association*, XI (1922), 426; Ralph H. Major, *A History of Medicine*, 2 vols. (Springfield, Ill., 1954), I, 457–60; Allen G. Debus, *The English Paracelsians: A Study of Iatrochemistry in England in 1640* (Ph.D. diss., Harvard, 1961), 257; Robert Multhauf, "Medical Chemistry and 'The Paracelsians,'" *Bulletin of the History of Medicine*, XXVIII (1954), 101–26.

5. P. O'Connell, "Composition and Therapeutical Uses of True James's Powder," *Chicago Medical Journal and Examiner*, XXXIX (1876), 160–66; R. Hingston Fox, "The Use of Antimony in Ancient and Modern Medicine," *Clinical Journal*, LXVI (1917), 129; James Walker, "An Account of an Uncommon Effect of Antimonial Wine," *Essays and Observations*, Philosophical Society of Edinburgh, II (1756) 254–56; James Parkinson, *The Chemical Pocket-Book; Or, Memoranda Chemica: Arranged in a Compendium of Chemistry: With Tables of Attractions, etc.* (Philadelphia, 1802), 91–94; A. Jacobi, "On the Oxysulphuret of Antimony as an Expectorant in Inflammatory

Diseases of the Infantile Respiratory Organs," *New York Journal of Medicine*, V (1856), 356–66.

6. Robert C. Cream, *Inaugural Dissertation on the Chemical History and Physiological and Therapeutical Action of Tartarized Antimony* (Edinburgh, 1835), 10–11; Edward Jenner, "A Process for Preparing Emetic Tartar by Recrystalization," *Transactions*, Society for the Improvement of Medical and Chirurgical Knowledge, I (1793), 30–33; Taylor, "Poisoning by Tartar Emetic," 379. The *U. S. D.* (1873) gave the following preparation:

ANTIMONII ET POTASSII TARTRAS
(TARTRATE OF ANTIMONY AND POTASSIUM.
TARTAR EMETIC)

Take of oxide of antimony, in very fine powder, two troyounces; Bitartrate of potassium, in very fine powder, two troyounces and a half; Distilled water eighteen fluid ounces. To the water, heated to the boiling point in a glass vessel, add the powders, previously mixed, and boil for an hour; then filter the liquid while hot, and set it aside that crystals may form. Lastly, dry the crystals, and keep them in a well-stopped bottle. By further evaporation the mother-water may be made to yield more crystals, which should be purified by a second crystalization.

7. Cream, *Inaugural Dissertation on the Chemical History and Physiological and Therapeutical Action of Tartarized Antimony*, 18.

8. The *U. S. D.* (1873) gave the following preparation:

VINUM ANTIMONII (ANTIMONIAL WINE)

Take tartrate of Antimony thirty-two grains; boiling distilled water a fluidounce; sherry wine a sufficient quantity. Dissolve the salt in the distilled water and, while the solution is hot, add sufficient sherry wine to make it measure a pint.

9. The *U. S. D.* (1873) gave the following preparation:

UNGUENTUM ANTIMONII (ANTIMONIAL OINTMENT)

Take of tartrate of antimony and potassium, in very fine powder, one hundred grains; lard four hundred grains. Rub the tartrate of antimony and potassium with the lard, gradually added, until they are thoroughly mixed.

10. The *U. S. D.* (1873) gave the following preparation:

EMPLASTRUM ANTIMONII (ANTIMONIAL PLASTER)

Take tartrate of antimony and potassium, in fine powder, a troyounce; burgundy pitch four troyounces; melt the pitch by means of a water-bath, and strain; then add the powder, and stir them well together until the mixture thickens on cooling.

11. A. Emil Hiss, *Thesaurus of Proprietary Preparations and Pharmaceutical Specialities, Including 'Patent' Medicines, Proprietary Pharmaceuticals, Open-Formula Specialities, Synthetic Remedies, etc.* (Chicago, 1898).

12. Quoted in William Balfour, *Illustrations of the Power of Emetic Tartar, in the Cure of Fever, Inflammation, and Asthma; and in Preventing Consumption and Apoplexy* (Edinburgh, 1819), 1–2.

13. Cream, *Inaugural Dissertation on the Chemical History and Physiological and Therapeutical Action of Tartarized Antimony*, 25; Alex Berman, "The Heroic Approach in Nineteenth Century Therapeutics," *American Journal of Hospital Pharmacy*, XI (1954), 321–27.

14. Taylor, "On Poisoning by Tartarized Antimony," 391; Thomas Marryatt, *Treatise on Therapeutics* (Bristol, 1758).

15. Quoted in Taylor, "On Poisoning by Tartarized Antimony," 392; Esmond R. Long, *A History of Pathology* (Baltimore, 1928), 122–23; Erwin H. Ackerknecht, *Medicine at the Paris Hospital, 1794–1848* (Baltimore, 1967), 61–72, 92–96; Fielding H. Garrison, *An Introduction to the History of Medicine* (Philadelphia, 1929), 408–12; Thomas J. Bole, "John Brown, Hegel and Speculative Concepts in Medicine," *Texas Reports on Biology and Medicine*, XXXII (1974), 287–97; Günter B. Risse, "The Brownian System of Medicine: Its Theoretical and Practical Implications," *Clio Medica*, V (1970), 45–51.

16. Quoted in Taylor, "On Poisoning by Tartarized Antimony," 394.

17. L. C. Boisliniere, "Pustular Eruption of the Skin from the Internal Use of Tartar Emetic," *St. Louis Medical and Surgical Journal*, XIV (1856), 20–21.

18. Taylor, "On Poisoning by Tartarized Antimony," 395.

19. John S. Wilson, "Specific Cutaneous Eruption, Produced by the Internal Use of Tartar Emetic," *Southern Medical and Surgical Journal*, VIII (1852), 343–45; William Griffith, "Effect of Tartar Emetic on the Genital Organs," *Provincial Medical and Surgical Journal*, V (1842), 127–28.

20. Boisliniere, "Pustular Eruption of the Skin from the Internal Use of Tartar Emetic," 21; P. M. Kollock, "On the Cutaneous Eruption Induced by the Internal Use of Tartar Emetic," *Southern Medical and Surgical Journal*, VIII (1852), 456–66.

21. N. R. Smithe, "On the Uses and Abuses of the Tartrate of Antimony," *Philadelphia Monthly Journal of Medicine and Surgery*, I (1827), 82–84; John T. Rees, *Remarks on the Medical Theories of Brown, Cullen, Darwin, and Rush* (Philadelphia, 1805); Richard H. Shryock, "The Advent of Modern Medicine in Philadelphia, 1800–1850," *Yale Journal of Biology and Medicine*, XIII (1941), 715–38;

Richard H. Shryock, "Benjamin Rush from the Perspective of the Twentieth Century," *Transactions, College of Physicians of Phila-delphia*, XIV (1946), 114–16; Major, *A History of Medicine*, II, 726–27; Günter B. Risse, "The Quest for Certainty in Medicine: John Brown's System of Medicine in France," *Bulletin of the History of Medicine*, XLV (1971), 1–12.

22. James Kitchen, "On the Administration of Tartarized Anti-mony, in Large Doses, in Some of the Phlegmasiae," *North American Medical and Surgical Journal*, V (1828), 303; René T. H. Laennec, *A Treatise on the Diseases of the Chest and on Mediate Auscultation* (New York, 1835).

23. Kitchen, "On the Administration of Tartarized Antimony, in Large Doses, in Some of the Phlegmasiae," 294; Long, *A History of Pathology*, 132–34.

24. William Balfour, *Illustrations of the Power of Emetic Tartar* (Lexington, Ky., 1823), 83.

25. Ibid., 8–10.

26. Ibid., 187–89.

27. Ibid., 12–13, 46.

28. Ibid., 186–87.

29. Ibid., 191–92.

30. Ibid., 199–200.

31. Ibid., 206, 211–12, 214–15.

32. Hugh Croskery, "On the Value of Tartar Emetic in Com-pression of the Brain, and in Controlling Convulsions and Mania-cal Excitements Dependent Thereon," *Irish Journal of Medicine and Practice*, XLIII (1867), 103. Actually the prescription of antimony in tropical disease was not an unreasonable one. Like its sister ele-ment arsenic, antimony proved valuable in cases where certain parasites were present in the body. By 1917, physicians were reg-ularly administering oxide of antimony and tartar emetic for try-panosomiasis, ulcerating granuloma, kala-azar, leishmaniasis, and malaria. See Fox, "The Use of Antimony in Ancient and Modern Medicine," 131; George C. Low, "The History of the Use of Intra-venous Injections of Tartar Emetic in Tropical Medicine," *Transac-tions, Society of Tropical Medicine and Hygiene*, X (1917), 37–40.

33. Evory Kennedy, "Observations on the Use of Tartar Emetic in Obstetric Practice," *American Journal of Medical Science*, XVII (1835), 301; William Read, "Effect of Tartrate of Antimony in Facil-itating Labor," *New England Journal of Medicine*, LV (1856–57), 505–6.

34. Kennedy, "Observations on the Use of Tartar Emetic in Obstetric Practice," 303–5.

35. Taylor, "On Poisoning by Tartarized Antimony," 373–75.

1850," *Yale Journal of Biology and Medicine*, XIII (1941), 726–27.

52. Alexander Means, "Calomel—Its Chemical Characteristics and Mineral Origin Considered in View of Its Curative Claims," *Southern Medical and Surgical Journal*, n.s. I (1845), 98.

53. J. Annesley, "Observations on the Use and Abuse of Calomel," *Transactions*, Medical and Physical Society of Calcutta, I (1825), 213–14; W. B. Watkins, "Some of the Indications and Contra-Indications for Calomel," *Texas Courier-Record of Medicine*, VIII (1890), 2; James Lind, *Essays on Diseases Incidental to Europeans in Hot Climates* (London, 1792), 99; James Lind, "An Account of the Efficacy of Mercury in the Cure of Inflammatory Diseases, and the Dysentery," *London Medical Journal*, VIII (1787), 43; Charles Mac-Lean, *Practical Illustrations of the Progress of Medical Improvement for the Last Thirty Years; Or, Histories of Cases of Acute Diseases, as Fevers, Dysentery, Hepatitis, and Plague, Treated According to the Principles of the Doctrine of Excitation* (London, 1818), 49–54; Sir James McGriegor, *Medical Sketches of the Expedition to Egypt from India* (London, 1804), 185; A. Campbell, "Fatal Effects of Calomel," *India Journal of Medical Science*, I (1834), 74; G. S. T. Cavanagh, "An Anti-Mercurial American Play," *Journal of the History of Medicine and Allied Sciences*, XXXIX (1974), 233–34.

54. Annesley, "Observations on the Use and Abuse of Calomel," 215; William Ferguson, "On the Mercurial Plan of Treatment of Dysentery," *Medico-Chirurgical Transactions*, II (1817), 181.

55. Annesley, "Observations on the Use and Abuse of Calomel," 223–24.

56. Means, "Calomel," 533; John Eberle, *A Treatise on the Practice of Medicine*, 2 vols. (Philadelphia, 1831), I, 240; James Thacher, *American Modern Practice; Or, A Simple Method of Prevention and Cure of Disease* (Boston, 1817), 589; Robley Dunglison, *The Practice of Medicine: A Treatise on Special Pathology and Therapeutics*, 2 vols. (Philadelphia, 1848), I, 113; Nathaniel Chapman, *A Compendium of Lectures on the Theory and Practice of Medicine* (Philadelphia, 1846), 133; Martyn Paine, *The Institutes of Medicine* (New York, 1860), 841; James C. Cross, "Note on the Sedative Action of Calomel," *Western and Southern Medical Recorder*, I (1842), 194–98.

57. "Discussions in the College of Physicians and Surgeons of Lexington, on the Action of Calomel in Health and Disease," 474.

58. Cross, "Note on the Sedative Action of Calomel," 193.

59. Means, "Calomel," 103.

60. Moore Hoyt, "Remarks on Calomel," *New York Medical and Physical Journal*, V (1826), 565, 569–71; John Armstrong, *Practical Illustrations on Typhus Fever, of the Common Continued Fever, and of Inflammatory Diseases* (Philadelphia, 1822), 328; Charles R. Curtis, "Why Such Quantities of Calomel are Consumed in the Western

States," *Western Medico-Chirurgical Journal*, II (1852), 231; Means, "Calomel," 106; Joseph Brown, "Dysentery," in John Forbes (ed.), *The Cyclopaedia of Practical Medicine*, 4 vols. (Philadelphia, 1850), I, 726; Michael O. Jones, "Climate and Disease: The Traveller Describes America," *Bulletin of the History of Medicine*, XLI (1967), 254–66.

61. William Hauser, "Cases Showing the Advantage of Heroic Doses of Calomel," *Atlanta Medical and Surgical Journal*, III (1857–58), 518–21; Watkins, "Indications and Contra-Indications for Calomel," 2.

62. Pickard and Buley, *The Midwest Pioneer: His Ills, Cures, and Doctors*, 105.

63. Curtis, "Why Such Quantities of Calomel are Consumed in the Western States," 233–35.

64. Ibid., 231.

65. "The Anatomy of Quackery," *Medical Circular*, II (1853), 266–67.

66. Samuel Jackson, "The Use of Calomel in Diseases of Children," *Transactions*, College of Physicians of Philadelphia, II (1853–56), 135–36; Marshall Hall, *Practical Observations and Suggestions*, 2 vols. (London, 1845–46), I, 193; John B. Beck, *Essays on Infant Therapeutics: To Which are Added Observations on Ergot, and an Account of the Origin of the Use of Mercury in Inflammatory Complaints* (New York, 1849); James J. Walsh, *History of Medicine in New York: Three Centuries of Progress*, 5 vols. (New York, 1919), II, 216; Charles West, *Lectures on the Diseases of Infancy and Childhood* (Philadelphia, 1850), 206, 308.

67. Hammond's Circular No. 6, quoted in U.S. Surgeon-General's Office, *The Medical and Surgical History of the War of Rebellion*, 3 vols. (Washington, D.C., 1870–88), vol. I, pt. 2, 719; Berman, "The Heroic Approach in Nineteenth Century Therapeutics," 321–27; Fort, "Uses and Abuses of Calomel," 84; George W. Adams, *Doctors in Blue: the Medical History of the Union Army in the Civil War* (New York, 1952), 39; Stewart Brooks, *Civil War Medicine* (Springfield, Ill., 1966), 63–73.

68. "Communication," *Chicago Medical Journal and Examiner*, VI (1863), 321; "Calomel and Tartar Emetic in the Army," *American Medical Times*, VI (1863), 297; "Calomel and Tartar Emetic as Remedial Agents," *Buffalo Medical and Surgical Journal*, III (1863), 32; J. F. Hibberd, "Circular No. 6 and the Profession," *Cincinnati Lancet and Observer*, VI (1863), 429; Morris Fishbein, "History of the American Medical Association," *JAMA*, CXXXII (1946), 1069; D. L. Griffiths, "Medicine and Surgery in the American Civil War," *Proceedings*, Royal Society of Medicine, LIX (1966), 204–8.

69. Fort, "Uses and Abuses of Calomel," 84; "Proceedings,"

36. See J. T. Morse, Jr., "The Wharton Trial," *American Law Review*, VI (1872), 647–68; S. C. Chew, "An Examination of the Medical Evidence in the Trial of Mrs. E. G. Wharton," *Medical Record*, VIII (1873), 332–38; John J. Reese, "A Review of the Recent Trial of Mrs. Elizabeth G. Wharton on the Charge of Poisoning General W. S. Ketchum," *American Journal of Medical Sciences*, LXIII (1872), 330; William E. A. Aiken, "On Some Supposed Fallacies in Determining the Presence of Tartar Emetic," *Richmond and Louisville Medical Journal*, XV (1873), 7–13; P. C. Williams, "A Correct Statement of the Chemical and Pharmaceutical Facts Developed during the Trials of Mrs. Wharton for the Alleged Murder of General Ketchum and Mr. Van Ness; With a Complete Exposure of the Inaccuracies, Indecencies, and Unworthy Devices of the So-Called Experts, Drs. H. C. Wood and J. J. Reese, Obtained from Philadelphia," *Richmond and Louisville Medical Journal*, XV (1873), 721–47.

37. For a history of the origin of calomel, see George Urdang, "The Early Chemical and Pharmaceutical History of Calomel," *Chyma*, I (1948), 94–108; George Urdang, "Origin of the Term Calomel," *Journal of the American Pharmaceutical Association*, IX (1948), 414–18; Edward Divers, "The Manufacture of Calomel in Japan," *Journal*, Tokyo University Faculty of Science, VII (1894), 1–2; Daniel Hanbury, "Notes on Chinese Materia Medica," in Joseph Ince (ed.), *Science Papers, Chiefly Pharmacological and Botanical of Daniel Hanbury* (London, 1876); C. H. Lawall and Joseph W. E. Harrison, "A Study of Calomel From the Physical and Chemical Standpoint," *Journal*, American Pharmaceutical Association, XXIV (1939), 97; Günter B. Risse, "Calomel and the American Medical Sects during the Nineteenth Century," *Mayo Clinic Proceedings*, XLVIII (1973), 57–64.

38. "Discussions in the College of Physicians and Surgeons of Lexington, on the Action of Calomel in Health and Disease," *Transylvania Journal of Medicine*, X (1837), 474–75; Lester King, "Rationalism in Early Eighteenth Century Medicine," *Journal of the History of Medicine and Allied Sciences*, XVIII (1963), 257–71.

39. J. M. Fort, et al., "Uses and Abuses of Calomel," *Texas Courier-Record of Medicine*, VI (1888–89), 56; Alfred Stillé, *Therapeutics and Materia Medica: A Systematic Treatise on the Action and Uses of Medicinal Agents*, 2 vols. (Philadelphia, 1860), II, 833.

40. Quoted in Elisha Bartlett, *Essay on the Philosophy of Medical Science* (Philadelphia, 1844), 115; William Seller, "On Some of the Metaphysical Aspects of Physiology," *Edinburgh Medical Journal*, V (1859), 1–12.

41. Richard H. Shryock, *Medicine in America: Historical Essays* (Baltimore, 1966), 207; Richard H. Shryock, "Benjamin Rush from the Perspective of the Twentieth Century," *Transactions*, College of

Physicians of Philadelphia, XIV (1946), 114–15; Günter B. Risse, "The Quest for Certainty in Medicine," XLV (1971), 1–12; Richard H. Shryock, "Empiricism versus Rationalism in American Medicine, 1650–1950," *Proceedings,* American Antiquarian Society, LXXIX (1969), 99–150; Richard H. Shryock, "The Medical Reputation of Benjamin Rush: Contrasts over Two Centuries," *Bulletin of the History of Medicine,* XLV (1971), 511–12.

42. Bartlett, *Essay on the Philosophy of Medical Science,* 114; Erwin H. Ackerknecht, "Elisha Bartlett and the Philosophy of the Paris Clinical School," *Bulletin of the History of Medicine,* XXIV (1950), 43–59; George M. Daniels, "Finalism and Positivism in Nineteenth Century American Physiological Thought," ibid., XXXVIII (1964), 343–63.

43. Bartlett, *Essay on the Philosophy of Medical Science,* 124, 128, 185, 224–39; Alex Berman, "Neo-Thomsonianism in the United States," *Journal of the History of Medicine and Allied Sciences,* X (1956), 133–55; Alex Berman, "The Thomsonian Movement and Its Relation to American Pharmacy and Medicine," *Bulletin of the History of Medicine,* XXV (1951), 405–38; Richard H. Shryock, *The Development of Modern Medicine: An Interpretation of the Social and Scientific Factors Involved* (Philadelphia, 1936), 160–61.

44. Bartlett, *Essay on the Philosophy of Medical Science,* 302, 305.

45. Ibid., 295; Owsei Temkin, "The Role of Surgery in the Rise of Modern Medical Thought," *Bulletin of the History of Medicine,* XXV (1951), 248–59; George Rosen, "The Philosophy of Ideology and the Emergence of Modern Medicine in France," ibid., XX (1946), 328–39; Phillis Allen, "Etiological Theory in America Prior to the Civil War," *Journal of the History of Medicine and Allied Sciences,* II (1947), 489–520; Shryock, *The Development of Modern Medicine,* 154–55.

46. Bartlett, *Essay on the Philosophy of Medical Science,* 232–33.

47. Ibid., 236–37; Lunsford Pitts Yandell, *A Memoir of the Life and Writings of Dr. John Esten Cooke* (Louisville, 1875), 5–6, 23.

48. John E. Cooke, *Treatise of Pathology and Therapeutics,* 2 vols. (Lexington, Ky., 1828), II, 242–54; Bartlett, *Essay on the Philosophy of Medical Science,* 238–39; Madge E. Pickard and Roscoe Carlyle Buley, *The Midwest Pioneer: His Ills, Cures, and Doctors* (Crawfordsville, Ind., 1945), 105.

49. "Allopathy," *Water Cure Journal,* VIII (1849), 159.

50. John Hunter, *A Treatise on the Venereal Disease* (Philadelphia, 1818), 7, 312–40.

51. J. W. P. Bates, "Calomel, Its Uses and Abuses," *Medical and Surgical Reporter,* XVI (1867), 191; David Hosack, *Lectures on the Theory and Practice of Physic* (Philadelphia, 1838), 364; Richard H. Shryock, "The Advent of Modern Medicine in Philadelphia, 1800–

Transactions, American Medical Association, XIV (1864), 23–24.

70. U.S. Surgeon-General's Office, *Medical and Surgical History of the War of the Rebellion*, I, 720–21; Philip D. Jordan, "The Secret Six: An Inquiry into the Basic Materia Medica of the Thomsonian System of Botanic Medicine," *Ohio History Quarterly*, LII (1943), 347–55.

71. Bates, "Calomel, Its Uses and Abuses," 189–91; George H. Tichenor, "Medicine during Reconstruction Period, 1865–1901 in the South," *Western Medical Times*, XLI (1922), 339–42.

72. Bates, "Calomel, Its Uses and Abuses," 190.

73. Watkins, "Indications and Contra-Indications for Calomel," 1.

74. J. R. H. Hatchett, "Calomel an Instantaneous Nervous Sedative," *The Southern Clinic*, VII (1884), 97–100.

75. Bartlett, *Essay on the Philosophy of Medical Science*, 237–38.

76. C. J. Funck, "Calomel," *Cincinnati Lancet-Clinic; A Weekly Journal of Medicine and Surgery*, XLIII (1899), 172–73.

77. Charles G. Cumston, "A Note on the History of Arsenic in Therapeutics," *Medical Record*, XCIX (1921), 679; "Arsenic in Its Historical Associations," *British Medical Journal*, I (1924), 1149; F. M. Sandwith, "Abstract of the Gresham Lectures on Drugs, Old and New," *Medical Magazine*, XXII (1913), 334.

78. W. F. Barclay, "Arsenic in Therapy," *Lancet-Clinic*, CIX (1913), 125–26.

79. Ralph St. J. Perry, "Arsenic—The Multipotent Drug," *American Journal of Clinical Medicine*, XIX (1912), 54–55; S. O. Habershon, "On the Medical Preparations of Arsenic," *Guy's Hospital Reports*, X (1864), 72; Lloyd Bullock, "On the Best Preparation of Arsenic for Internal Administration," *Lancet*, II (1850), 674–75.

80. Homer W. Smith, "Arsenic Therapy," *Journal*, American Pharmaceutical Association, XI (1922), 424; Gordon Sharp, "Notes on the History and Romance of Arsenic," *Pharmaceutical Journal*, XXVIII (1908), 232–34; Frank Charteris, "The Action and Uses of Arsenic," *Medical Brief*, XXX (1902), 1473.

81. G. N. Hill, "Observations on the Use of Arsenic," *Edinburgh Medical and Surgical Journal*, V (1809), 21–23, 27, 55–61, 312–14.

82. D. Theodore Coxe, "Remarks on the Remedial Value of Arsenic," *North American Medical and Surgical Journal*, VIII (1829), 42–43.

83. Romberg, quoted in James Begbie, "Arsenic: Its Physiological and Therapeutical Effects; With Reflections on the Relations of Certain Diseases, Their Common Origin, and Treatment," *Edinburgh Medical Journal*, III (1858), 970.

84. Thomas Hunt, "On the Administration of Arsenic," *Lancet*, I (1847), 91–92.

85. Begbie, "Arsenic: Its Physiological and Therapeutical Effects," 962–63.

86. Isaac E. Taylor, "On the Use of the Liquor of Hydriodate of Arsenic and Mercury in Cutaneous and Uterine Affections," *American Journal of the Medical Sciences*, n.s. V (1843), 319–25.

87. Arthur P. Burns, "Arsenic in Menorrhagia, Leucorrhea, etc.," *American Journal of the Medical Sciences*, XXXVIII (1859), 393–95; Perry, "Arsenic—the Multipotent Drug," 59.

88. John Jenkinson, "On the Cases in Which the Use of Arsenic is Indicated," *Edinburgh Medical and Surgical Journal*, V (1809), 311.

89. W. B. Kesteven, "On Arsenic-Eating," *Association Medical Journal*, IV (1856), 721; James F. W. Johnston, *The Chemistry of Common Life*, 2 vols. (London, 1855), II, 202.

90. Johnston, *The Chemistry of Common Life*, II, 203–4, 207.

91. Kesteven, "On Arsenic-Eating," 733, 757; Craig MacLagan, "On the Arsenic-Eaters of Styria," *Edinburgh Medical Journal*, X (1864), 201; A. Gattinger, "The Effects of Arsenious Acid upon the Animal Organism," *Nashville Journal of Medicine and Surgery*, II (1867), 141.

92. Charles Boner, "Poison-Eaters," *Chambers's Journal*, V (1856), 90.

93. P. A. Jewett, "Arsenic-Eating," *Proceedings*, Connecticut State Medical Society, LXXXVIII (1879), 80; "Arsenic Eating and Arsenic Poisoning," *British and Foreign Medical-Chirurgical Review*, XXIX (1862), 144.

94. F. A. H. LaRue, "An Arsenic-Eater," *Boston Medical and Surgical Journal*, LXXIV (1866), 439–42; John Aule, "A Study of the Pharmacology and Therapeutics of Arsenic," *New York Medical Journal*, LII (1891), 394; Iretus G. Cardner, "Studies in Materia Medica. Arsenic in Consumption, and Generally in Diseases Where There Is a Tendency to Death by Asthenia; Its Physiological and Psychological Action," *International Record of Medicine*, IX (1869), 127–28.

95. "Arsenic Smoked with Tobacco," *Association Medical Journal*, CXXII (1855), 429.

96. Thomas Hunt, "Memoir on the Medicinal Action of Arsenic," *Transactions*, Provincial Medical and Surgical Association, XVI (1849), 402.

97. Boner, "Poison-Eaters," 90; "Arsenic Eating and Arsenic Poisoning," 149; John H. Winslow, *Darwin's Victorian Malady: Evidence for Its Medically Induced Origin* (Philadelphia, 1971), ch. 4.

98. Daniel G. Brinton and George H. Napheys, *Laws of Health in Relation to the Human Form* (Springfield, Mass., 1870), 239–40.

99. C. F. Brown, "Arsenic as a Prophylactic," *Provincial Medical Journal*, XII (1893), 9–11.

100. A. P. Merrill, "On Arsenic as a Remedy," *American Practitioner*, I (1870), 322–25; Coleman Rogers, "On Some of the Therapeutical Uses of Arsenic," ibid., IX (1874), 223–25; C. Durselen, "Arsenic in Certain Affections," *Detroit Review of Medicine and Pharmacy*, X (1875), 336–38; Arthur Leared, "Use of Arsenic in Certain Painful Affections of the Stomach and Bowels," *Medical Times and Gazette*, II (1870), 94–95.

101. Perry, "Arsenic—The Multipotent Drug," 59; W. F. Barclay, "Arsenic in Therapy," *Lancet-Clinic*, CIX (1913), 125.

102. See Wallace C. Abbott, *Abbott's Alkaloidal Digest* (Chicago, 1906).

CHAPTER FOUR

Transcendental Medicine

1. "Modern Faith Healing," *British Medical Journal*, II (1911), 1555; Isaac H. Flack [Harvey Graham], *Eternal Eve: The History of Gynecology and Obstetrics* (Garden City, N.Y., 1951), 459–61; Walter Pagel, "Religious Motives in the Medical Biology of the 17th Century," *Bulletin of the History of Medicine*, III (1935), 97–128; Sir William Osler, *The Evolution of Modern Medicine: A Series of Lectures* (New Haven, 1921), 140; Eric Maple, *Magic, Medicine and Quackery* (London, 1968), 132–36; Charles Mackay, *Extraordinary Popular Delusions and the Madness of Crowds* (Boston, 1932), 317; Baron Jean Dupotet de Sennevoy, *An Introduction to the Study of Animal Magnetism* (London, 1838), 315, 319–21; Alexander Jacques François Bertrand, *On Magnétisme animal en France* (Paris, 1826), 18; Allen G. Debus, "Harvey and Fludd: The Irrational Factor in the Rational Science of the 17th Century," *Journal of the History of Biology*, III (1970), 81–105; James J. Walsh, *Cures: The Story of the Cures That Fail* (New York, 1923), 78, 81; Michael H. Stone, "Mesmer and His Followers: The Beginnings of Sympathetic Treatment of Childhood Emotional Disorders," *History of Childhood Quarterly*, I (1974), 659–79.

2. "Modern Faith Healing," 79; W. P. Hartford, "Subjective Therapeutics," *Medical Record*, LIV (1898), 157; Joseph Jastrow, "Malicious Animal Magnetism," *Milwaukee Medical Journal*, XVIII (1910), 358; Fred Kaplan, "The Mesmeric Mania: The Early Victorians and Animal Magnetism," *Journal of the History of Ideas*, XXX (1974), 691–702; Rudolf Tischner, *Franz Anton Mesmer* (Munich, 1928); Margaret L. Goldsmith, *Franz Anton Mesmer: The History of an Idea* (London, 1934); Donald M. Walmsley, *Anton Mesmer* (Lon-

don, 1967); Robert Darnton, *Mesmerism, and the End of the Enlightenment in France* (Cambridge, Mass., 1968).

3. "Modern Faith Healing," 199–200; Maple, *Magic, Medicine and Quackery*, 137.

4. "Modern Faith Healing," 1559.

5. Frank Podmore, *Mesmerism and Christian Science: A Short History of Mental Healing* (Phila., 1909), 219; Douglas Guthrie, *A History of Medicine* (London, 1945), 460; José Custodio de Faria, *De la cause du sommeil lucide; ou étude de la nature de l'homme* (Paris, 1819); Joseph P. F. Deleuze, *Histoire critique du magnétisme animal* (Paris, 1813); Nicholas Bergasse, *Observations de M. Bergasse sur un écrit du Docteur Mesmer* (London, 1785); George Winter, *History of Animal Magnetism* (Bristol, 1801); James Braid, *Neurypnology; or, the Rationale of Nervous Sleep, Considered in Relation with Animal Magnetism* (London, 1843); John Elliotson, *Human Physiology* (London, 1840); Jon Palfreman, "Mesmerism and the English Medical Profession: A Study of Conflict," *Ethics in Science and Medicine*, IV (1977), 51–66.

6. Podmore, *Mesmerism and Christian Science*, 148; Bernard Wolfe and Raymond Rosenthal, *Hypnotism Comes of Age: Its Progress from Mesmer to Psychoanalysis* (New York, 1949); Henri F. Ellenberger, "Mesmer and Puysegur: From Magnetism to Hypnotism," *Psychoanalysis and Psychoanalytic Review*, LII (1965), 137–53; Madge E. Pickard and Roscoe Carlyle Buley, *The Midwest Pioneer: His Ills, Cures, and Doctors* (Crawfordsville, Ind., 1945), 226; C. D. T. James, "Mesmerism: A Prelude to Anaesthesia," *Proceedings*, Royal Society of Medicine, LXVIII (1975), 446–47.

7. George Bush, *Mesmer and Swedenborg: Or, the Relation of the Developments of Mesmerism to the Doctrines and Disclosures of Swedenborg* (New York, 1847), 159–205; Ilza Veith, "From Mesmerism to Hypnotism," *Modern Medicine* (1959), 195–206; Robert H. Collyer, *Lights and Shadows of American Life* (Boston, 1844?); La Roy Sunderland, *Pathetism: Man Considered to His Form, Life, Sensation, Soul, Mind, Spirit; Giving the Rationale of Those Laws Which Produce the Mysteries, Miseries, Felicities, of Human Nature!* (Boston, 1847); Charles Morley, *Elements of Animal Magnetism: Or Process and Application for Relieving Human Suffering* (New York, 1847); Andrew Jackson Davis, *The Magic Staff: An Autobiography* (New York, 1876); Andrew Jackson Davis, *The Principles of Nature, Her Divine Revelations, and a Voice to Mankind* (New York, 1847).

8. Lester King, "Stahl and Hoffman: A Study in 18th Century Animism," *Journal of the History of Medicine and Allied Sciences*, XIX (1964), 118–30; Lester King, "Basic Concepts of Early 18th Century Animism," *American Journal of Psychiatry*, CXXIV (1967), 797–802; L. J. Rather, "G. E. Stahl's Psychological Physiology,"

Bulletin of the History of Medicine, XXXV (1961), 37–49; Worthington Hooker, *Lessons from the Story of Medical Delusions* (New York, 1850), 9.

9. "Hahnemann and Homeopathy," *Medical Gazette*, III (1869), 100; Sir Michael Foster, *Lectures on the History of Physiology during the Sixteenth, Seventeenth and Eighteenth Centuries* (New York, 1970), 168–71, 173, 260.

10. Quoted in "Hahnemann and Homeopathy," 109; Thomas Bradford, *The Life and Letters of Dr. Samuel Hahnemann* (Phila., 1895), 38; Robert E. Dudgeon, *Lectures on the Theory and Practice of Homeopathy* (Manchester, 1854), xxi; Wilhelm Ameke, *History of Homeopathy: Its Origin, Its Conflicts* (London, 1885), 99.

11. "Hahnemann and Homeopathy," 109. Hahnemann derived the idea of drug experimentation from Baron Anton Stoerck (1731–1803), director of the Vienna faculty of medicine who had carried out numerous experiments in the area of pharmacology. See Bradford, *Life and Letters of Dr. Samuel Hahnemann*, 42.

12. Quoted in John P. Harrison, "On the Absurdities and Dangers of the Empirical Mode of Practice, Denominated Homeopathy," *Western Lancet*, V (1847), 326.

13. Quoted in John McNaughton, "Homeopathy," *Transactions*, Medical Society of the State of New York, IV (1838), 8.

14. William E. Quinn, "The Medical Profession, the Causes of Its Division into Discordant Elements and the Reasons I Am Not a Homeopath," *Journal of Medicine and Science*, V (1899), 401; Bradford, *Life and Letters of Dr. Samuel Hahnemann*, 136; Linn J. Boyd, *A Study of the Simile in Medicine* (Phila., 1936), 2, 9, 13, 50; Osler, *The Evolution of Modern Medicine*, 140–41.

15. Samuel Hahnemann, *Organon of Homeopathic Medicine* (New York, 1843), 104; Alexander N. Dougherty, "Popular Insanity as Exemplified in the Favor Accorded to Homeopathy," *New Jersey Medical Recorder*, I (1848), 21, 27; A. B. Arnold, "Homeopathy," *Transactions*, Medical and Chirurgical Faculty of the State of Maryland (1878), 20.

16. Quoted in Arnold, "Homeopathy," 23, 28.

17. Dougherty, "Popular Insanity as Exemplified in the Favor Accorded Homeopathy," 28.

18. Arnold, "Homeopathy," 21.

19. Hahnemann, *Organon*, 338; McNaughton, "Homeopathy," 14.

20. Hahnemann, *Organon*, 210–11; Boyd, *A Study of Simile in Medicine*, 114–18; "Hahnemann and Homeopathy," 197; Thomas W. Blatchford, "Homeopathy Illustrated," *Transactions*, Medical Society of the State of New York, V (1843), 368; Bradford, *Life and*

Letters of Dr. Samuel Hahnemann, 52; Dudgeon, *Lectures on the Theory and Practice of Homeopathy*, 12, 133, 137–90.

21. John B. Roberts, "The Present Attitude of Physicians and Modern Medicine Towards Homeopathy," *Transactions*, Medical Society of the State of Pennsylvania, XXXVI (1895), 55; Bradford, *Life and Letters of Dr. Samuel Hahnemann*, 457–58.

22. Henry H. Hemenway, "Modern Homeopathy and Medical Science," *Journal*, American Medical Association, XXII (1894), 369.

23. Blatchford, "Homeopathy Illustrated," 381; Gottlieb H. G. Jahr, *New Homeopathic Pharmacopoeia and Poslogy, or the Preparation of Homeopathic Medicines and the Administration of Doses* (Phila., 1842), 35; T. W. Gordon, "Beauties of Homeopathy Exemplified," *Atlanta Medical and Surgical Journal*, II (1856), 193; Aleksiei G. Eustatiev, *Homeopathia Revealed: A Brief Exposition of the Whole System Adapted to General Comprehension* (New York, 1846), 35; Dudgeon, *Lectures on the Theory and Practice of Homeopathy*, 351.

24. John W. Sevier, "Homeopathy," *Nashville Journal of Medicine and Surgery*, VII (1854), 372.

25. Quoted in Charles W. Earle, "Homeopathy as It Was and as It Is," *Chicago Medical Examiner*, XII (1871), 521; Samuel Hahnemann, *The Chronic Diseases: Their Specific Nature and Homeopathic Treatment* (New York, 1845), 126–35.

26. Samuel Swan, *Catalogue of Morbific Products, Nosodes, and Other Remedies in High Potencies* (New York, 1886); Harris L. Coulter, "Homeopathic Influences in 19th Century Allopathic Therapeutics: A Historical and Philosophical Study," *Journal*, American Institute of Homeopathy, LXV (1972), 207–44; "Hahnemann and Homeopathy," 229.

27. J. P. Harrison, "On the Absurdities and Dangers of the Empirical Mode of Practice, Denominated Homeopathy," *Western Lancet*, V (1856–57), 329–30; Samuel Hahnemann, *Materia Medica Pura* (New York, 1846), 19; Samuel Willard, "Fallacies of Homeopathy," *St. Louis Medical and Surgical Journal*, VI (1848), 8; Arnold, "Homeopathy," 29.

28. Blatchford, "Homeopathy Illustrated," 399; John B. Roberts, *Modern Medicine and Homeopathy* (Phila., 1895), 56; E. Fischer-Homberger, "Eighteenth Century Nosology and Its Survivors," *Medical History*, XIV (1970), 397–402; James J. Robertson, "The Pseudo-Sciences—Homeopathy," *Medical Times and Gazette*, n.s. III (1851), 224; Harrison, "On the Absurdities and Dangers of the Empirical Mode of Practice, Denominated Homeopathy," 332.

29. Earle, "Homeopathy as It Was and as It Is," 525–27; Blatchford, "Homeopathy Illustrated," 218–19.

30. Dougherty, "Popular Insanity as Exemplified in the Favor

Accorded to Homeopathy," 39; Günter B. Risse, "Philosophical Medicine in Nineteenth Century Germany: An Episode in the Relations between Philosophy and Medicine," *Journal of Medicine and Philosophy*, I (1976), 72–92; Richard H. Shryock, "Empiricism versus Rationalism in American Medicine, 1650–1950," *Proceedings*, American Antiquarian Society, LXXIX (1969), 118–20.

31. Dougherty, "Popular Insanity as Exemplified in the Favor Accorded to Homeopathy," 39; Charles Rosenberg, "The American Medical Profession: Mid–19th Century," *Mid-America*; XLIV (1962), 168–70; David H. Donald, *An Excess of Democracy: The American Civil War and the Social Process* (Oxford, 1960); Frederick C. Waite, "American Sectarian Medical Colleges before the Civil War," *Bulletin of the History of Medicine*, XIX (1946), 162–66; Lewis B. Flinn, "Homeopathic Influence in the Delaware Community: A Retrospective Reassessment," *Delaware Medical Journal*, XLVIII (1976), 418–28.

32. William F. Norwood, *Medical Education in the United States before the Civil War* (Phila., 1944), 416–17; Harris L. Coulter, "Political and Social Aspects of Nineteenth Century Medicine in the United States: Formation of the AMA and Its Struggle with Homeopathic and Eclectic Physicians," (Ph.D. diss., Columbia, 1970), 147.

33. Robertson, "The Pseudo-Sciences—Homeopathy," 224; Bradford, *Life and Letters of Dr. Samuel Hahnemann*, 285; William Harvey King (ed.), *History of Homeopathy and Its Institutions in America; Their Founders, Benefactors, Faculties, Officers, Hospitals, Alumni, etc.*, 4 vols. (New York, 1905), II, 13–14; John F. Gray, *The Early Annals of Homeopathy in New York: A Discourse before the Homeopathic Societies of New York and Brooklyn on the 10th of April, 1863* (New York, 1863); Pickard and Buley, *The Midwest Pioneer: His Ills, Cures and Doctors*, 208; William H. Holcombe, *How I Became a Homeopath* (New York, 1866), 10–11.

34. Quoted from the *Water-Cure Journal* in Harry B. Weiss and Howard R. Kemble, *The Great American Water-Cure Craze: A History of Hydropathy in the United States* (Trenton, 1967), 54.

35. Quoted in William A. Purrington, "Christian Science and Its Legal Aspects," *Medical Era*, XVII (1899), 94–95; Sir Arthur Newsholme, *Evolution of Preventive Medicine* (Baltimore, 1927), 156.

36. A. H. Crosby, "Orthodoxy and Heterodoxy in Medicine," *Transactions*, New Hampshire Medical Society, LXXXVII (1877), 86.

37. McNaughton, "Homeopathy," 24–25; Jacques M. Quen, "Elisha Perkins, Physician, Nostrum-Vendor, or Charlatan?" *Bulletin of the History of Medicine*, XXXVII (1963), 159–66; Edwin Lee, *Animal Magnetism and Homeopathy* (London, 1838); Grete de Francesco, *The Power of the Charlatan* (New Haven, 1939), 253; Walter R.

Steiner, "The Conflict of Medicine and Quackery," *Annals of Medical History*, VI (1924), 60–70; Hooker, *Lessons from the Story of Medical Delusions*, 18.

38. L. A. Dugas, "A Clinical Lecture at the Augusta Hospital upon the Subject of Homeopathy," *Southern Medical and Surgical Journal*, XVI (1860), 250.

39. Edward Waldo Emerson, "The Man as Doctor," *New England Journal of Medicine*, CVI (1882), 534–45.

40. A. D. Lippe, "Liberty of Medical Opinion and Action," *Hahnemannian Monthly*, VI (1870), 154.

41. Jahr, *New Homeopathic Pharmacopoeia and Posology, or the Preparation of Homeopathic Medicines and the Administration of Doses*, 36.

42. Martin Kaufman, *Homeopathy in America: The Rise and Fall of a Medical Heresy* (Baltimore, 1971), 69–74.

43. A. Behr, "Review of the So-Called Science of Homeopathy," *St. Louis Medical and Surgical Journal*, XI (1853), 33; Dudgeon, *Lecture on the Theory and Practice of Homeopathy*, 493–99.

44. Mary A. Brinkmann, "The Relation of Homeopathy to Gynaecology; Or, Sectarianism in Medicine," *Homeopathic Journal of Obstetrics*, XII (1890), 164–74.

45. Arnold, "Homeopathy," 20.

46. Willis J. Beach, "A Protest against the Recent Action of the New York Medical Society with Regard to Consultations," *Connecticut State Medical Society*, n.s. II (1882), 100.

47. William W. Parker, "Rise and Decline of Homeopathy," *Transactions*, Medical Society of Virginia (1890), 163.

48. A. B. Palmer, "The Fallacies of Homeopathy," *North American Review*, CXXXIV (1882), 310–11; Quinn, "The Medical Profession, the Causes of Its Division into Discordant Elements and the Reasons I Am Not a Homeopath," 405–7.

49. Quoted in J. B. Roberts, "Points of Similarity between Us and Homeopathic Physicians," *JAMA*, XX (1893), 582.

50. Ibid., 583.

51. B. Jackson, "Against Sectarianism in Medicine," *Medical News*, LV (1889), 426; John B. Roberts, *Modern Medicine and Homeopathy* (Phila., 1895), 11; Earle, "Homeopathy as It Was and as It Is," 539–40.

52. S. W. Wetmore, "What Is Modern Homeopathy?" *American Observer and Medical Monthly*, XV (1878), 140–41; Edward J. Forster, *A Sketch of the Medical Profession. From the Professional and Industrial History of Suffolk County* (Boston, 1894), 219–20; King, *History of Homeopathy and Its Institutions in America*, I, 76–111, 210–40, 322–40.

53. J. S. Lynch, "The Conflict of Rational, Scientific Medicine with Homeopathy," *Medical Chronicle*, I (1882), 2; Albert H. Buck,

The Dawn of Modern Medicine: An Account of the Revival of the Science and Art of Medicine Which Took Place in Western Europe during the Latter Half of the Eighteenth Century and the First Part of the Nineteenth (New Haven, 1920), 27–28; Coulter, "Political and Social Aspects of Nineteenth Century Medicine in the United States: Formation of the AMA and Its Struggle with Homeopathic and Eclectic Physicians," 223.

54. George B. Peck, "Homeopathy in the United States," *Hahnemannian Monthly*, XXXV (1900), 560; A. K. Crawford, "Hahnemann and Homeopathy," *Clinique*, XVIII (1897), 562; Morris Fishbein, "The Rise and Fall of Homeopathy," *American Mercury*, II (1924), 150–54.

55. James C. Wood, "Relations of Homeopathy to Allied Systems of Therapeutics," *Hahnemannian Monthly*, XXXIV (1899), 609–10; Hahnemann, *The Chronic Diseases: Their Specific Nature and Homeopathic Treatment*, 177–81; Bradford, *Life and Letters of Dr. Samuel Hahnemann*, 44–47; Dudgeon, *Lectures on the Theory and Practice of Homeopathy*, xxiii; Thomas D. Washburn, "The Relation of the Profession to the Secular Press and the Rostrum," *Medical Examiner*, XXI (1874), 510; John Duffy (ed.), *The Rudolph Matas History of Medicine in Louisiana*, 2 vols. (Baton Rouge, La., 1958), II, 37.

56. Roberts, "Points of Similarity between Us and Homeopathic Physicians," 581; Daniel B. St. John Roosa, *A Doctor's Suggestions to the Community: Being a Series of Papers upon Various Subjects from a Physician's Standpoint* (New York, 1880), 62.

57. Quoted in Quinn, "The Medical Profession, the Causes of Its Division into Discordant Elements and the Reasons I am Not a Homeopath," 409.

58. Roosa, *A Doctor's Suggestions to the Community*, 62–63; John B. Huber, "Faith Cures and the Law," *Medical Record*, LIX (1901), 606; Raymond J. Cunningham, "From Holiness to Healing: The Faith Cure in America, 1872–1892," *Church History*, XLIII (1974), 499–513.

59. Henry H. Goddard, "The Effects of Mind on Body as Evidenced by Faith Cures," *American Journal of Psychology* (1898–99), 437; Milton O. Kepler, "Medicine and Religion: A Brief Historical Survey of Their Interrelationship," *Nebraska State Medical Journal*, LIII (1968), 585–89.

60. J. M. Buckley, "Faith-Healing and Kindred Phenomena," *Century Magazine*, II (1886), 781–82. Buckley was editor of the *Christian Advocate*.

61. Quoted in James J. Lloyd, "Faith Cures," *Medical Record*, XXIX (1886), 350; R. Kelso Carter, "Divine Healing, or 'Faith-Cure,'" *Century Magazine*, II (1886), 780.

62. Quoted in Lloyd, "Faith Cures," 350.

63. J. C. Bierwirth, "The Relations of the So-Called 'Christian Science Cure' and 'Faith Cure,'" *New York Medical Journal*, L (1889), 713–16; Leander E. Whipple, *The Philosophy of Mental Healing: A Practical Exposition of Natural Restorative Power* (New York, 1893), 105–6; William A. Purrington, "Manslaughter, Christian Science, and the Law," *Medical Record*, LIV (1898), 761.

64. William I. Gill, "Faith Cure," *New England Magazine*, V (1887), 448; Cunningham, "From Holiness to Healing: The Faith Cure in America, 1872–1892," 499–501; Buckley, "Faith-Healing and Kindred Phenomena," 875; James M. Buckley, *Faith-Healing, Christian Science, and Kindred Phenomena* (New York, 1892); Donald B. Meyer, *The Positive Thinkers: A Study of the American Quest for Health and Personal Power from Mary Baker Eddy to Norman Vincent Peale* (Garden City, N.Y., 1965), 43; Walsh, *Cures: The Story of the Cures That Fail*, 10, 22.

65. Robert E. Campbell, "Homeopathy," *Atlanta Medical and Surgical Journal*, II (1856), 196–97; Eustatiev, *Homeopathy Revealed: A Brief Exposition of the Whole System Adapted to General Comprehension*, 73–74; Elisha Bartlett, *An Essay on the Philosophy of Medical Science* (Phila., 1844), 244–45.

66. John Fiske, *Studies in Religion: Being the Destiny of Man; the Idea of God; Through Nature to God; Life Everlasting* (Boston, 1902), 266; Gail T. Parker, *Mind Cure in New England; From the Civil War to World War I* (Hanover, N.H., 1973), 60–61, 79.

67. Goddard, "The Effects of Mind and Body as Evidenced by Faith Cures," 446–47; Jastrow, "Malicious Animal Magnetism," 359; Annetta Dresser, *The Philosophy of P. P. Quimby, With Selections from His Manuscripts and a Sketch of His Life* (Boston, 1895); Robert Peel, *Mary Baker Eddy: The Years of Discovery* (New York, 1966), 152–54, 297–303; Meyer, *The Positive Thinkers*, 33–34; Ilza Veith, "From Hypnotism to Suggestion," *Modern Medicine* (1959), 304–14.

68. Quoted in Morris Fishbein, *Fads and Quackery in Healing: An Analysis of the Foibles of the Healing Cults, With Essays on Various Other Peculiar Notions in the Health Field* (New York, 1932), 45.

69. Mary Baker Eddy, *Science and Health with Key to the Scriptures* (Boston, 1875), 172; Bryon R. Wilson, *Sects and Society: A Sociological Study of the Elim Tabernacle, Christian Science, and Christadelphians* (Berkeley, 1961), ch. 7; Raymond J. Cunningham, "Christian Science and Mind Cure in America: A Review Article," *Journal of the History of the Behavioral Sciences*, XI (1975), 299–311.

70. Hildegarde H. Longsdorf, "Christian Science and Its Relation to the Medical Profession," *Transactions*, Medical Society of the State of Pennsylvania (1894), 153–54; Peel, *Mary Baker Eddy*, 111, 135–36, 172.

71. Eddy, *Science and Health With Key to the Scriptures*, 157.

72. Mary Baker Eddy, *Message to the Mother Church, Boston, Massachusetts, 1901* (Boston, 1901), 18.

73. Mary Baker Eddy, *Christian Healing and the People's Idea of God* (Boston, 1915), 12.

74. Eddy, *Message to the Mother Church*, 18.

75. Eddy, *Science and Health with Key to the Scriptures*, 149; Parker, *Mind Cure in New England*, 13–14, 128.

76. Carol Norton, "Christian Science and the Law," *Medico-Legal Journal*, XVII (1899), 186–87.

77. Mary Baker Eddy, *The People's Idea of God; Its Effects on Health and Christianity* (Boston, 1912), 1, 3–4; Eddy, *Christian Healing and the People's Idea of God*, 15, 18.

78. Aurelius J. L. Gliddon, *Faith Cures: Their History and Mystery* (London, 1890), 136.

79. Eddy, *The People's Idea of God*, 16.

80. Goddard, "The Effects of Mind on Body as Evidenced by Faith Cures," 434; Norton, "Christian Science and the Law," 188; Frank L. Riley, *Spiritual Healing* (Los Angeles, 1917); John B. Huber, "The *Medical News* Investigation into the Claims of Christian Science," *Medical News*, LXXIV (1899), 107.

81. Eddy, *Message to the Mother Church*, 19–20; Stephen Gottschalk, *The Emergence of Christian Science in American Religious Life* (Berkeley, 1974), xxii.

82. Jastrow, "Malicious Animal Magnetism," 356, 359; Wilson, *Sects and Society*, 139–40.

83. J. B. Huber, "Christian Science from a Physician's Point of View," *Popular Science Monthly*, LV (1899), 763; Norton, "Christian Science and the Law," 186–87; Louis S. Reed, *The Healing Cults: A Study of Sectarian Medical Practice: Its Extent, Causes, and Control* (Chicago, 1932), 73.

84. Samuel Clemens, *Christian Science; With Notes Containing Corrections to Date* (New York, 1907), 1–28, 87, 110; Gottschalk, *The Emergence of Christian Science in American Religious Life*, 42.

85. Rev. Warren Felt Evans, *The Mental-Cure, Illustrating the Influence of the Mind on the Body, Both in Health and Disease, and in the Psychological Method of Treatment* (Boston, 1869), 23, 266; A. F. Hoch, *The Natural Law of Mind Healing and Mind Creating of Sickness, Disease and Deformity* (Los Angeles, 1915); Parker, *Mind Cure in New England*, 41–48, 53–55, 60–61.

86. Rev. Warren Felt Evans, *Esoteric Christianity and Mental Therapeutics* (Boston, 1886), 37, 144–45; Emanuel Swedenborg, *Angelic Wisdom Concerning the Divine Love and the Divine Wisdom* (New York, 1885); Emanuel Swedenborg, *Angelic Wisdom Concerning the Divine Providence* (New York, 1892); Bush, *Mesmer and*

Swedenborg: Or, the Relation of the Developments of Mesmerism to the Doctrines and Disclosures of Swedenborg, 21–53.

87. Rev. Warren Felt Evans, *Soul and Body; Or, the Scriptural Science of Health and Disease* (Boston, 1876), 34–35. Like Mrs. Eddy, the Rev. Evans was once a disciple of Quimby.

88. Ibid., 35–38; Charles W. Close, *Phrenopathy; Or, Rational Mind Cure* (Bangor, Maine, 1900), 19–20.

89. Evans, *Esoteric Christianity and Mental Therapeutics*, 6–7, 152; Close, *Phrenopathy; Or, Rational Mind Cure*, 39–48; Harriet Hale Rix, *Christian Mind-Healing: A Course of Lessons in the Fundamentals of New Thought* (Los Angeles, 1914), 65; Reed, *The Healing Cults*, 79.

90. Evans, *Soul and Body*, 127, 135–36.

91. R. Lauder, "Therapeutic Value of Faith Cure," *Proceedings*, Connecticut State Medical Society, n.s. IV (1888), 110.

92. B. D. Eastman, "Psychic Healing," *Kansas Medical Journal*, IX (1897), 575–80.

93. W. F. Hartford, "Subjective Therapeutics," *Medical Record*, LIV (1898), 158–59.

94. Goddard, "The Effects of Mind on Body as Evidenced by Faith Cures," 500.

95. Ibid., 481, 500.

96. Ibid., 445.

97. Geoffrey Rhodes, *Mind Cures* (London, 1915), 161–63; Charles F. Winbigler, *Handbook of Instructions for Healing and Helping Others; Containing Scriptural, Psycho-Therapeutic, Psychological, and Optimistic Principles, Simply Stated and Thoroughly Tested* (Los Angeles, 1916), 10, 15–16; S. P. Fullinwider, "Neurasthenia: The Genteel Caste's Journey Inward," *Rocky Mountain Social Science Journal*, XI (1974), 1–9.

98. Samuel McComb, "Nervousness—A National Menace," *Everybody's Magazine*, XXII (1910), 258–62; Robert MacDonald, *Mind, Religion and Health; With an Appreciation of the Emmanuel Movement; How Its Principles Can be Applied in Promoting Health and in the Enriching of Our Daily Life* (New York, 1908); John Greene, "The Emmanuel Movement, 1906–1929," *New England Quarterly*, VII (1943), 494–532; Barbara Sicherman, "The Uses of a Diagnosis: Doctors, Patients, and Neurasthenia," *Journal of the History of Medicine and Allied Sciences*, XXXII (1977), 33–54.

99. McComb, "Nervousness—A National Menace," 262–63.

100. Ibid., 264; Samuel McComb, "My Experience With Nervous Sufferers," *Harper's Bazaar*, XLIV (1910), 29; Henry E. Sigerist, *Civilization and Disease* (Ithaca, N.Y., 1943), 144–45.

101. Stow Persons, *American Minds: A History of Ideas* (New York, 1958), 425; Ellwood Worcester, Samuel McComb, and Dr. Isidor H. Coriat, *Religion and Medicine: The Moral Control of Nervous Disorders*

(New York, 1908); L. Gilbert Little, *Nervous Christians* (Nebraska, 1956); Meyer, *The Positive Thinkers*, 250–56; Gilbert V. Seldes, *The Stammering Century* (New York, 1928), chs. 22–25; Lyman P. Powell, *The Emmanuel Movement in a New England Town: A Systematic Account of Experiments and Reflections Designed to Determine the Proper Relationship between the Minister and the Doctor in the Light of Modern Needs* (New York, 1909); Gottschalk, *The Emergence of Christian Science in American Religious Life*, 214–15.

CHAPTER FIVE

Midwives in Britches

1. Joseph Adams, "On Midwives and Accoucheurs," *Medical and Physical Journal*, XXXV (1816), 84–88; "Women Midwives," *Medical Times and Gazette*, I (1872), 686–87; Clement Godson, "On the Evolution of Obstetrics and Gynecology," *British Gynecological Journal* (1895–96), 15; J. Elise Gordon, "The Midwife in Biblical History and Legend," *Midwife and Health Visitor*, IV (1968), 423–26. "During the Roman period it is known that midwives studied medicine, usually under the tutelage of a capable female practitioner. . . . The Greeks differentiated between amateur and professional midwives, the latter of whom were entrusted with considerable responsibility, since they were preferred as abortionists. Rome also, when Hellenized, possessed a class of skilled midwives who, according to Soranus, were skilled in both the theory and practice of their art." See James V. Ricci, *The Genealogy of Gynaecology: History of the Development of Gynaecology throughout the Ages, 2000 B.C.–1800 A.D.* (Phila., 1950), 84; J. Elise Gordon, "Some Women Practitioners of Past Centuries," *Practitioner*, CCVIII (1972), 561–67.

2. William Goodell, "When and Why Were Male Physicians Employed as Accoucheurs?" *American Journal of Obstetrics and Diseases of Women and Children*, IX (1876), 388; James H. Aveling, "English Midwives: Their History and Prospects," *Lancet*, I (1872), 501; Godson, "On the Evolution of Obstetrics and Gynecology," 15; Lucille B. Pinto, "The Folk Practice of Gynecology and Obstetrics in the Middle Ages," *Bulletin of the History of Medicine*, XLVII (1973), 513–23; Ricci, *The Genealogy of Gynaecology*, 237–47.

3. William Hamilton, *The History of Medicine, Surgery, and Anatomy, from the Creation of the World to the Commencement of the Nineteenth Century*, 2 vols. (London, 1831), II, 142. Most medical historians agree that although Clément was accorded the title of accoucheur, a Monsieur Boucher was actually responsible for the early deliveries of the Duchesse de la Vallière. See George Ban-

croft-Livingston, "Louise de la Vallière and the Birth of the Man-Midwife," *Journal of Obstetrics and Gynecology of the British Empire*, LXIII (1956), 261–67; J. K. Kelly, "Gynecology One Hundred Years Ago," *Glasgow Medical Journal*, LII (1899), 103–13.

4. "Celebrated Midwives of the Seventeenth and Beginning of the Eighteenth Centuries," *St. Thomas's Hospital Gazette*, V (1895), 35.

5. Goodell, "When and Why Were Male Physicians Employed as Accoucheurs?" 382–85; William Goodell, *A Sketch of the Life and of the Writings of Louyse Bourgeois, Midwife to Marie de Medici, the Queen of Henry IV of France* (Phila., 1876); Richard L. Petrelli, "The Regulation of French Midwifery during the Ancien Régime," *Journal of the History of Medicine and Allied Sciences*, XXVI (1971), 283.

6. Aveling, "English Midwives," 534; Isaac H. Flack [Harvey Graham], *Eternal Eve: The History of Gynecology and Obstetrics* (Garden City, N.Y., 1951), ch. 8; Douglas Guthrie, *A History of Medicine* (London, 1945), 236; P. W. Van Peyma, "The Midwife," *Buffalo Medical Journal*, LXVI (1910–11), 447; J. E. Gordon, "British Midwives through the Centuries," *Midwife and Health Visitor*, III (1967), 275.

7. Herbert R. Spencer, *The History of British Midwifery from 1600 to 1800: The Fitz Patrick Lectures for 1927* (London, 1927), 163; J. M. M. Kerr, R. W. Johnstone, and Miles H. Phillips (eds.), *Historical Review of British Obstetrics and Gynecology, 1800–1950* (Edinburgh, 1954), 332; Guthrie, *History of Medicine*, 237; Pierre V. Renouard, *History of Medicine, from Its Origin to the Nineteenth Century, with Appendix, Containing a Philosophical and Historical Review of Medicine to the Present Time* (Cincinnati, 1856), 463; Walter Radcliffe, *Milestones in Midwifery* (Bristol, 1967), 12; J. W. Huffman, "The Great Eighteenth Century Obstetric Atlases and Their Illustrator," *Obstetrics and Gynecology*, XXXV (1970), 971–76; Leonard E. Laufe, *Obstetrics Forceps* (New York, 1968), 1–11; Wyndham E. B. Lloyd, *A Hundred Years of Medicine* (London, 1936), 200; James M. Dunlop, "Midwifery: Ancient and Modern," *History of Medicine*, VI (1975), 55.

8. F. H. Garrison, "Samuel Bard and the King's College School," *Bulletin*, New York Academy of Medicine, I (1925), 85–91; John B. Blake, "Women and Medicine in Ante-Bellum America," *Bulletin of the History of Medicine*, XXXIX (1965), 108–10; Walter Channing, *Remarks on the Employment of Females as Practitioners in Midwifery. By a Physician* (Boston, 1820); Lewis C. Scheffey, "The Earlier History and the Transition Period of Obstetrics and Gynecology in Philadelphia," *Annals of Medical History*, III (1940), 215–18; I. Snapper, "Midwifery, Past and Present," *Bulletin*, New York Academy of Medicine, XXXIX (1963), 518–21.

9. W. Robert Penman, "The Public Practice of Midwifery in Philadelphia," *Transactions and Studies*, College of Physicians of Philadelphia, XXXVII (1969), 124–32; Herbert Thoms, "The Beginnings of Obstetrics in America," *Yale Journal of Biology and Medicine*, IV (1932), 672–74; Esmond F. Cody, "The Registered Midwife: A Necessity," *Boston Medical and Surgical Journal*, CLXVII (1913), 416; Douglas M. Haynes, "The Vanishing Obstetrician," *Southern Medical Journal*, LXI (1968), 469; J. Glaister, *Dr. William Smellie and His Contemporaries: A Contribution to the History of Midwifery in the Eighteenth Century* (Glasgow, 1894); Herbert Thoms, *Chapters in American Obstetrics* (Springfield, Ill., 1933), 16–17; Irving S. Cutter and Henry R. Viets, *A Short History of Midwifery* (Phila., 1964), 144–45, 156, 167.

10. Goodell, "When and Why Were Male Physicians Employed as Accoucheurs?" 390; "Midwives and Midwifery," *Lancet*, I (1842), 762; J. G. F. Holstori, "History of Midwifery in Ohio," *Transactions*, Ohio Medical Society (1857), 63–64.

11. Quoted in "Celebrated Midwives of the Seventeenth and Eighteenth Centuries," 35; J. H. Young, "James Hamilton (1767–1839) Obstetrician and Conversationalist," *Medical History*, VII (1963), 62–72; Godson, "On the Evolution of Obstetrics and Gynecology," 15; Gordon, "British Midwives through the Centuries," 278; Sir Charles Illingworth, "William Hunter's Influence on Obstetrics," *Scottish Medical Journal*, XV (1970), 58–60.

12. Quoted in Edward Mailins, "An Address on Midwifery and Midwives," *British Medical Journal*, I (1901), 1530; Philip J. Klukoff, "Smollett's Defence of Dr. Smellie in *The Critical Review*," *Medical History*, XXIV (1970), 31–41.

13. Halford quoted in Kerr, Johnstone, and Phillips (eds.), *Historical Review of British Obstetrics and Gynecology*, 332.

14. John Blunt (pseud.), *Man-Midwifery Dissected; Or the Obstetric Family-Instructor. For the Use of Married Couples, and Single Adults of Both Sexes* (London, 1793), 69–70.

15. George Morant, *Hints to Husbands: A Revelation of the Man-Midwife's Mysteries* (London, 1857), 7, 24–25, 46, 52, 56. See also Orson S. Fowler, *Maternity: Or, the Bearing and Nursing of Children* (New York, 1856), 183; William F. Mengert, "The Origins of the Male Midwife," *Annals of Medical History*, n.s. IV (1932), 453–65; James A. Mowris, *An Expose of Surgical Seduction! As Practiced by Physicians Who Specialize on Female Disease* (Syracuse, N.Y., 1871), 4.

16. Samuel Bard, *A Compendium of the Theory and Practice of Midwifery* (New York, 1807), 181; William Potts Dewees, *Compendious System of Midwifery, Chiefly Designed to Facilitate the Inquiries of Those Who May be Pursuing This Branch of Study* (Phila., 1824), 190–91.

17. "Report of the Trial: The People Versus Dr. Horatio N.

Loomis, For Libel. Tried at the Erie County Oyer and Terminer, June 24, 1850, . . . Buffalo, 1850," in *The Male Mid-Wife and the Female Doctor: The Gynecology Controversy in Nineteenth Century America* (New York, 1974), 13, 50.

18. Quoted in James H. Aveling, *English Midwives: Their History and Prospects* (London, 1872), 52–53; Thomas R. Forbes, *The Midwife and the Witch* (New Haven, 1966), 112–32; R. V. Schnucker, "The English Puritans and Pregnancy, Delivery and Breast Feeding," *History of Childhood Quarterly*, I (1974), 637–58; Aristotle (pseud.), *Aristotle's Master-Piece Completed* (New York, 1793), 58–61, 110–20; Aristotle (pseud.), *Aristotle's Compleat and Experienc'd Midwife* (London, 1700), 53, 57, 75, 96–97; Thoms, "The Beginnings of Obstetrics in America," 665–75; Cutter and Viets, *A Short History of Midwifery*, 143–44; Walton B. McDaniel, "The Medical and Magical Significance in Ancient Medicine of Things Connected with Reproduction and Its Origins," *Journal of the History of Medicine and Allied Sciences*, III (1948), 525–46.

19. Jane B. Donegan, "Midwifery in America, 1760–1860: A Study in Medicine and Mortality" (Ph.D. diss., Syracuse Univ., 1972), 58–59, 82–83; T. Gaillard Thomas, "A Century of American Medicine, 1776–1876: Obstetrics and Gynecology," *American Journal of the Medical Sciences*, LXXIII (1876), 134; Richard W. and Dorothy C. Wertz, *Lying-in: A History of Childbirth in America* (New York, 1977), 1–21.

20. Beatrice Mongeau et al., "The Granny Midwife; Changing Roles and Functions of a Folk Practitioner," *American Journal of Sociology*, LXVI (1960–61), 500.

21. John Duffy, "Anglo-American Reaction to Obstetrical Anesthesia," *Bulletin of the History of Medicine*, XXXVIII (1964), 32–44; B. E. Cotling, "Anaesthetics in Midwifery," *Boston Medical and Surgical Journal*, LIX (1858–59), 369–70.

22. Mongeau et al., "The Granny Midwife," 503; Van Peyma, "The Midwife," 485–86; Robert A. Ross, "The Midwife in North Carolina since 1587," in Dorothy Long (ed.), *Medicine in North Carolina: Essays in the History of Medical Science and Medical Service, 1524–1960*, 2 vols. (Raleigh, N.C., 1972), II, 659–61; Thomas N. Ivey, "Medicine in the Pioneer West—1850–1900," *North Carolina Medical Journal*, XXVI (1965), 162.

23. C. S. Bacon, "Failures of Midwives in Asepsis," *JAMA*, XXVIII (1897), 248; Helen Olson Halvorsen and Lorraine Fletcher, "Nineteenth Century Midwife: Some Recollections," *Oregon Historical Quarterly*, LXX (1969), 39–49; Holstori, "History of Midwifery in Ohio," 49; Helinina Jeidell and Wilma M. Fricke, "The Midwives of Anne Arundel County, Maryland," *Johns Hopkins Hospital Bulletin*, XXIII (1912), 281.

24. Carolyn C. Van Blarcom, "Midwives in America," *American Journal of Public Health*, IV (1914), 198; Holstori, "History of Midwifery in Ohio," 57; J. H. Pryor, "The Status of the Midwife in Buffalo," *New York Medical Journal*, XL (1884), 130.

25. Samuel Wright, "An Experimental Inquiry into the Physiological Actions of Ergot of Rye," *Edinburgh Medical and Surgical Journal*, LII (1840), 22–23; A. K. Gardner, "An Essay on Ergot, with New Views of Its Therapeutic Action," *New York Journal of Medicine*, n.s. XI (1853), 207; E. N. Chapman, "Ergot: Its Natural History and Uses as a Therapeutic Agent," *Medical and Surgical Reporter*, n.s. V (1861), 416; L. Spaulding, "Letter on Ergot," *New England Journal of Medicine and Surgery*, VII (1818), 146; Oliver Prescott, "A Dissertation on the Natural History and Medicinal Effects of the Secale Cornutum, or Ergot," *Medical Communications*, Massachusetts Medical Society, III (1822), 84; Frank L. Bové, *The Story of Ergot* (New York, 1970), 273.

26. William Commons, "Ergot; Its Use and Abuse," *Transactions*, Indiana State Medical Society, XXX (1880), 64.

27. John B. Beck, "Observations on Ergot," *Transactions*, Medical Society of the State of New York, V (1841), 185.

28. Ibid., 185.

29. David Hosack, "Observations on Ergot," *New York Medical and Physical Journal*, I (1822), 205–8.

30. W. G. Maxwell, "Contrariety of Opinions Regarding Ergot of Rye," *India Journal of Medical and Physical Sciences*, II (1837), 725; Chapman, "Ergot: Its Natural History and Uses," 421; Etienne Evetzky, "The Physiological and Therapeutical Action of Ergot," *New York Medical Journal and Obstetrical Review*, XXXIV (1881), 114.

31. Holstori, "History of Midwifery in Ohio," 63; Peal, "A Century of Obstetrics," 85–86; Douglas M. Hoynes, "The Vanishing Obstetrician," *Southern Medical Journal*, LXI (1968), 470; Owen H. Wagensteen, "Nineteenth Century Wound Management of the Parturient Uterus and Compound Fracture: The Semmelweis-Lister Priority Controversy," *Bulletin*, New York Academy of Medicine, XLVI (1970), 577–78; Flack, *Eternal Eve*, 376–79, 406–10; J. J. Nierstrasz, "General Pathology and Therapy of Inflammations in the 1860s," *Janus*, LIV (1967), 168–82; Charles J. Cullingworth, *Charles White, F.R.S.: A Great Provincial Surgeon and Obstetrician of the Eighteenth Century* (London, 1904).

32. John Stevens, *Man-Midwifery Exposed; Or the Danger and Immorality of Employing Men in Midwifery Proved: And the Remedy for the Evil Found. Addressed to the Society for the Suppression of Vice* (London, 1849), 35–36.

33. Fielding H. Garrison, *An Introduction to the History of Medicine* (Phila., 1929), 435; I. Snapper, "Midwifery, Past and Present," *Bul-*

letin, New York Academy of Medicine, XXXIX (1963), 524–25.

34. Arturo Castiglioni, *A History of Medicine* (New York, 1958), 630, 725; Oliver W. Holmes, "On the Contagiousness of Puerperal Fever," *New England Journal of Medicine,* I (1842–43), 503–30; Ignác F. Semmelweis, *Die Aetiologie, der Begriff und die Prophylaxis des Kindbettfiebers* (Budapest, 1861). Those who early noted the infectious nature of the disease include Alexander Gordon of Aberdeen in 1795, Thomas Denman of Edinburgh in 1801, Robert Collins of Dublin in 1835, and Gabriel Andral, the teacher of Oliver Wendell Holmes. See Virginia Parker, "Oliver Wendell Holmes: Man of Medicine, Man of Letters," *Bulletin,* Medical Library Association, LIV (1966), 145.

35. Harry Wain, *A History of Preventive Medicine* (Springfield, Ill., 1970), 221, 224; Gail Pat Parsons, "The British Medical Profession and Contagion Theory: Puerperal Fever as a Case Study, 1830–1860," *Medical History,* XXII (1978), 138–50.

36. Hodge quoted in Fred L. Adair, *The Country Doctor and the Specialist* (Maitland, Fla., 1968), 102–3; Meigs quoted in Thoms, *Chapters in American Obstetrics,* 58; J. Wister Meigs, "Puerperal Fever and Nineteenth Century Contagionism: The Obstetrician's Dilemma," *Transactions and Studies,* College of Physicians of Philadelphia, XLII (1975), 273–75; Karl M. Vogel, "Oliver Wendell Holmes and the Medical Student," *Medical Record,* XCVII (1920), 1069.

37. Lloyd, *A Hundred Years of Medicine,* 202.

38. W. S. Smith, "Careless and Unscientific Midwifery," *Maryland Medical Journal,* XXXIII (1895–96), 147.

39. Van Peyma, "The Midwife," 484; Jean Donnison, *Midwives and Medical Men: A History of Inter-Professional Rivalries and Women's Rights* (New York, 1977), 8.

40. R. W. Lobenstine, "The Influence of the Midwife," *American Journal of Obstetrics and Diseases of Women,* LXIII (1911), 877, 880; Ira S. Wile, "Immigration and the Midwife Problem," *New England Journal of Medicine,* CLXVII (1912), 115.

41. Van Blarcom, "Midwives in America," 198.

42. Carolyn C. Van Blarcom, "A Possible Solution to the Midwife Problem," *Proceedings,* National Conference of Charities and Corrections, XXXVII (1910), 350–51.

43. Ibid., 356.

44. S. W. Newmayer, "The Status of Midwifery in Pennsylvania and a Study of the Midwives of Philadelphia," *Monthly Cyclopedia and Medical Bulletin,* I (1911), 716.

45. J. Whitridge Williams, "Medical Education and the Midwife Problem in the United States," *JAMA,* LVIII (1912), 5; Francis E. Kobrin, "The American Midwife Controversy: A Crisis of Profes-

sionalization," *Bulletin of the History of Medicine*, XL (1966), 350–63; Judy B. Litoff, *American Midwives: 1860 to the Present* (Westport, Conn., 1978).

46. Williams, "Medical Education and the Midwife Problem," 6–7.

47. Cody, "The Registered Midwife," 416.

48. "An Abstract of the Laws and Regulations With Reference to Midwives Abroad," *Medical Examiner*, I (1876), 109; Petrelli, "Regulation of French Midwifery during the Ancien Régime," 276–91.

49. F. G. Champhees, "Inaugural Address," *Transactions*, Obstetrical Society of London, XXXVII (1896), 93–94.

50. S. Josephine Baker, "Schools for Midwives," *American Journal of Obstetrics and Diseases of Women*, LXV (1912), 259–60. Carl Siegmund Franz Credé (1819–92), professor of obstetrics and gynecology at Leipzig, introduced a method of massaging the uterus after delivery to encourage expulsion of the placenta. See his *Die Verhütung der Augenentzündung der Neugeborenen* (Berlin, 1884); Flack, *Eternal Eve*, 552–55.

51. Quoted in Aveling, "English Midwives," 500; "Melioration of Midwives," *Obstetrical Journal of Great Britain and Ireland*, I (1873), 689–98; Thomas R. Forbes, "The Regulation of English Midwives in the Sixteenth and Seventeenth Centuries," *Medical History*, VII (1964), 236; Petrelli, "Regulation of French Midwifery during the Ancien Régime," 285.

52. James H. Aveling, "On the Instruction, Examination, and Registration of Midwives," *British Medical Journal*, I (1873), 308; Andrew Boorde, *The Breuiary of Helthe, for all maner of syckenesses and diseases which may be in man, or woman doth folowe* (London, 1547); Forbes, "Registration of English Midwives," 235–44; Charles M. Crombie, *Remarks on Midwifery to Midwives: An Introductory Address* (Aberdeen, 1872), 20–23. Proposals for the instruction and licensing of midwives in England:

Andrew Boorde	1547	Anonymous	1740
Peter Chamberlen	1616	George Counsell	1752
Peter Chamberlen, Dr.	1633	Elizabeth Nihell	1760
Percival Willughby	1660	Fores, S. W.	1793
Elizabeth Cellier	1687	Margaret Stephen	1795
Mawbray, Dr.	1725	Soc. of Apothecaries	1813
John Douglas, Dr.	1736	Ladies' Obstet. College	1864
Bracken, Dr.	1737	Nightingale, Miss	1871
Sarah Stone	1737	Obstet. Soc. Lond.	1871
Manningham, Sir R.	1739	Gen. Med. Council	1872

53. "Melioration of Midwives," 617–20; Spencer, *The History of British Midwifery from 1650 to 1800*, 144.

54. Jean Donnison, "Medical Women and Lady Midwives: A Case Study in Medical and Feminist Politics," *Women's Studies*, III (1976), 229–50; Aveling, "On the Instruction, Examination and Registration of Midwives," 308–9.

55. Aveling, ibid., 310.

56. F. G. Champhees, "Inaugural Address," 89–91; Sir John Peel, "A Century of Obstetrics," *Practitioner*, CCI (1968), 90; Gordon, "British Midwives through the Centuries," 280–81; Kerr, Johnstone, and Phillips (eds.), *Historical Review of British Obstetrics and Gynecology*, 334.

57. Van Blarcom, "A Possible Solution to the Midwife Problem," 352; Taliaferro Clark, "Training of Midwives," *Chicago Medical Recorder*, XLVI (1924), 297–99; Victoria E. M. Bennett, *Lectures to Practicing Midwives* (London, 1909), 1–15; Sir Comyns Berkeley, *A Handbook for Midwives and Maternity Nurses* (London, 1909); Donnison, *Midwives and Medical Men*, 159–75.

58. T. Darlington, "The Present Status of the Midwife," *American Journal of Obstetrics*, LXIII (1911), 871.

59. James L. Kortright, "Should Midwives Be Registered?" *Transactions*, Medical Society of the State of New York (1893), 417; Georgina Grothan, "Evil Practices of the So-Called Midwife," *Practical Therapeutics*, VIII (1895–96), 177.

60. Henry J. Garriques, "Midwives," *Medical News*, LXXII (1898), 233.

61. Ibid., 235; S. C. Young, "Obstetrical Reflections Suggested by Passages in the First Chapter of Exodus," *New Orleans Medical and Surgical Journal*, XVII (1860), 836; J. Henry Fruitnight, "The Status of the Midwife, Legal and Professional," *American Journal of Neurology and Psychiatry*, III (1884), 530; Madeline Simms, "Midwives and Abortion in the 1930s," *Midwife and Health Visitor*, X (1974), 114; Horatio R. Storer and Franklin Heard, *Criminal Abortion: Its Nature, Its Evidence, and Its Law* (Boston, 1868), 99–100; Andrew Nebinger, *Criminal Abortion: Its Extent and Prevention* (Phila., 1870), 10–19; James C. Mohr, *Abortion in America: The Origins and Evolution of National Policy* (New York, 1878), 53–60.

62. Elbridge T. Gerry, "Midwives as Illegal Practitioners," *Medical Record*, LIV (1898), 938–39; Sims, "Midwives and Abortion in the 1930s," 115; R. Sauer, "Attitudes to Abortion in America, 1800–1973," *Population Studies*, XXVIII (1974), 53–67; Donegan, *Midwifery in America, 1760–1860: A Study in Medicine and Morality*, 239.

63. Darlington, "Present Status of the Midwife," 870; Lee W. Thomas, "The Supervision of Midwives in New York City," *Monthly Bulletin*, New York City Department of Health, IV (1919), 117.

64. Thomas J. Hillis, "Remarks on the Midwifery Question: The Availability and Simplicity of the Midwife, the Secret of Her Hold on the Masses," *Medical Record*, LX (1899), 783.

65. Grace Abbott, "The Midwife in Chicago," *American Journal of Sociology*, XX (1915), 694.

66. Wile, "Immigration and the Midwife Problem," 113; Florence S. Wright, "The Midwives and Our Foreign Born in America," *Public Health Nurse*, XI (1919), 661.

67. "The Education of Midwives," *Transactions*, Medical Association of Alabama (1890), 115.

68. Jeidell and Fricke, "The Midwives of Anne Arundel County, Maryland," 279–80; Ross, "Midwife in North Carolina Since 1587," 660–61; Lloyd C. Taylor, *The Medical Profession and Social Reform, 1885–1945* (New York, 1974), 67.

69. Robert C. Eve, "Licensing of Midwives," *Charlotte Medical Journal*, VI (1895), 990–95.

70. Taylor, *Medical Profession and Social Reform, 1885–1945*, 65; Frances Bradley, "Save the Country Baby," *Survey*, LI (1923), 321–23; id., "All in a Day's Work," *Survey*, LXV (1930), 38; Alex S. Freedman, "The Passing of the Arkansas Granny Midwife," *Kentucky Folklore Record*, XX (1976), 101–3.

71. Rudolph W. Holmes, "Midwife Practice—An Anachronism," *Illinois Medical Journal*, XXXVII (1920), 30.

72. Quoted in Darlington, "Present Status of the Midwife," 872.

73. Baker, "Schools for Midwives," 262–63.

74. Grothan, "Evil Practices of the So-Called Midwife," 178.

75. Van Blarcom, "A Possible Solution to the Midwife Problem," 351; James L. Huntington, "The Regulation of Midwifery," *Boston Medical and Surgical Journal*, CLXVII (1912), 86; John A. Foote, "Legislative Measures against Maternal and Infant Mortality: The Midwife Practice Laws of the States and Territories of the United States," *American Journal of Obstetrics and Diseases of Women*, LXXX (1919), 535.

76. James L. Huntington, "Midwives in Massachusetts," *New England Journal of Medicine*, CLXVII (1912), 542–43.

77. Newmayer, "Status of Midwifery in Pennsylvania and a Study of the Midwives of Philadephia," 714, 717.

78. Kortright, "Should Midwives be Registered?" 419; Grothan, "Evil Practices of the So-Called Midwife," 177.

79. C. S. Bacon, "The Midwife Question in America," *JAMA*, XXIX (1897), 1092.

80. William W. Lobenstine, "Attempts at Regulation of Midwife Practice," *American Journal of Obstetrics and Diseases of Women*, LXIII (1911), 898–901.

81. E. R. Hardin, "The Midwife Problem," *Southern Medical Journal*, XVIII (1925), 347; "Discussion on Proposed Legislation against Midwives," *Medical Record*, LIII (1898), 211; Harold Bailey, "Control of Midwives," *American Journal of Obstetrics and Gynecology*, IX (1923), 294.

82. W. H. Mays, "Midwives," *Western Lancet*, LXXX (1879), 447–49; "Discussion on Proposed Legislation against Midwives," 211.

83. Pryor, "Status of the Midwife in Buffalo," 131.

84. Garriques, "Midwifery," 235.

85. Thomas J. Hillis, "Some Remarks on the Midwifery Question—Must the Midwife Perish?" *Medical Record*, LIV (1898), 472.

86. Ibid., 474–75.

87. Ibid., 474; Henry Bennet, "Women as Practitioners of Midwifery," *Lancet*, I (1870), 887–88.

88. Hillis, "Remarks on the Midwifery Question," 787–88. For rebuttal, see E. Jarett, "The Midwife or the Woman Doctor," *Medical Record*, LIV (1898), 610–11.

89. Charles E. Ziegler, "The Elimination of the Midwife," *JAMA*, LX (1913), 32–34.

90. Ibid., 34.

91. Ibid., 35.

92. Ibid., 36.

93. Quoted in ibid., 36.

94. Quoted in ibid., 37.

95. Ibid., 37–38; Charles E. Ziegler, "How Can We Best Solve the Midwifery Problem," *American Journal of Public Health*, XII (1922), 410.

96. George W. Kosmak, "Certain Aspects of the Midwife Problem in Relation to the Medical Profession and the Community," *Medical Record*, LXXXV (1914), 1015; James M. H. Rowland, "Summary of Obstetrical Service in Baltimore from the Late 1880s to 1926," *Maryland State Medical Journal*, XXIV (1975), 46–49.

97. Charles V. Chapin, "The Control of Midwifery," *Medical Progress*, XXXIX (1923), 76–79; John B. Wheeler, *Memoirs of a Small-Town Surgeon* (New York, 1935), 45–46; Charles E. Rosenberg, "Social Class and Medical Care in Nineteenth Century America: The Rise and Fall of the Dispensary," *Journal of the History of Medicine and Allied Sciences*, XXIX (1974), 32–54; Gert H. Brieger, "The Use and Abuse of Medical Charities in Late Nineteenth Century America," *American Journal of Public Health*, LXVII (1977), 264–67; George Rosen, "The Efficiency Criterion in Medical Care, 1900–1920," *Bulletin of the History of Medicine*, L (1976), 28–44.

CHAPTER SIX

Most Noble Art, Imperfect Science

1. William F. Norwood, *Medical Education in the United States before the Civil War* (Phila., 1944), 32–33; Charles M. Andrews, *Colonial Folkways: A Chronicle of American Life in the Reign of the Georges* (New Haven, 1920), 92–93, 146–48, 189; Simon Flexner and James T. Flexner, *William Henry Welch and the Heroic Age of American Medicine* (New York, 1941), 61–63; George W. Corner, "Apprenticed to Aesculapius: The American Medical Student, 1765–1965," *Proceedings*, American Philosophical Society, CVI (1965), 249–51.

2. Nathan S. Davis, *Contributions to the History of Medical Education and Medical Institutions in the United States of America, 1776–1876* (Washington, D.C., 1877), 26.

3. William Smith, *The History of the Province of New York, from the First Discovery to the Year 1732* (London, 1757), 212.

4. Abraham Flexner, *Medical Education: A Comparative Study* (New York, 1925), 14; Whitfield J. Bell, Jr., "Medical Practice in Colonial America," *Bulletin of the History of Medicine*, XXXI (1957), 442–53; John Duffy, *The Healers: Rise of the Medical Establishment* (New York, 1976), 62–63.

5. Samuel Lewis, "List of the American Graduates in Medicine at the University of Edinburgh from 1705 to 1866 with their Theses," *New England History and Genealogical Register*, XLII (1888), 159–65; J. G. Wilson, "The Influence of Edinburgh on American Medicine in the 18th Century," *Proceedings*, Institute of Medicine of Chicago, VII (1929), 129–38; Whitfield J. Bell Jr., "Some American Students of 'that shining oracle of physics,' Dr. William Cullen of Edinburgh," *Proceedings*, American Philosophical Society, XCIV (1950), 275–81; Grace Goldin, "A Walk through a Ward in the 18th Century," *Journal of the History of Medicine and Allied Sciences*, XXII (1967), 121–38; Anand C. Chitnis, "Medical Education in Edinburgh, 1790–1826, and Some Victorian Consequences," *Medical History*, XVII (1973), 173–85; Sir George N. Clark, *A History of the Royal College of Physicians of London*, 2 vols. (London, 1964–66); John D. Comrie, *History of Scottish Medicine*, 2 vols. (London, 1932); J. D. H. Widdess, *The Royal College of Surgeons in Ireland and Its Medical School, 1784–1966* (Edinburgh, 1967); Whitfield J. Bell, Jr., "Dr. James Rush on His Philadelphia, Edinburgh, and London Teachers," *Journal of the History of Medicine and Allied Sciences*, XIX (1964), 419–21; Douglas Guthrie, "The Influence of the Leyden School upon Scottish Medicine," *Medical History*, III (1959), 108–22.

6. Frederick C. Waite, "Medical Degrees Conferred in the

American Colonies and in the United States in the 18th Century," *Annals of Medical History*, IX (1937), 316; Norwood, *Medical Education in the U.S. before the Civil War*, 381; Whitfield J. Bell, Jr., "The American Philosophical Society and Medicine," *Bulletin of the History of Medicine*, XL (1966), 112–23; Charles G. Cumston, "The Origins of Medical Instruction in the United States of America," *International Record of Medicine*, CXXVI (1927), 441–44; William S. Middleton, "John Morgan, Father of Medical Education in North America," *Annals of Medical History*, IX (1927), 13–26; George W. Corner, "Beginnings of Medical Education in Philadelphia, 1765–1776," *JAMA*, CXCIV (1965), 719–21; David Riesman, "The Dublin Medical School and Its Influence upon Medicine in America," *Annals of Medical History*, IV (1922), 86–96; F. C. Wood, "The College of Physicians of Philadelphia," *Transactions and Studies*, College of Physicians of Philadelphia, XXXV (1967), 67–73; Edward B. Krumbhaar, "The Early History of Anatomy in the United States," *Annals of Medical History*, IV (1922), 271–86.

7. Francis R. Packard, "How London and Edinburgh Influenced Medicine in Philadelphia in the 18th Century," *Annals of Medical History*, IV (1922), 219–44; Whitfield J. Bell, Jr., "Philadelphia Medical Students in Europe, 1750–1800," *Philadelphia Magazine of History and Biography*, LXVII (1943), 1–29; Michael Kraus, "American and European Medicine in the 18th Century," *Bulletin of the History of Medicine*, VIII (1940), 679–95; Robert W. I. Smith, *English-Speaking Students of Medicine at the University of Leyden* (Edinburgh, 1932); Lyman H. Butterfield (ed.), "Letters of Benjamin Rush," *Memoirs*, American Philosophical Society, XXX, 2 vols. (Phila., 1951), II, 1184–85; Corner, "Apprenticed to Aesculapius," 251; Saul Jarcho, "The Legacy of British Medicine to American Medicine, 1800–1850," *Proceedings*, Royal Society of Medicine, London, LXVIII (1975), 737–38; Harold J. Abrahams and Wyndham D. Miles, "Reminiscences of Olden Times," *Transactions and Studies*, College of Physicians of Philadelphia, XXXIX (1971), 132–36.

8. Norwood, *Medical Education in the U.S. before the Civil War*, 32; Abraham Flexner, *Medical Education in the United States and Canada: A Report to the Carnegie Foundation for the Advancement of Teaching* (New York, 1910), 4–5; Davis, *Contributions to the History of Medical Education and Medical Institutions in the U.S.A.*, 25–26.

9. Henry B. Shafer, *The American Medical Profession, 1783 to 1850* (New York, 1936), 55; Norwood, *Medical Education in the U.S. before the Civil War*, 405; Harold J. Abrahams, *Extinct Medical Schools of 19th Century Philadelphia* (Phila., 1966), 23; John B. Wheeler, *Memoirs of a Small-Town Surgeon* (New York, 1935), 1–2.

10. Wheeler, *Memoirs of a Small-Town Surgeon*, 4; Richard H.

Shryock, "The Advent of Modern Medicine in Philadelphia, 1800–1850," *Yale Journal of Biology and Medicine*, XIII (1941), 727–28.

11. Abrahams, *Extinct Medical Schools of 19th Century Philadelphia*, 23; Norwood, *Medical Education in the U.S. before the Civil War*, 38.

12. Norwood, *Medical Education in the U.S. before the Civil War*, 380–81.

13. Charles G. Sellers, *Jacksonian Democracy* (Washington, D.C., 1958); James H. Young, "American Medical Quackery in the Age of the Common Man," *Mississippi Valley Historical Review*, XLVII (1961), 582.

14. Rosemary Stevens, *American Medicine and the Public Interest* (New Haven, 1971), 20–21; Charles Rosenberg, "The American Medical Profession: Mid-19th Century," *Mid-America*, XLIV (1962), 168–70.

15. Shafer, *American Medical Profession*, 42; Kenneth M. Lynch, "Medical Schooling in South Carolina," *Journal*, South Carolina Medical Association, LXI (1965), 71–74; J. M. Mason, "Early Medical Education in the Far South," *South Atlantic Quarterly*, XXIX (1930), 166–71; B. B. Mitchell, "Southern versus Northern Practice," *Medical Examiner*, n.s. IV (1848), 591; Michael O. Jones, "Climate and Disease: The Traveller Describes America," *Bulletin of the History of Medicine*, XLI (1967), 254–66; William Currie, *An Historical Account of the Climates and Diseases of the United States of America; And of the Remedies and Methods of Treatment* (Phila., 1792).

16. Quoted in Richard H. Shryock, "The American Physician in 1846 and 1946," *JAMA*, CXXXIV (1947), 418; Shafer, *American Medical Profession*, 40; Richard H. Shryock, "Medical Practice in the Old South," *South Atlantic Quarterly*, XXIX (1930), 166–71; Barnes Riznik, *Medicine in New England, 1790–1840* (Sturbridge, Mass., 1965), 8.

17. Only after Dunglison published his *Medical Student* in 1837 was there any guide to schools, faculty, and course requirements. At best there were only self-serving circulars sent out by schools. See Shafer, *American Medical Profession*, 47; Abrahams, *Extinct Medical Schools of 19th Century Philadelphia*, 24.

18. Saul Jarcho, "The Legacy of British Medicine to American Medicine, 1800–1850," *Proceedings*, Royal Society of Medicine, London, LVIII (1975), 739; Duffy, *The Healers*, 172–73; Douglas Carroll, "Medical Students 1818 and 1834," *Maryland State Medical Journal*, XXIII (1974), 37–42; Douglas Carroll, "Medicine in Maryland, 1634 to 1835," *Maryland State Medical Journal*, XX (1971), 59–63.

19. Frederick C. Waite, "American Sectarian Medical Colleges before the Civil War," *Bulletin of the History of Medicine*, XIX (1946), 148–66; Martin Kaufman, "American Medical Diploma Mills,"

Medical Faculty Bulletin, Tulane University, XXVI (1967), 53–57; Alex Berman, "A Striving for Scientific Respectability: Some American Botanics and the 19th Century Plant Materia Medica," *Bulletin of the History of Medicine*, XXX (1956), 7–31; Alex Berman, "The Thomsonian Movement and Its Relation to American Pharmacy and Medicine," *Bulletin of the History of Medicine*, XXV (1951), 405–28, 519–38; Alex Berman, "Neo-Thomsonianism in the United States," *Journal of the History of Medicine and Allied Sciences*, X (1956), 133–55; Philip D. Jordan, "The Secret Six: An Inquiry into the Basic Materia Medica of the Thomsonian System of Botanic Medicine," *Ohio Historical Quarterly*, LII (1943), 347–55; Harry B. Weiss and Howard R. Kemble, *The Great American Water-Cure Craze: A History of Hydropathy in the United States* (Trenton, 1967).

20. Shafer, *American Medical Profession*, 43–47; Flexner, *Medical Education in the U.S. and Canada*, vii; Norwood, *Medical Education in the U.S. before the Civil War*, 382–83.

21. Donald E. Konold, *A History of American Medical Ethics, 1847–1912* (Madison, Wis., 1962), 7; Rosenberg, "American Medical Profession," 164; Kenneth M. Lynch, "Medical Schooling in South Carolina," *Journal*, South Carolina Medical Association, LXI (1965), 72–73; Martin Kaufman, "American Medical Diploma Mills," 53; Duffy, *The Healers*, 177.

22. John W. S. Gouley, *Conferences on the Moral Philosophy of Medicine, Prepared by an American Physician* (New York, 1906), 44; Stevens, *American Medicine and the Public Interest*, 26–27; Shafer, *American Medical Profession*, 36–37.

23. Davis, *Contributions to the History of Medical Education and Medical Institutions in the U.S.A.*, 41; Stevens, *American Medicine and the Public Interest*, 24; J. M. Toner, "Statistical Sketch of the Medical Profession in the United States," *Indiana Journal of Medicine*, IV (1873), 5, 7, 14–17; J. M. Toner, "Statistics of the Medical Profession in the United States," *New England Journal of Medicine*, LXXXV (1871), 7; Edward C. Atwater, "The Medical Profession in a New Society, Rochester, New York (1811–1860)," *Bulletin of the History of Medicine*, XLVII (1973), 122–35.

24. J. Howe Adams, "The Physicians of the United States," *Medical Times*, XXXV (1907), 105–8.

25. Flexner, *Medical Education in the U.S. and Canada*, 6–7.

26. William R. Hurley, *The Relation of the Physician to the Public: An Address* (Knoxville, Tenn., 1858), 11.

27. Emil Amberg, "The Young Physician," *Philadelphia Medical Journal*, IX (1902), 546.

28. Flexner, *Medical Education in the U.S. and Canada*, 8; William S. Miller, "Medical Schools in Wisconsin: Past and Present," *Wisconsin Medical Journal*, XXXV (1936), 477; Harry Bloch, "Medical Re-

search and Education in 19th Century America," *New York State Journal of Medicine*, LXXIV (1974), 1071–74; David Riesman, "Clinical Teaching in America with Some Remarks on Early Medical Schools," *Transactions and Studies*, College of Physicians of Philadelphia, VII (1939), 89–110; Irving A. Beck, "An Early American Journal Keyed to Medical Students: A Pioneer Contribution of Elisha Bartlett," *Bulletin of the History of Medicine*, XL (1966), 124–34; James J. Walsh, *History of Medicine in New York*, 2 vols. (New York, 1919), I, 258; Harold J. Abrahams, "Chemistry at Extinct Medical Schools of 19th Century Philadelphia," *Transactions and Studies*, College of Physicians of Philadelphia, XL (1972), 73–79.

29. Virginia Parker, "Oliver Wendell Holmes: Man of Medicine; Man of Letters," *Bulletin*, Medical Library Association, LIV (1966), 142–47; Oliver Wendell Holmes, *The Position and Prospects of the Medical Student: An Address Delivered before the Boylston Society of Harvard University, January 12, 1844* (Boston, 1844), 4–22. George Rosen, "The Philosophy and Ideology and the Emergence of Modern Medicine in France," *Bulletin of the History of Medicine*, XX (1946), 328–39; Shryock, "Advent of Modern Medicine in Philadelphia," 728–35; Samuel Jackson, *Address to the Medical Graduates of the University of Pennsylvania* (Phila., 1840); Russell M. Jones, "An American Medical Student in Paris, 1831–1833," *Harvard Library Bulletin*, XV (1967), 59–81; Ferdinand C. Stewart, *Hospitals and Surgeons of Paris: An Historical and Statistical Account of the Civil Hospitals of Paris* (New York, 1843); J. Chalmers da Costa, "The French School of Surgery in the Reign of Louis Philippe," *Annals of Medical History*, IV (1922), 77–79; Erwin H. Ackerknecht, "Elisha Bartlett and the Philosophy of the Paris Clinical School," *Bulletin of the History of Medicine*, XXIV (1950), 43–60; Russell M. Jones, "American Doctors in Paris, 1820–1860," *Journal of the History of Medicine and Allied Sciences*, XXV (1970), 143–57; George E. Gifford, Jr. (ed.), "An American in Paris, 1841–1842: Four Letters from Jeffries Wyman," ibid., XXII (1967), 274–85; Walter R. Steiner, "Dr. Pierre-Charles-Alexandre Louis, a Distinguished Parisian Teacher of American Medical Students," *Annals of Medical History*, II (1940), 451–60.

30. Edward Waldo Emerson, "The Man as Doctor," *Boston Medical and Surgical Journal*, CVI (1882), 533–34.

31. Godman quoted in "Memoir of Dr. John D. Godman," *Waldie's Select Circulating Library*, I (1833), 296; Stephanie Morris, "John Davidson Godman (1794–1830): Physician and Naturalist," *Transactions and Studies*, College of Physicians of Philadelphia, XLI (1974), 295–303. See also Thomas Sewall, *Memoir of Dr. Godman: Being an Introductory Lecture* (New York, 1832); Emmet F. Horine, "Early Medicine in Kentucky and the Mississippi Valley: A Tribute

to Daniel Drake, M.D.," *Journal of the History of Medicine*, III (1948), 263–78; Shryock, "Advent of Modern Medicine in Philadelphia," 725–26.

32. John K. Mitchell, *On the Usefulness of the Medical Profession beyond the Limits of the Profession: A Lecture Introductory to the Course of Practice of Medicine in Jefferson Medical College of Philadelphia* (Phila., 1842), 7; John K. Mitchell, *Impediments to the Study of Medicine: A Lecture, Introductory to the Course of Practice of Medicine* (Phila., 1850), 21.

33. Mitchell, *On the Usefulness of the Medical Profession beyond the Limits of the Profession*, 9.

34. Ibid., 24; Samuel W. Butler, *Doctors' Commons: An Ethic Address Delivered before the District Medical Society, for the County of Burlington, January 10, 1854* (Burlington, N.J., 1854), 9; A. E. Dobis, *Education and Social Movements, 1700–1850* (London, 1919); J. W. Wilson, "The Old Medical School at Brown University," *Books at Brown*, Friends of the Library of Brown University, XXII (1968), 11–17; Edward D. Branch, *The Sentimental Years, 1836–1860* (New York, 1934), 270–72; Konold, *History of American Medical Ethics*, 2–3; J. W. Wilson, "The First Natural History Lectures at Brown University, 1786, by Dr. Benjamin Waterhouse," *Annals of Medical History*, IV (1942), 396.

35. Silas W. Mitchell, *Two Lectures on the Conduct of the Medical Life* (Phila., 1893), 18; Donald Ball, "Silas Weir Mitchell," *Practitioner*, CCXVII (1976), 117–24.

36. Traill Green, "The True Physician, A Student of Natural and Medical Science: An Address to the Medical Society of Pennsylvania," *Transactions*, Medical Society of the State of Pennsylvania, V (1868), 45; George G. Simpson, "The Beginnings of Vertebrate Paleontology in North America," *Proceedings*, American Philosophical Society, LXXXVI (1942), 130–88; William M. and Mabel S. C. Smallwood, *Natural History and the American Mind* (New York, 1941); Edward Lurie, *Louis Agassiz: A Life in Science* (Chicago, 1960); Dirk J. Struik, *Yankee Science in the Making* (New York, 1962); Clark A. Elliott, "The American Scientist in Antebellum Society: A Quantitative View," *Social Studies of Science*, V (1975), 93–108; George H. Daniels, *American Science in the Age of Jackson* (New York, 1968); Donald de B. Bever, "The American Scientific Community, 1800–1860: A Statistical-Historical Study," (Ph.D. diss., Yale, 1966); George H. Daniels, "The Process of Professionalization in American Science: The Emergent Period, 1820–1860," *Isis*, LVIII (1967), 151–67; Richard M. Jellison, "The American Physician as Scientist in the 19th Century: An Interpretation," *Pagine di storia della medicine*, XIV (1970), 68–81. Some of the early physicians included John E. Holbrook in herpetology and ichthyology, Asa Gray

in botany, Samuel G. Morton in craniology, Josiah C. Nott in ethnology, Joseph Le Conte in geology, Richard Harlan in anatomy. G. E. Gifford, "Medicine and Natural History—Crosscurrents in Philadelphia in the Nineteenth Century," *Transactions and Studies, College of Physicians of Philadelphia*, XLV (1978), 139–49.

37. George H. Daniels, *Science in American Society: A Social History* (New York, 1971), 43–44; Phyllis A. Richmond, "The 19th Century American Physician as a Research Scientist," *International Record of Medicine*, CLXXI (1958), 493.

38. Stevens, *American Medicine and the Public Interest*, 13; Alan D. Aberbach, "Samuel Latham Mitchell: A Physician in the Early Days of the Republic," *Bulletin*, New York Academy of Medicine, XL (1964), 501–10.

39. Quoted in Fredric T. Lewis, "The Preparation for the Study of Medicine," *Popular Science Monthly*, LXXV (1909), 65.

40. Amberg, "The Young Physician," 547.

41. R. H. Babcock, "The Ethics of Medical Advertising," *Journal of Sociologic Medicine*, IV (1899), 213.

42. Richard D. Arnold, *The Reciprocal Duty of Physicians and of the Public toward Each Other: An Address Delivered before the Medical Society of the State of Georgia at Its Second Annual Meeting, Held at Atlanta on the 9th of April, 1851* (Savannah, 1851), 21.

43. Henry H. Tucker, *The True Physician: An Address Delivered before the Graduating Class of the Medical College of Georgia, at Its Annual Commencement, March 1st, 1867* (Georgia, 1867), 10.

44. Roberts Bartholow, "Some Points in Medical Politics," *Maryland Medical Journal*, VIII (1882), 509; "The Physician," *Arena*, VI (1892), 98–100.

45. George E. Frothingham, *A Lecture on the Code of Medical Ethics, Delivered before the Students' Medical Social Science Association, December 15, 1885* (Tecumseh, Mich., 1886), 26–27.

46. John S. Billings, "Address to the Graduating Class of Bellevue Hospital Medical College," *Medical News*, XL (1882), 285; Samuel Chew, *Lectures on Medical Education: Or, On the Proper Method of Studying Medicine* (Phila., 1864), xiii, 104–6, 115.

47. Stevens, *American Medicine and the Public Interest*, 10.

48. Norwood, *Medical Education in the U.S. before the Civil War*, 422–23; Shafer, *American Medical Profession*, 92–93.

49. Eugene P. Link, "Yale, Pennsylvania, and the Founding of the A. M. A.," *New York State Journal of Medicine*, LXVII (1967), 946–51; B. Stookey, "Origins of the First National Medical Convention, 1826–1846," *JAMA*, CLXXVII (1961), 133; James G. Burrow, *A M A; Voice of American Medicine* (Baltimore, 1963), 1–51.

50. William Maxwell Wood and Ninian Pinkney, "A Statement in Relation to the U.S. Naval Medical Corps," *Transactions*, American Medical Association, I (1848), 301–4; Flexner, *Medical Education in*

the U.S. and Canada, 170; Arnold, *Reciprocal Duty of Physicians and of the Public toward Each Other*, 17.

51. A. H. Stevens, et al., "Report of the Committee on Education," *Transactions*, American Medical Association, I (1848), 335–47; Shafer, *American Medical Profession, 1783 to 1850*, 51, 93–94; Konold, *History of American Medical Ethics*, 17.

52. Morris Fishbein, "History of the American Medical Profession," *JAMA*, CXXXII (1946), 921.

53. Konold, *History of American Medical Ethics*, 19.

54. Quoted in Arnold, *Reciprocal Duty of Physicians and of the Public toward Each Other*, 9.

55. Henry S. Hewitt, *The Relations and Reciprocal Obligations between the Medical Profession and the Educated and Cultured Classes: An Oration Delivered before the Alumni Association of the Medical Department of the University of the City of New York, February 23, 1869* (New York, 1869), 7.

56. Arnold, *Reciprocal Duty of Physicians and of the Public toward Each Other*, 15.

57. H. R. Storer, "The Mutual Relations of the Medical Profession, Its Press, and the Community," *Transactions*, Gynecological Society of Boston, IV (1871), 5.

58. H. Bert Ellis, "What Should Be the Physician's Position in the Body Politic?" *JAMA*, XLII (1904), 1214; Robert Hudson, "Abraham Flexner in Perspective: American Medical Education, 1865–1910," *Bulletin of the History of Medicine*, XLVI (1972), 547; Charles McIntire, *The Percentage of College-Bred Men in the Medical Profession* (Phila., 1883).

59. Augustus H. Burbank, "Our Mutual Relations as Medical Men," *Transactions*, Maine Medical Association, XI (1892), 38.

60. Arnold, *Reciprocal Duty of Physicians and of the Public toward Each Other*, 13.

61. Harry Bloch, "Medical Research and Education in 19th Century America," *New York State Journal of Medicine*, LXXIV (1974), 1071–74; Samuel Jackson, *On the Methods of Acquiring Knowledge: An Introductory Lecture to the Course of the Institutes of Medicine, for the Session of 1838–1839* (Phila., 1838).

62. Henry J. Bigelow, *Medical Education in America: Being an Annual Address Read before the Massachusetts Medical Society, June 7, 1871* (Cambridge, Mass., 1871), 62–63; Theodor Billroth, *The Medical Sciences in the German Universities: A Study in the History of Civilization* (New York, 1924).

63. Richard H. Shryock, *Medical Licensing in America, 1650–1965* (Baltimore, 1967), 56–57; T. N. Bonner, *American Doctors and German Universities: A Chapter in International Intellectual Relations, 1870–1914* (Lincoln, Neb., 1963), 23; Charles Rosenberg, "The Practice of Medicine in New York a Century Ago," *Bulletin of the*

History of Medicine, XLI (1967), 251; Shryock, "Advent of Modern Medicine in Philadelphia," 734–35.

64. Stevens, *American Medicine and the Public Interest*, 24; Rosenberg, "The Practice of Medicine in New York a Century Ago," 240–41; Flexner, *Medical Education in the U.S. and Canada*, 9; Lord Cohen of Birkenhead, "Medical Education in Great Britain and Ireland," *Practitioner*, CCI (1968), 179–93; William F. Norwood, "The Mainstream of American Medical Education, 1765–1965," *Annals*, New York Academy of Sciences, CXXVIII (1965), 463–72.

65. Charles J. Whallen, "The Doctor as a Politician," *JAMA*, XXXII (1899), 758–59; Amberg, "The Young Physician," 546–47.

66. C. F. Andrew, "The Physician in Politics," *Rocky Mountain Medical Journal*, IV (1907), 240.

67. Quoted in T. Puschmann, *A History of Medical Education from the Most Remote to the Most Recent Times* (London, 1891), 535; Samuel E. Morison, *The Development of Harvard University since the Inauguration of President Eliot, 1869–1929* (Cambridge, Mass., 1930); Bernard J. Stern, *American Medical Practice in the Perspectives of a Century* (New York, 1945), 87; Leslie B. Arey, "The Origin of the Graded Medical Curriculum," *Journal of Medical Education*, LI (1976), 1010–12.

68. James H. Means, *The Association of Medical Physicians: Its First Seventy-Five Years* (New York, 1961), 17; Stern, *American Medical Practice in the Perspectives of a Century*, 87; Charles W. Eliot, "Discussion of Report of the Committee on Preliminary Education," *Bulletin*, American Medical Association, III (1908), 262; Abraham Flexner, *Daniel Coit Gilman, Creator of the American Type of University* (New York, 1946), 110–54; Frederic T. Lewis, "Preparation for the Study of Medicine," 65–74.

69. Frank J. Weed, "Address," reprinted in *Bulletin*, Cleveland Medical Library, XIV (1967), 64; Leslie L. Hanawalt, "A Short History of Wayne State University School of Medicine," *Michigan Medicine*, LXVII (1968), 30–32.

70. Lloyd C. Taylor, *The Medical Profession and Social Reform, 1885–1945* (New York, 1974), 1–14; Flexner, *Medical Education in the U.S. and Canada*, 12; Walter J. Meek, "The Beginnings of American Physiology," *Annals of Medical History*, X (1928), 111–25.

71. Sir Douglas Hubble, "William Osler and Medical Education," *Journal*, Royal College of Physicians of London, IX (1975), 269–78; E. L. Strohl, "Osler in American Medicine," *Proceedings*, Institute of Medicine of Chicago, XXVI (1966), 142–44; H. Cushing, *The Life of Sir William Osler* (New York, 1940); A. E. Rodin, "The Influence of Experience in Pathology on Two 19th Century Practitioners," *Texas Reports on Medicine and Biology*, XXXII (1974), 135–40; Richard H. Shryock, *The Unique Influence of the Johns Hopkins University on American Medicine* (Copenhagen, 1953), 31–

32; Thomas B. Turner, "History of Medical Education at Johns Hopkins," *Johns Hopkins Medical Journal*, CXXXIX (1976), 27–36.

72. Amberg, "The Young Physician," 546.

73. Shryock, *Medical Licensing in America*, 45–46.

74. Bigelow, *Medical Education in America*, 16.

75. Ibid., 14, 17.

76. Quoted in Fishbein, "History of the American Medical Profession," 637; Roberts Bartholow, "Some Points in Medical Politics," *Maryland Medical Journal*, VIII (1882), 509.

77. J. L. Orton, "The Medical Profession as a Public Trust," *JAMA*, XV (1890), 666–70; Lyman Beecher Todd, "The Public and the Medical Profession—Their Reciprocal Relations, Duties, and Responsibilities," *American Practitioner and News*, XI (1891), 390.

78. The call for reform of medical colleges came from J. M. Biddle of Jefferson Medical College of Philadelphia, William H. Mussey of Miami Medical College in Cincinnati, John T. Hodgen of St. Louis Medical College, J. Adams Allen of Rush Medical College, W. T. Briggs of the medical department of the University of Nashville, and J. M. Bodine of the medical department of the University of Louisville. See Dean F. Smiley, "History of the Association of American Medical Colleges," *Journal of Medical Education*, XXXII (1957), 512.

79. Shryock, *Medical Licensing in America*, 54–55; Frank S. Hough, "Doctor in Politics," *Physician and Surgeon*, XVI (1894), 491.

80. Amberg, "The Young Physician," 545.

81. Shryock, *Medical Licensing in America*, 47–56; Abrahams, *Extinct Medical Schools of 19th Century Philadelphia*, 23–24; John B. Bardo, "A History of the Legal Regulation of Medical Practice in New York State," *Bulletin*, New York Academy of Medicine, XLIII (1967), 924–40. By 1905 the National Confederation of State Medical Examining and Licensing Boards adopted the standards set by the AAMC, including a curriculum of 4,000 hours. See Smiley, "History of the AAMC," 518.

82. Kaufman, "American Medical Diploma Mills," 53–57; Leo T. Abbott, "Medical and Dental Diploma Mills in Vermont in the 1880s and 1890s," *Vermont History*, XXXVII (1969), 194–206; Eileen R. Cunningham, "A Short Review of the Development of Medical Education and Schools of Medicine," *Annals of Medical History*, VII (1935), 238; "Fraudulent Medical Institutions," *JAMA*, XXII (1894), 464–65; "Free Trade in Diplomas," *Boston Medical and Surgical Journal*, XVIII (1883), 234–35.

83. Elton Rayack, *Professional Power and American Medicine: The Economics of the American Medical Association* (Cleveland, 1967), 66–70; Smiley, "History of the AAMC," 518–19; Shryock, *Medical Licensing in America*, 63–64; Robert Hudson, "Abraham Flexner in

Perspective: American Medical Education, 1865–1910," *Bulletin of the History of Medicine*, XLVI (1972), 545–61.

84. Esmond R. Long, *A History of American Pathology* (Springfield, Ill., 1962), 182; Hudson, "Abraham Flexner in Perspective," 556.

85. Pritchett in intro. to Flexner, *Medical Education in the U.S. and Canada*, x; Shryock, *Medical Licensing in America*, 61–62.

86. Henry Miller, "Fifty Years after Flexner," *Lancet*, II (1966), 647–54; Howard S. Berliner, "A Larger Perspective on the Flexner Report," *International Journal of Health Sciences*, V (1975), 573–92; H. David Banta, "Medical Education: Abraham Flexner—A Reappraisal," *Social Science and Medicine*, V (1971), 655–61.

87. Flexner, *Medical Education in the U.S. and Canada*, 154.

88. Randolph Winslow quoted in Jarcho, "Legacy of British Medicine to American Medicine," 740.

89. Flexner, *Medical Education in the U.S. and Canada*, 155.

90. Ibid., 18–19, 146, 151.

91. Shryock, *Medical Licensing in America*, 64; Donna B. Munger, "Robert Brookings and the Flexner Report: A Case Study of the Reorganization of Medical Education," *Journal of the History of Medicine and Allied Sciences*, XXIII (1968), 356–71.

92. Flexner, *Medical Education in the U.S. and Canada*, 14–17, 167.

93. J. F. Stevens, "Nebraska College of Medicine Closes Voluntarily," *JAMA*, LII (1909), 1862; Norman Barnesby, *Medical Chaos and Crime* (New York, 1910), 65–66.

94. "Report of the Committee on Medical Legislation," *JAMA* XLV (1905), 260.

CHAPTER SEVEN

The Business and Ethics of Medicine

1. Charles Phelps, "The Causes of a Decline in the Average Income of General Practitioners of Medicine," *Transactions*, New York State Medical Association, XIV (1897), 30.

2. George W. Cook, "The History of Medical Ethics," *New York Medical Journal*, CI (1886), 140–46, 205–7; James J. Walsh, "Early Chapters in Medical and Surgical Ethics," *Hospital Progress*, II (1921), 403–6; Chauncey D. Leake, "Percival's Code: A Chapter in the Historical Development of Medical Ethics," *JAMA*, LXXXI (1923), 366–71; Chester R. Burns, "Medical Ethics in the United States before the Civil War," (Ph.D. diss., Johns Hopkins University, 1969), 108–9; Donald E. Konold, *A History of American Medical*

Ethics, 1847–1912 (Madison, Wis., 1962), 2; Morris Fishbein, "An Historical Appraisal: The Medical Society of New Jersey," *Journal, Medical Society of New Jersey*, LXIII (1966), 230; Ivan Waddington, "The Development of Medical Ethics—A Sociological Analysis," *Medical History*, XIX (1975), 36–51.

   3. Chauncey D. Leake, "What Was Kappa Lambda?" *Annals of Medical History*, IV (1922), 192–206; Lee D. Van Antwerp, "Kappa Lambda, Elf or Ogre?" *Bulletin of the History of Medicine*, XVII (1945), 327–50; Edward C. Atwater, "The Medical Profession in New York Society; Rochester, New York (1811–1860)," *Bulletin of the History of Medicine*, XLVII (1973), 232–33; Chauncey D. Leake, "Percival's Medical Ethics: Promise and Problems," *California Medicine*, CXIV (1971), 68–70.

   4. Chester R. Burns, "Malpractice Suits in American Medicine before the Civil War," *Bulletin of the History of Medicine*, XLIII (1969), 41–56; Morris Fishbein, "History of the American Medical Association," *JAMA*, CXXXII (1946), 783–85; Eugene P. Link, "Yale, Pennsylvania, and the Founding of the American Medical Association," *New York State Journal of Medicine*, LXVII (1967), 946–51; Henry B. Shafer, *The American Medical Association, 1783 to 1850* (New York, 1936), 92; Elton Rayack, *Professional Power and American Medicine: The Economics of the American Medical Association* (Cleveland, 1967), 2–3.

   5. Morris Fishbein, *A History of the American Medical Association from 1847 to 1947* (Philadelphia, 1947), 35–40. The Committee included John Bell, Isaac Hays, and G. Emerson of Philadelphia; W. W. Morris of Delaware; T. C. Dunn of Rhode Island; A. Clarke of New York; and R. D. Reynold of Georgia. Hays was editor of the *American Journal of Medical Science* from 1827 to 1879. See Konold, *History of American Medical Ethics*, 10; John W. S. Gouley, *Conferences on the Moral Philosophy of Medicine, Prepared by an American Physician* (New York, 1906), 156; Austin Flint, *Medical Ethics and Etiquette: The Code of Ethics Adopted by the American Medical Association, with Commentaries by Austin Flint* (New York, 1883), 5.

   6. C. H. Todd, "Medical Ethics," *Transactions*, Kentucky State Medical Association, XXI (1876), 67; "A Commentary upon Medical Ethics," *Nashville Journal of Medicine and Surgery*, V (1853), 265–74, 399–44; C. T. Quintard, "Graduating Pledge—Code of Ethics, etc.," *Memphis Medical Recorder*, II (1853–1854), 108–12; P. Hamilton, "An Essay on Medical Ethics," *Transactions*, Belmont Medical Society (1852–53), 3–9; Ayres P. Merrill, *A Public Lecture on Medical Ethics, and the Mutual Relations of Patient and Physician* (Memphis, 1857); J. F. M. Geddings, "President's Address," *Transactions*, South Carolina Medical Association (1877), x–xviii.

   7. M. B. Wright, "Report of Special Committee on Medical Eth-

ics," *Transactions*, Ohio State Medical Society (1855), 37; Fishbein, *History of the American Medical Association*, 38; Burns, "Medical Ethics in the U.S. before the Civil War," 231–33.

8. "Code of Ethics," *Medical Gazette*, III (1869), 150.

9. Ibid., 216, 186; Louis Bauer, "The AMA: Its Relations to Medical Education; Its Code of Ethics and the Workings Thereof," *St. Louis Periscope and Clinical Review*, IV (1879), 89; G. S. Franklin, "Shall the Code of Ethics be Perpetuated?" *Lancet-Clinic*, XXX (1876), 990.

10. "Code of Ethics," 126.

11. F. A. Seymour, "The Code: An Interpretation," *Southern California Practitioner*, VI (1891), 326–27.

12. Bauer, "The AMA," 89.

13. "Code of Ethics," 136, 138.

14. Wright, "Report of Special Committee on Medical Ethics," 48, 50.

15. Franklin, "Shall the Code of Ethics be Perpetuated?" 988–89; Bauer, "The AMA," 89; Seale Harris, *Woman's Surgeon: The Life Story of J. Marion Sims* (New York, 1950), 86–87, 175–76, 182–83, 273–75.

16. Ezra M. Hunt, *Professional Ethics: An Essay Read before the Medical Society of New Jersey at the Annual Meeting, May 27, 1873* (Newark, N.J., 1873), 14–15.

17. Wright, "Report of Special Committee on Medical Ethics," 38–40; Horatio C. Meriam, "Professional Atmosphere and Morals: Or, Patents and Secrets vs. a Liberal Profession," *Dental Cosmos*, XXXI (1889), 422; Konold, *History of American Medical Ethics*, 20.

18. E. L. Hayford, "Physicians' Fees and Collections," *Clinical Review*, XII (1900), 456; Charles A. Robertson, *Medical Ethics and Medical Dissensions: A Paper Read before the Albany County Medical Society* (Albany, 1871), 29.

19. "The Pecuniary Conditions of the Medical Profession in the United States," *New England Journal of Medicine*, IV (1831), 9–10; James J. Walsh, "Physicians' Fees Down the Ages," *International Clinics*, XX (1910), 262–63; L. P. Meredith, *Examination, Appreciation, and Fees* (Cincinnati, 1874), 18.

20. Charles R. Cullen, "Medical Paupers," *Transactions*, Medical Society of Virginia (1887), 237–42; Michael M. Davis, *America Organizes Medicine* (New York, 1941), 165.

21. Franklin Tuthill, *First Years of Practice: An Address to the Graduating Class of the New York Medical College, March, 1854* (New York, 1855), 8.

22. Poem by F. L. J. quoted in John Jay Taylor, *The Physician as a Business Man: Or, How to Obtain the Best Financial Results in the Practice of Medicine* (Philadelphia, 1891), 99.

23. Walsh, "Physicians' Fees Down the Ages," 273; John Duffy, *The Rudolph Matas History of Medicine in Louisiana*, 2 vols. (Baton Rouge, 1958–62), II, 402; Konold, *History of American Medical Ethics*, 64; John Duffy, *The Healers: Rise of the Medical Establishment* (New York, 1976), 178–79.

24. J. J. Conner, "The Financial Relations of the Medical Profession to the People and Public," *JAMA*, XXXVI (1901), 1384.

25. Hayford, "Physicians' Fees and Collections," 458; Atwater, "The Medical Profession in a New York Society," 221–35; Barnes Riznik, "The Professional Lives of Early Nineteenth Century New England Doctors," *Journal of the History of Medicine and Allied Sciences*, XIX (1964), 1–16.

26. Konold, *History of American Medical Ethics*, 56; Taylor, *The Physician as a Business Man*, 52–55; Thomas D. Mitchell, *Annual Address to the College of Physicians and Surgeons of Lexington, in Which the Principles and Practice of Medical Ethics are Illustrated and Urged as Essential to the Welfare of the Profession* (Lexington, Ky., 1839), 27; H. M. F. Behneman, "Leaves from a Doctor's Notebook," *Maryland State Medical Journal*, XVII (1968), 63–66; Richard H. Shryock, "An American Physician in 1846 and in 1946," *JAMA*, CXXXIV (1947), 419; Conner, "The Financial Relations of the Medical Profession to the People and Public," 1385; G. Willis Bass, "The Doctor's Income," *Northwestern Lancet*, XIII (1893), 21–23; Joseph Fairhall, "The Physician as a Businessman," *Fort Wayne Medical Journal and Magazine*, XIX (1899), 78.

27. Hayford, "Physicians' Fees and Collections," 458; Shafer, *American Medical Profession*, 154–55; Duffy, *The Healers*, 71–73.

28. Hayford, "Physicians' Fees and Collections," 459; Straub Sherrer, "The Contract Physician: His Use and Abuse," *Pennsylvania Medical Journal*, VIII (1904–5), 104–7; Richard H. Shryock, "Medical Practice in the Old South," *South Atlantic Quarterly*, XXIX (1930), 172–73; Jerome L. Schwartz, "Prepayment Medical Clinics of the Mesabi Iron Range: 1904–1964," *Journal of the History of Medicine and Allied Sciences*, XXXIX (1965), 450–75; Pierce Williams, *The Purchase of Medical Care through Fixed Periodic Payment* (New York, 1932); R. Ginger, "Company-Sponsored Welfare Plans in the Anthracite Industry before 1900," *Bulletin*, Business Historical Society, XXVII (1953), 112–20.

29. Duffy, *Rudolph Matas History of Medicine*, II, 400–401; Konold, *History of American Medical Ethics*, 58.

30. Lillian Bryant, "The City Practitioner," *McClure's Magazine*, XXV (1905), 323–26; Walter Lindley, "The Contract System," *Pacific Medical Journal*, XX (1877–78), 103–4.

31. G. Frank Lydston, "Opening Address at the Chicago College of Physicians and Surgeons, Session of 1892–1893," *Western Medi-*

cal Reporter, XIV (1892), 265–66; F. T. Rogers, "The Ethical Advertiser," *Atlantic Medical Weekly*, X (1898), 194.

32. Tuthill, *First Years of Practice*, 16; Thomas D. Washburn, "The Relation of the Profession to the Secular Press and the Rostrum," *Medical Examiner*, XXI (1874), 516; Nelson Fanning, "The Public Press and the Medical Profession: Their Relations and Duties to Each Other," *American Medical Monthly*, XIII (1860), 11–15; M. M. Chipman, "Medical Advertising," *San Francisco Western Lancet*, VIII (1879–80), 343–45.

33. E. Ingals, "Professional Advertisements," *Chicago Medical Journal and Examiner*, XXXVII (1878), 302–7; R. H. Babcock, "The Ethics of Medical Advertising," *Journal of Sociologic Medicine*, IV (1899), 207–8; Henry Rider-Taylor, "Newspapers vs. the Doctors," *Texas Medical Journal*, IX (1893–94), 206–11; F. T. Rogers, "The Ethical Advertiser," *Atlantic Medical Weekly*, X (1898), 195.

34. Henry H. Tucker, *The True Physician: An Address Delivered before the Graduating Class of the Medical College of Georgia, at its Annual Commencement, March 1st, 1867* (Georgia, 1867), 7; Abraham Blinderman, "Medical Advertisements: Rhetoric in American Newspapers, 1861–1865," *New York State Journal of Medicine*, LXXIV (1974), 1474–77.

35. Charles R. Mabee, *The Physicians' Business and Financial Adviser* (Cleveland, 1900), 16; Rogers, "Ethical Advertiser," 197; Solomon S. Cohen, "The Relation of the Physician to the Public Press," *Journal of Sociologic Medicine*, III (1897), 102–4, 106–7.

36. Konold, *History of American Medical Ethics*, 22.

37. E. E. Munger, "The Physician and the Newspaper," *JAMA*, XLIX (1907), 656.

38. Editorial, "Altruism in the Medical Profession," *American Gynecological and Obstetrical Journal*, XV (1899), 426; Duffy, *The Healers*, 184–86.

39. William B. Lyman, "The Psychology of the Medical Profession," *St. Paul Medical Journal*, III (1901), 293–94.

40. H. G. Taylor, "The Unity of the Medical Profession," *Transactions*, Medical Society of New Jersey (1879), 83, 85; John M. Farrington, "The Brotherhood of the Medical Profession," *Charlotte Medical Journal*, IX (1896), 589–92.

41. Ashbel Woodward, "Medical Ethics," *Proceedings*, Connecticut State Medical Society (1860–63), 27–30.

42. Bauer, "The AMA," 84–90; Alexander Y. P. Garnett, *Exposition of Facts to the Medical Profession of Washington and Georgetown, D.C.* (Washington, D.C., 1877).

43. Julius Homberger, *Batpaxomyomaxia: A Fight on "Ethics"* (New Orleans, 1869), 13–14.

44. Mabee, *The Physicians' Business and Financial Adviser*, 12; Silas

W. Mitchell, *The Early History of Instrumental Precision in Medicine: An Address before the Second Congress of American Physicians and Surgeons, September 23, 1891* (New York, 1891), 3.

45. "Report of the Committee on Specialities, and the Propriety of Specialist Advertising," *Transactions*, American Medical Association, XX (1869), 111–13; Bernard J. Stern, *American Medical Practice in the Perspectives of a Century* (New York, 1945), 48–49.

46. George McComb, "The Divided Fee," *Vermont Medical Monthly*, XI (1905), 182; Robert L. Gillespie, "Division of Fee," *Medical Sentinel*, IX (1901), 248.

47. McComb, "The Divided Fee," 183.

48. G. Frank Lydston quoted in Gillespie, "Division of Fee," 245–46; J. C. Morfit, "Graft in Medicine," *Missouri Medicine*, II (1905–6), 771–76.

49. G. F. Lydston, "Further Remarks on the Bisection of Fees, Surgical Drummers and Drumming Surgeons," *Philadelphia Medical Journal*, VI (1900), 1077.

50. H. M. Lymann, "On the Code of Ethics," *Chicago Medical Journal and Examiner*, XXXVII (1878), 502–14.

51. Sennex, "Consultation with Homeopaths," *Boston Medical and Surgical Journal*, LVIII (1858), 192.

52. Harris L. Coulter, "Political and Social Aspects of Nineteenth Century Medicine in the United States: Formation of the A. M. A. and Its Struggle with Homeopathic and Eclectic Physicians," (Ph.D. diss., Columbia, 1970), 151, 162.

53. Ibid., 189–90, 259.

54. An example of this thinking is Isaac Wood, *An Inaugural Address Delivered before the New York Academy of Medicine* (New York, 1850).

55. Edward S. Dunster, *An Argument Made before the American Medical Association at Atlanta, Georgia, May 7, 1879, against the Proposed Amendment to the Code of Ethics Restricting the Teaching of Students of Irregular or Exclusive Systems of Medicine* (Ann Arbor, 1879), 24–25; Konold, *History of American Medical Ethics*, 27.

56. Coulter, "Political and Social Aspects of Nineteenth Century Medicine in the U.S.," 357, 368; William H. Holcombe, *How I Became a Homeopath* (Chicago, 1866), 12–15.

57. Coulter, "Political and Social Aspects of Nineteenth Century Medicine in the U.S.," 4; Burke A. Hinsdale, *History of the University of Michigan* (Ann Arbor, 1906), 106–10.

58. Quoted in Dunster, *An Argument Made before the American Medical Association*, 5; Fishbein, *History of the American Medical Association*, 91.

59. Quoted in Dunster, *An Argument Made before the American Medical Association*, 7.

60. Ibid., 9.

61. Ibid., 18.

62. Quoted in ibid., 22.

63. Ibid., 21–22.

64. Coulter, "Political and Social Aspects of Nineteenth Century Medicine in the U.S.," 391.

65. Nathan S. Davis, *The New York State Medical Society and Ethics* (New York, n.d.), 3; Henry G. Piffard, "The Status of the Medical Profession in the State of New York," *New York Medical Journal*, XXXVII (1883), 400–403; T. W. Dwight, "Concerning Freedom in Consultations," *Medical Record*, XXI (1882), 523–24; Martin Burke, "A Reply to 'Concerning Freedom in Consultations,'" ibid., 585–86.

66. R. C. M'Ewen, "The New York Code," *Medical and Surgical Reporter*, XLVII (1882), 88.

67. Coulter, "Political and Social Aspects of Nineteenth Century Medicine in the U.S.," 418. According to Coulter, the division of "highs" and "lows" within homeopathy had actually served as catalyst for the New York feud. "In 1879," Coulter wrote, "two graduates of Homeopathic colleges applied for admission to the Medical School of the County of New York, promising not to practice 'sectarian' medicine. In anticipation of this move the County Society had already applied to the State Society for a clarification of the reluctant portion of the Code of Ethics, receiving the reply that the County Society was quite competent to interpret the code itself."

68. John B. Roberts, "The Present Attitude of Physicians and Modern Medicine toward Homeopathy," *Transactions*, Medical Society of State of Pennsylvania, XXXVI (1895), 68.

69. "News Item," *Medical News*, XLII (1883), 750–51.

70. W. J. Beach, "A Protest against the Recent Action of the New York Medical Society with Regard to Consultations," *Proceedings*, Connecticut State Medical Society, n.s. II (1882), 99; Roberts, "The Present Attitude of Physicians and Modern Medicine toward Homeopathy," 68; A. A. Carroll, "Consultation with Irregulars," *Medical Record*, XXI (1882), 276–77. The AMA Code of Ethics stated, "no one can be considered a regular practitioner or a fit associate in consultation, whose practice is based on an exclusive dogma, to the rejection of the accumulated experience of the profession, and of the aids actually furnished by anatomy, physiology, pathology, and organic chemistry." (Art. 4.) In contrast the homeopaths had their own code of ethics, which stated, "no difference in views on objects of medical principles or practice should be allowed to influence a physician against consenting to a consultation with a fellow practitioner. . . . No tests of orthodoxy in medical practice should be applied to limit the freedom of consultations. Medicine is a pro-

gressive science. Its history shows that what is heresy in one century may, probably will, be orthodoxy in the next. No greater misfortune can befall the medical profession than the action of an influential association or academy establishing a creed or standard of orthodoxy or 'regularity.'" (Art. 4.) See Charles H. Leonard (ed.), *The Code of Medical Ethics (American Medical Association, American Institute of Homeopathy, Natural Eclectic Society) and Advertiser* (Detroit, 1878), 45.

71. Thaddeus Donahue, "Are Consultations with Different Schools of Medicine Injurious to the Public Welfare?" *Transactions*, Tennessee State Medical Association (1886), 146–47; Frank Hamilton, *Conversations between Drs. Warren and Putnam on the Subject of Medical Ethics with an Account of the Medical Empiricisms of Europe and America* (New York, 1884), 13–14, 16–17, 39. This position was expressed decades earlier, when Thomas D. Mitchell remarked that "physicians cannot consult for the benefit of a patient, if there be not between them, at least a semblance of moral agreement, an apparent assimilation in the fundamental principles of honor and honesty." See his *Annual Address to the College of Physicians and Surgeons of Lexington*, 14.

72. Henry I. Bowditch, "The Past, Present, and Future Treatment of Homeopathy, Eclecticism, and Kindred Delusions," *Transactions*, Rhode Island Medical Society, III (1885), 300–301.

73. Konold, *History of American Medical Ethics*, 72; "Differences Between Doctors," *Harper's Weekly*, XXXVII (1893), 1086. This interpretation was revised in 1950 to allow for the instruction of optometrists and in 1959 to include osteopathic students.

74. Quoted in L. Harrison Mettler, "Druggists and Physicians," *Medical Register*, I (1887), 256.

75. George B. H. Swayze, "The Professional Relations between the Physician and Druggist," *Philadelphia Medical Times*, XI (1881), 292; N. Vossmeyer, "The History of Opium and Opiates," *Texas State Journal of Medicine*, LXV (1969), 76–85; David L. Dykstra, "The Medical Profession and Patent and Proprietary Medicines during the Nineteenth Century," *Bulletin of the History of Medicine*, XXIX (1955), 401–19.

76. W. H. Saylor, "The Relations That Exist between Physicians and Druggists," *Proceedings*, Oregon State Medical Association, XI (1884), 90; Frederic H. Gerrish, "The Ownership of Prescriptions," *Boston Medical and Surgical Journal*, CIII (1880), 561–62; Charles E. Rosenberg, "The Practice of Medicine in New York a Century Ago," *Bulletin of the History of Medicine*, XLI (1967), 246.

77. Saylor, "Relations That Exist between Physicians and Druggists," 253.

78. William H. Hefland, "James Morrison and His Pills," *Trans-*

actions, British Society for the History of Pharmacy, I (1974), 101–35; James Harvey Young, *The Toadstool Millionaires: A Social History of Patent Medicines in America before Federal Regulation* (Princeton, 1961); Stewart H. Holbrook, *The Golden Age of Quackery* (New York, 1959); Dorothea D. Reeves, "Come All for the Cure-All: Patent Medicines, Nineteenth Century Bonanza," *Harvard Library Bulletin*, XV (1967), 253–72.

79. "Report of the Committee of the Philadelphia Medico-Legal Society," *Medical and Surgical Reporter*, XLIII (1880), 76–78.

80. A Junior M.D., "Physician and Pharmacist," *Medical Record*, XVIII (1880), 217.

81. "Physician and Pharmacist," ibid., 219; J. K. Crellin, "The Growth of Professionalism in 19th Century British Pharmacy," *Medical History*, XI (1967), 215.

82. F. E. Varney, "Should Physicians Dispense Their Medicines?" *Transactions*, Maine Medical Association, XII (1896), 330–34; A. W. Herzog, "Shall Physicians Dispense Their Own Medicines?" *New York Medical Journal*, LIII (1891), 287–88; B. A. C., "Physician and Pharmacist," *Medical Record*, XVIII (1880), 218.

83. V. H. Dumbeck, "Pharmacists vs. Physicians," *Peoria Medical Monthly*, II (1881), 252.

84. "Dosimetry as a Prophylactic Method against Disease," *Dosimetric Medical Review*, I (1887), 69–70; Adolphe Burggraeve, "The Principles of Dosimetry," *Dosimetric Medical Review*, II (1888), 289–90; Editorial Announcement, *Dosimetric Medical Review*, I (1887), 6; L. A. Merriam, "Therapeutic Uses of Some of the Salts of Strychnine," *Dosimetric Medical Review*, II (1888), 175.

85. Editorial Announcement, *Dosimetric Medical Review*, I (1887), 8.

86. Albert Salivas, "Dosimetry and Homeopathy," *Dosimetric Medical Review*, IX (1895), 123.

87. Otto Juettner, "The Physician His Own Druggist," *Dosimetric Medical Review*, VII (1893), 371.

88. Wallace C. Abbott, *Abbott's Alkaloidal Digest* (Chicago, 1906), 1.

89. Charles H. La Wall, *The Curious Lore of Drugs and Medicines: Four Thousand Years of Pharmacy* (Garden City, N.Y., 1927), 504–5.

90. Charles L. Greene, "The Relation of Druggist and Physician," *JAMA*, XIX (1892), 720.

91. Bernard de Mandeville, *A Treatise of the Hypochondriack and Hysterick Passions Vulgarly Call'd the Hypo in Men and Vapours in Women; In Which the Symptoms, Causes, and Cure of Those Diseases are Set Forth after a Method Entirely New* (London, 1711), 224–25.

92. V. M. Reichard, "The Physician's Debt to His Profession," *Maryland Medical Journal*, IV (1906), 24–25.

93. Ibid., 25–26.
94. Silas W. Mitchell, *Two Lectures on the Conduct of the Medical Life* (Philadelphia, 1893), 3.
95. Ibid., 13.
96. Norman Barnesby, *Medical Chaos and Crime* (London, 1910), 39.
97. F. A. Seymour, "The Code," 321–36.
98. J. S. Nowlin, "Open Consultation and Consultation With Irregulars," *Nashville Journal of Medicine and Surgery*, n.s. XXXII (1883), 132; Lymann, "On the Code of Ethics," 507; Robert M. MacIver, "The Social Significance of Professional Ethics," *Annals*, American Academy of Political and Social Science, CI (1922), 5–11; Parsons Talcot, "The Professions and Social Structure," *Social Forces*, XVII (1939), 457–67; Nathan E. Wood, *Dollars to Doctors: Or, Diplomacy and Prosperity in Medical Practice* (Chicago, 1903), 30, 129, 136.

CHAPTER EIGHT

Evolutionary Medicine

1. Significant works dealing with the present chapter include Sir Hedley Atkins, "The Darwinian Influence on Medical Science," *Transactions*, Medical Society of London, LXXXIX (1972–73), 1–19; Sol Tax (ed.), *Evolution After Darwin: The University of Chicago Centennial*, 3 vols. (Chicago, 1960); Bernard Towers, "The Impact of Darwin's *Origin of Species* on Medicine and Biology," in Frederick N. Poynter (ed.), *Medicine and Science in the 1860s* (London, 1968), 45–55; E. Mendelsohn, "Physical Models and Physiological Concepts: Explanation in Nineteenth Century Biology," *British Journal of the History of Science*, II (1965), 201–19; Robert S. Drews, "The Role of the Physician in the Development of Social Thought," *Bulletin of the History of Medicine*, VIII (1940), 874–908.
2. William Hooker, *Physician and Patient: Or, a Practical View of the Mutual Duties, Relations and Interests of the Medical Profession and the Community* (London, 1850), 389–90.
3. Rufus W. Clark, *The Sources of a Physician's Power: An Address Delivered at the Commencement of the Albany Medical College, May 28, 1863* (Albany, 1863), 20, 27.
4. Clarence J. Blake, "The Citizen-Doctor," *Yale Medical Journal*, V (1898), 4, 17.
5. H. A. Boardman, *The Claims of Religion upon Medical Men* (Phila., 1844), 7.
6. Stephen S. N. Greeley, *The Aims, Duties, Responsibilities, and El-*

ements of Success, in Medical Practice: An Address, Delivered at the 34th Commencement of the Berkshire Medical College, Pittsfield, Massachusetts, November 25, 1856* (Pittsfield, Mass., 1856), 14–15.

7. Boardman, *Claims of Religion upon Medical Men*, 7.

8. Thomas S. Powell, "The True Physician," *Transactions*, Medical Society of Georgia (1878), 170.

9. Ezra Mundy Hunt, *A Physician's Counsels to His Professional Brethren* (Phila., 1859), 25–26.

10. Elias R. Beadle, *The Sacredness of the Medical Profession: A Sermon Delivered before the Students of Jefferson Medical College and the Medical Department of the University of Pennsylvania, Sabbath Evening, November 19, 1865* (Phila., 1865), 18.

11. Silas W. Mitchell, *Two Lectures on the Conduct of the Medical Life* (Phila., 1893), 11–12.

12. E. S. Gaillard, "Medical and General Science as Vindicators of the Mosaic Record, and as Repudiators of the Modern Doctrines of Development and Selection," *Richmond and Louisville Medical Journal*, XIV (1872), 428, 452.

13. John S. Andrews, "Review of the Darwinian Theory," *Massachusetts Eclectic Society*, I (1872), 503.

14. Louis Agassiz, *Methods of Study in Natural History* (Boston, 1863), 317–18; Edward Lurie, *Louis Agassiz: A Life in Science* (Chicago, 1960), 286, 289, 290–300, 381–87.

15. Hiram Christopher, "Genesis," *St. Louis Medical and Surgical Journal*, XXXIV (1878), 4.

16. Louis Agassiz, *Essay on Classification* (London, 1859), 175.

17. Christopher, "Genesis," 415.

18. Eugene Grissom, "Medical Science in Conflict with the Theory of Evolution," *Denver Medical Times*, XV (1895–96), 283–84; Amos Sawyer, "Thoughts on Evolution," *Medical Review*, X (1884), 403–6, 417–20.

19. Grissom, "Medical Science in Conflict with the Theory of Evolution," 285.

20. Gaillard, "Medical and General Science as Vindicators of the Mosaic Record," 164.

21. Quoted in Grissom, "Medical Science in Conflict with the Theory of Evolution," 285; Ernst H. P. A. Haeckel, *The Evolution of Man: A Popular Exposition of the Principal Points of Human Ontogeny and Phylogeny*, 2 vols. (New York, 1876), I, 455.

22. Grissom, "Medical Science in Conflict with the Theory of Evolution," 286.

23. Edward Waldo Emerson, "The Man as Doctor," *New England Journal of Medicine*, CVI (1882), 529.

24. Alexander Dickson, "On Evolution," *Edinburgh Medical Journal*, XXX (1884), 1–5.

25. Quoted in Erwin H. Ackerknecht, *Rudolph Virchow: Doctor, Statesman, Anthropologist* (Madison, 1953), 202.

26. Grissom, "Medical Science in Conflict with the Theory of Evolution," 322.

27. T. B. Greenley, "The Evolution and Descent of Man," *American Practitioner and News*, XVII (1894), 291–92.

28. "Theories of Evolution," *American Journal of Insanity*, XXVIII (1871), 127, 129.

29. Quoted in P. Dougherty, "Evolution vs. Special Creation," *Charlotte Medical Journal*, VIII (1896), 760.

30. Quoted in "Theories of Evolution," 129.

31. Samuel Haughton, "Teleology and Evolution," *British Medical Journal*, II (1871), 149; J. W. Eastwood, "On Darwinism in Its Relation to the Higher Faculties," *Edinburgh Medical Journal*, XIX (1873–74), 101–11; C. Shepard, "The Evolution of Man, and Our Relation to Him as Physicians," *Transactions*, Michigan State Medical Society (1887), 29–44; James T. Whittacker, "The Evolution of Life," *Cincinnati Lancet and Observer*, XX (1877), 978–90; Lawrence Irwell, "General Evolution and Natural Selection as Exemplified by Man," *Medical Record*, LIX (1898), 86–88.

32. Stanford Chaille, "Evolution and Human Anatomy," *Medical Record*, XV (1879), 169.

33. P. Dougherty, "Medical Science in Conflict with the Theory of Evolution," *Denver Medical Times*, XV (1896), 351.

34. Edward D. Cope, *The Origin of the Fittest: Essays on Evolution* (New York, 1887), 2.

35. Packard first used the term in his *Standard Natural History* (Boston, 1885), iii. See also Lester Ward, "Neo-Darwinism and Neo-Lamarckism," *Proceedings*, Washington Biological Society, VI (1891), 53; L. H. Bailey, "Neo-Lamarckism and Neo-Darwinism," *American Naturalist*, XXVIII (1894), 661–78.

36. Edward D. Cope, *The Primary Factors of Organic Evolution* (Chicago, 1896), 4–5.

37. Alpheus Packard, *Lamarck, the Founder of Evolution: His Life and Work, with Translations of His Writings on Organic Evolution* (New York, 1901), 391, 402.

38. Ward, "Neo-Darwinism and Neo-Lamarckism," 12.

39. Cope, *Primary Factors of Organic Evolution*, 4–5.

40. Edward D. Cope, "On the Origin of Genera," *Proceedings*, Philadelphia Academy of Natural Sciences (1868), 244, 299–300.

41. Cora H. Flagg, "The Pathology of Evolution," *Medical Record*, LII (1897), 450, 452.

42. Sir John Bland-Sutton, *Evolution and Disease* (New York, 1890), 2. See also Sir Arthur Keith, "Man's Posture: Its Evolution

and Disorders," *British Medical Journal*, I (1923), 451, 499, 545, 624, 699.

43. Flagg, "Pathology of Evolution," 451–52; R. B. Bucke, "Mental Evolution in Man," *Medical Record*, LII (1897), 417; Marion H. Carter, "Darwin's Idea of Mental Development," *American Journal of Psychiatry*, IX (1897–98), 534–59.

44. G. Frank Lydston, "The Evolutionary Aspect of Infectious Diseases, with Especial Reference to the Local Venereal Diseases," *JAMA*, XXXVIII (1902), 1290. Supplementary articles on germ theory include J. K. Crellin, "The Dawn of the Germ Theory: Particles, Infection and Biology," in Poynter (ed.), *Medicine and Science in the 1860s*, 57–76; K. D. Keele, "The Sydenham-Boyle Theory of Morbific Particles," *Medical History*, XVIII (1974), 240–48; G. H. Brieger, "American Surgery and Germ Theory of Disease," *Bulletin of the History of Medicine*, XL (1966), 135–45; Karel B. Absolon, Mary J. Absolon, and Ralph Zientek, "From Antisepsis to Asepsis; Louis Pasteur's Publication on 'The Germ Theory and Its Application to Medicine and Surgery,'" *Review of Surgery*, XXVII (1970), 245–58; Walter Pagel, "The Speculative Basis of Modern Pathology: Jahn, Virchow and the Philosophy of Pathology," *Bulletin of the History of Medicine*, XVIII (1945), 3–40; R. A. Buerki, "Reception of the Germ Theory of Disease in the American Journal of Pharmacy," *Pharmacy in History*, XIII (1971), 158–68; A. Scott Earle, "The Germ Theory in America: Antisepsis and Sepsis," *Surgery*, LXV (1969), 508–22; E. R. L. Gaughran, "From Superstition to Science: The History of a Bacterium," *Transactions*, New York Academy of Science, XXXI (1969), 3–24; E. H. Ackerknecht, "Anticontagionism between 1821 and 1867," *Bulletin of the History of Medicine*, XXII (1948), 562–93; William Bulloch, *The History of Bacteriology* (London, 1938); Jacques Nicolle, *Louis Pasteur: A Master of Scientific Inquiry* (London, 1961), 54–68, 120–37, 167–71.

45. Lydston, "Evolutionary Aspect of Infectious Diseases," 1368–69; G. Frank Lydston, *The Surgical Diseases of the Genito-Urinary Tract: Venereal and Sexual Diseases* (Phila., 1899), 52–53, 267–68; id., *Addresses and Essays* (Chicago, 1890), 2–3; Phyllis A. Richmond, "American Attitudes toward the Germ Theory of Disease (1860–1880)," *Journal of the History of Medicine and Allied Sciences*, IX (1954), 435, 444–45; Edgar E. Hume, *Max Von Pettenkofer—His Theory of the Etiology of Cholera, Typhoid Fever and Other Intestinal Diseases: A Review of His Arguments and Evidence* (New York, 1927); John Farley, "The Spontaneous Generation Controversy (1859–1880): British and German Reactions to the Problem of Abiogenesis," *Journal of the History of Biology*, V (1972), 285–319.

46. Lydston, "Evolutionary Aspect of Infectious Diseases," 1287–88; id., *Surgical Diseases of the Genito-Urinary Tract*, 116–

17. Lydston agreed with English pathologist Henry C. Bastion, who reasoned that germ theory did not restrict completely the possibility of spontaneous generation; if it was plausible that spontaneous generation occurred sometime in "the beginning," it could surely be repeated under similar circumstances. See Henry C. Bastion, *Evolution and the Origin of Life* (London, 1874); Crellin, "Dawn of the Germ Theory," 66–68.

47. Lydston, "Evolutionary Aspect of Infectious Diseases," 1369. See also Sir Benjamin W. Richardson, *Lecture on the Poisons of the Spreading Disease: Their Nature and Mode of Distribution* (London, 1867).

48. Lydston, "Evolutionary Aspect of Infectious Diseases," 1288; id., *Addresses and Essays*, 17–24.

49. Winfield S. Hall, "Altruism in the Medical Profession," *Bulletin*, American Academy of Medicine, VII (1905), 230. It was Herbert Spencer who had defined evolution as a "change from an indefinite incoherent homogeneity to a definite coherent heterogeneity, through continuous differentiations and integrations." As translated by one medical skeptic, it became: "Evolution is a change from a nohowish, untalkaboutable, all-alikeness, to a somehowish, and in-general-talkaboutable, not-at-all-alikeness, by continuous somethingelseifications and sticktogetherations." See "Definition of Evolution," *Canadian Journal of Medical Science*, V (1880), 21.

50. J. S. Foote, "The Ethics of Evolution," *Western Medical Review*, IV (1899), 13.

51. Howard D. Kramer, "Agitation for Public Health Reform," *Journal of the History of Medicine and Allied Sciences*, III (1948), 473–88; IV (1949), 78–89; W. H. Sanders, "The Relations of the Medical Profession to the State and the People," *Transactions*, Medical Association of the State of Alabama, XXXVI (1884), 344–78; J. Croyny, "President's Address: The Medical Profession and the Public," *Transactions*, New York State Medical Association (1888), 30; George Conrad, "Duty of the State toward the Medical Profession," *Physician and Surgeon*, VII (1885), 289–99; Richard H. Shryock, "The Origins and Significance of the Public Health Movement in the United States," *Annals of Medical History*, I (1929), 645–65.

52. Woods Hutchinson, "Health Insurance, or Our Financial Relations to the Public," *JAMA*, VII (1886), 477.

53. Nathan Allen, "Influence of Medical Men," *New England Medical Monthly*, XI (1882–83), 546; John Duffy, "Social Impact of Disease on the Late Nineteenth Century," *Bulletin*, New York Academy of Medicine, XLVII (1971), 797–810; R. M. MacLeod, "Law, Medicine and Public Opinion: The Resistance to Compulsory

Health Legislation, 1870–1907," *British Journal of Administration Law* (1967), 108.

54. Allen, "Influence of Medical Men," 547; J. H. Beech, "The Ex-Officio Duties of the Physician," *Toledo Medical and Surgical Journal*, II (1878), 202; George Rosen, "What is Social Medicine? A Genetic Analysis of the Conflict," *Bulletin of the History of Medicine*, XXI (1947), 674–733.

55. W. Laighton, "On the Duties of Physicians," *Transactions*, New Hampshire Medical Society (1859), 53; Lawson Tait, "Has the Law of Natural Selection by Survival of the Fittest Failed in the Case of Man?" *Irish Journal of Medical Science*, XLVII (1869), 102–13.

56. A. W. Martin, "The Elimination of the Unfit by the State," *Public Health*, XX (1907–8), 36.

57. Ibid., 186.

58. Charles Darwin, *The Descent of Man, and Selection in Relation to Sex* (London, 1871), 501. See also William R. Greg, *Enigmas of Life* (Boston, 1873); Erwin Ray Lankester, *On Comparative Longevity in Man and the Lower Animals* (London, 1870); Sir Francis Galton, *Hereditary Genius: An Inquiry into Its Laws and Consequences* (New York, 1870); Alfred Wallace, *Contributions to the Theory of Natural Selection* (London, 1870).

59. Darwin, *Descent of Man*, 500–505; Edward D. Cope, "Two Perils of the Indo-European," *Open Court*, III (1890), 2052.

60. Karl Pearson, *Darwinism, Medical Progress and Eugenics* (London, 1912), 29; Bernard J. Norton, "Karl Pearson and Statistics: The Social Origins of Scientific Innovation," *Social Studies of Science*, VIII (1978), 3–34; Lindley Darden, "William Bateson and the Promise of Mendelism," *Journal of the History of Biology*, X (1977), 87–106.

61. E. O. Sisson, "Heredity and Evolution, as They Should Be Viewed by the Medical Profession," *Medical Review*, XXX (1894), 307–8.

62. Ibid., 306.

63. C. J. Devendorf, "The Relations of the Physician to Mankind," *Physician and Surgeon*, XV (1893), 243.

64. Henry D. Chapin, "The Survival of the Unfit," *Popular Science Monthly*, XLI (1892), 185; W. F. Thoms, "Health in Country and Cities. Illustrated by Tables of the Death Rates, Sickness Rates, etc. . . ." *Transactions*, American Medical Association, XVII (1866), 422–34; Robert Ernst, *Immigrant Life in New York City, 1825–1863* (New York, 1949).

65. Henry Beates, "The Proper Attitude of the Medical Profession, as Such, to Existing Political Parties," *Lancet Clinic*, n.s. LIII (1904), 225.

66. Swan M. Burnett, "The Physician as a Man and a Citizen," *JAMA*, XVI (1891), 145; Mazyck P. Ravenel (ed.), *A Half Century of Public Health: Jubilee Historical Volume of the American Public Health Association, in Commemoration of the 50th Anniversary Celebration of Its Foundation* (New York, 1921), 181–96, 133–60, 361–411; L. Emmett Holt, "Infant Mortality and Its Reduction, Especially in New York City," *JAMA*, LIV (1910), 682–90.

67. Beates, "Proper Attitude of the Medical Profession," 225; R. Hubbard, "The Mutual Relations of the Public and the Regular Medical Profession," *Proceedings*, Connecticut State Medical Society (1878), 30–36; J. H. Blenk, "The Medical Profession and Its Social Mission," *New Orleans Medical and Surgical Journal*, LIX (1907), 580–85.

68. E. T. Devine, "The Medical Profession and Social Reform," *Journal of Sociologic Medicine*, VI (1902–3), 82; Charles J. Whallen, "The Doctor as a Politician," *JAMA*, XXXII (1899), 756–58.

69. John S. Billings, "Address to the Graduating Class of Bellevue Hospital Medical College," *Medical News*, XL (1882), 286.

70. N. S. Davis, "The Mutual Relations and Consequent Mutual Duties of the Medical Profession and the Community," *Chicago Medical Examiner*, I (1860), 326.

71. H. Bert Ellis, "What Should Be the Physician's Position in the Body Politic?" *JAMA*, XLII (1904), 1212.

72. Donly C. Hawley, "The Relation of the Physician to Politics," *Journal of Sociologic Medicine*, VI (1902–3), 235.

73. Burnett, "Physician as a Man and a Citizen," 146–47.

74. Erwin H. Ackerknecht, *Rudolph Virchow: Doctor, Statesman, Anthropologist* (Madison, 1953), 46.

75. Burnett, "Physician as a Man and a Citizen," 147.

76. Charles A. Reed, "The Doctor in Politics," *JAMA*, XLII (1904), 212; George D. Tarnowsky, "The Duty of the Physician to the Public as a Politician," *Illinois Medical Journal*, VI (1904), 605.

77. Quoted in John Punton, "The Civic Duties and Responsibilities of the Physician to His Community, State, and Nation," *Alienist and Neurologist*, XVIII (1879), 410.

78. Ellis, "What Should Be the Physician's Position in the Body Politic?" 1214; Charles E. Rosenberg, "The Practice of Medicine in New York a Century Ago," *Bulletin of the History of Medicine*, XLI (1967), 223–53.

79. E. T. Devine, "The Medical Profession and Social Reform," *Journal of Sociologic Medicine*, VI (1902–3), 82, 86–87; George Rosen, *A History of Public Health* (New York, 1958), 234.

80. J. G. Orton, "The Medical Profession as a Public Trust," *JAMA*, XV (1890), 671.

81. W. A. Jones, "The Doctor in Politics," *Northwestern Lancet,*

XVI (1896), 397; Erastus O. Haven, *The Relation of the Medical Profession to Science: An Address to the Graduating Class of the Department of Medicine and Surgery, of the University of Michigan, March 30, 1864* (Ann Arbor, 1864), 15.

82. C. F. Andrew, "The Physician in Politics," *Rocky Mountain Medical Journal*, IV (1907), 239–40; Thomas D. Washburn, "The Relation of the Profession to the Secular Press and the Rostrum," *Medical Examiner*, XXI (1874), 516.

83. Reed, "Doctor in Politics," 212; Jonathan D. Wirtschafter, "The Genesis and Impact of the Medical Lobby: 1898–1906," *Journal of the History of Medicine and Allied Sciences*, XIII (1958), 15–49.

84. Reed, "Doctor in Politics," 214; Beates, "Proper Attitude of the Medical Profession," 226.

85. Reed, "Doctor in Politics," 215.

86. Claude Bernard, *An Introduction to the Study of Experimental Medicine* (New York, 1927), 1, 3.

87. Ibid., 205.

88. Ibid., 220–21.

89. Henry Maudsley, "The Medical Profession in Modern Thought," *Popular Science Monthly*, X (1876–77), 337–38.

90. Ibid., 333–34.

91. Ibid., 338–40.

92. Abraham Flexner, *Medical Education: A Comparative Study* (New York, 1925), 7–12.

CHAPTER NINE

Problems and Prospects

1. Henry Maudsley, "The Medical Profession in Modern Thought," *Popular Science Monthly*, X (1876–77), 348.

Selected Bibliography

THIS BOOK has been researched chiefly from primary sources—books, pamphlets, and journal articles of the nineteenth century. Although medical journals were a major source, I have not attempted to include them in this bibliography. The notes for each chapter should provide the interested reader with those journal materials which are considered relevant. I have included, however, a complete list of books and pamphlets, as well as certain general works that afford insights into the period and subject as a whole.

Abbott, Wallace C. *Abbott's Alkaloidal Digest.* Chicago, 1906.
Abrahams, Harold J. *Extinct Medical Schools of Nineteenth Century Philadelphia.* Philadelphia, 1966.
Ackerknecht, Erwin H. *History and Geography of the Most Important Diseases.* New York, 1965.
———. *Medicine at the Paris Hospital, 1794–1848.* Baltimore, 1967.
———. *Rudolph Virchow: Doctor, Statesman, Anthropologist.* Madison, Wis., 1953.
———. *A Short History of Medicine.* New York, 1955.
Ackerknecht, Erwin H., and Henri V. Vallois. *Franz Joseph Gall, Inventor of Phrenology and His Collection.* Madison, Wisconsin, 1956.
Adair, Fred L. *The Country Doctor and the Specialist.* Maitland, Fla., 1968.
Adams, Francis, ed. and trans. *The Extant Works of Aretaeus, the Cappadocian.* London, 1856.
———. *The Genuine Works of Hippocrates.* London, 1849.
Adams, George W. *Doctors in Blue: The Medical History of the Union Army in the Civil War.* New York, 1952.
Adams, M. *Eyes for the Blind!!! Man-Midwifery Exposed! Or What It Is and What It Ought to Be; Proving the Practice to Be Injurious and Disgraceful to Society.* London, 1830.

Addison, Thomas. *A Collection of the Published Writings of the Late Thomas Addison, M.D., Physician to Guy's Hospital.* London, 1868.

Address to the Physicians of Philadelphia on the Present Decline of the Medical Character, and the Means of Advancing Professional Respectability. Philadelphia, n.d.

Agassiz, Louis. *Essay on Classification.* London, 1859.

———. *Methods of Study in Natural History.* Boston, 1863.

Alcott, William A. *Forty Years in the Wilderness of Pills and Powders: Or the Cogitations and Confessions of an Aged Physician.* New York, 1859.

Allbutt, Sir Thomas C. *Greek Medicine in Rome.* London, 1921.

Allen, Paul W. *Eclectic Medicine: The Lessons of Its Past and the Duties of Its Future.* N.p., 1868.

———. *Medical Sectarianism.* Cincinnati, 1854.

Ameke, Wilhelm. *History of Homeopathy: Its Origin, Its Conflicts.* London, 1885.

American Medical Association. *Nostrums and Quackery and Pseudo-Medicine.* 3 vols. Chicago, 1911–36.

Andrews, Charles M. *Colonial Folkways: A Chronicle of American Life in the Reign of the Georges.* New Haven, 1920.

Aristotle. *The Works of Aristotle,* edited by D'Arcy W. Thompson. Vol. 4, *Historia Animalum.* Oxford, 1910.

——— (pseud.). *Aristotle's Compleat and Experienc'd Midwife.* London, 1700.

———. *Aristotle's Master-piece Completed.* New York, 1793.

Armstrong, John. *Practical Illustrations of Typhus Fever, of the Common Continued Fever, and of Inflammatory Diseases.* Philadelphia, 1822.

Arnold, Richard D. *The Reciprocal Duty of Physicians and of the Public toward Each Other: An Address Delivered before the Medical Society of the State of Georgia at Its Second Annual Meeting, Held at Atlanta on the 9th of April, 1851.* Savannah, 1851.

Astruc, Jean. *Elements of Midwifery.* London, 1766.

Atkins, Gaius G. *Modern Religious Cults and Movements.* New York, 1923.

Atkinson, Eric M. *Behind the Mask of Medicine.* New York, 1941.

Atkinson, William B. *The Physicians and Surgeons of the United States.* Philadelphia, 1878.

Aveling, James H. *The Chamberlens and the Midwifery Forceps.* London, 1882.

———. *English Midwives; Their History and Prospects.* London, 1872.

Baas, Johann Hermann. *Outlines of the History of Medicine and the*

Babb, Lawrence. *The Elizabethan Malady: A Study of Melancholia in English Literature from 1580 to 1642.* East Lansing, Mich., 1951.

Bagchi, Kumar N. *Poisons and Poisoning: Their History and Romance and Their Detection in Crimes*. Calcutta, 1969.

Balfour, William. *Illustrations of the Power of Emetic Tartar, in the Cure of Fever, Inflammation, and Asthma; And in Preventing Consumption and Apoplexy*. Edinburgh, 1819.

―――. *Illustrations of the Power of Emetic Tartar*. Lexington, Ky., 1823.

Bard, Samuel. *A Compendium of the Theory and Practice of Midwifery*. New York, 1807.

Barnesby, Norman. *Medical Chaos and Crime*. New York, 1910.

Bartholow, Roberts. *Annual Oration on the Degree of Certainty in Therapeutics, Delivered before the Medical and Chirurgical Faculty at its 78th Annual Session*. Baltimore, 1876.

Bartlett, Elisha. *An Essay on the Philosophy of Medical Science*. Philadelphia, 1844.

Bartol, Cyrus A. *The Relation of the Medical Profession to the Ministry*. Boston, 1854.

Bastion, Henry C. *Evolution and the Origin of Life*. London, 1874.

―――. *The Evolution of Life*. London, 1907.

―――. *The Nature and Origin of Living Matter*. London, 1905.

Bates, Ralph S. *Scientific Societies in the United States*. Cambridge, Mass., 1965.

Bauer, Julius. *Constitutional Principles in Clinical Medicine*. New York, 1934.

―――. *Genetics in Cancer*. Lancaster, Pa., 1934.

Bauer, Louis H., ed. *Seventy-Five Years of Medical Progress, 1878–1953*. Philadelphia, 1954.

Baxter, Jedediah H. *Statistics, Medical and Anthropological of the Provost-Marshall-General's Bureau*. 2 vols. Washington, D.C., 1875.

Bayfield, Samuel. *A Treatise of Practical Cupping: Comprising an Historical Relation of the Operation through Ancient and Modern Times; With a Copious and Minute Description of the Several Methods of Performing It; Intended for the Instruction of the Medical Student and of Practitioners in General*. London, 1823.

Bayne-Jones, Stanhope. *The Evolution of Preventive Medicine in the United States Army, 1607–1939*. Washington, D.C., 1968.

Beadle, Elias R. *The Sacredness of the Medical Profession: A Sermon Delivered before the Students of Jefferson Medical College and the Medical Department of the University of Pennsylvania, Sabbath Evening, November 19, 1865*. Philadelphia, 1865.

Beall, Otho T., and Richard H. Shryock. *Cotton Mather: First Significant Figure in American Medicine*. Baltimore, 1954.

Beard, George M. *American Nervousness, Its Causes and Consequences, a Supplement to Nervous Exhaustion (Neurasthenia)*. New York, 1881.

Beaver, Donald de Blasitis. "The American Scientific Community,

1800–1860: A Statistical-Historical Study." Ph.D. diss., Yale, 1966.

Beck, John B. *Essays on Infant Therapeutics: To Which Are Added Observations on Ergot, and an Account of the Origin of the Use of Mercury in Inflammatory Complaints.* New York, 1849.

————. *An Inaugural Dissertation on Infanticide.* New York, 1817.

————. *Lectures on Materia Medica and Therapeutics.* New York, 1861.

————. *Medicine in the American Colonies.* Reprint of 2nd ed. Albuquerque, 1966.

Beck, Theodoric R. *Elements of Medical Jurisprudence.* 2 vols. Albany, 1823.

Bell, Whitfield J. *Early American Science and Opportunities for Study.* Williamsburg, Va., 1955.

————. *John Morgan, Continental Doctor.* Philadelphia, 1965.

Beneke, Friedrich W. *Die anatomischen grundlagen der constitution sanomalieen des menschen.* Marburg, 1878.

Bennett, Victoria E. M. *Lectures to Practicing Midwives.* London, 1909.

Berdoe, Edward. *The Origin and Growth of the Healing Art.* London, 1893.

Bergasse, Nicolas. *Observations de M. Bergasse, sur un écrit du Docteur Mesmer.* London, 1785.

Berkeley, Sir Comyns. *A Handbook for Midwives and Maternity Nurses.* London, 1909.

Berlant, Jeffrey L. *Profession and Monopoly: A Study of Medicine in the United States and Great Britain.* Berkeley, 1975.

Bernard, Claude. *An Introduction to the Study of Experimental Medicine.* New York, 1927.

Bertrand, Alexandre Jacques François. *Du Magnétisme animal en France.* Paris, 1826.

Bibby, Harold C. *Scientist Extraordinary: The Life and Scientific Work of Thomas Henry Huxley, 1825–1895.* New York, 1972.

Biedl, Artur. *The Internal Secretory Organs: Their Physiology and Pathology.* London, 1912.

Bigelow, Henry J. *Medical Education in America: Being the Annual Address Read before the Massachusetts Medical Society, June 7, 1871.* Cambridge, Mass., 1871.

Bigelow, Jacob. *Brief Expositions of Rational Medicine.* Boston, 1858.

Billroth, Theodor. *The Medical Sciences in the German Universities: A Study in the History of Civilization.* New York, 1924.

Binet, Alfred and Charles Féré. *Animal Magnetism.* New York, 1888.

Bittinger, Joseph B. *The True Mission of the Physician.* Cleveland, 1856.

Blake, John B. *Education in the History of Medicine: Report of a Macy Conference.* New York, 1968.

Bland-Sutton, Sir John. *Evolution and Disease*. New York, 1890.

Blanton, Wyndham B. *Medicine in Virginia in the Seventeenth Century*. Richmond, 1930.

———. *Medicine in Virginia in the Nineteenth Century*. Richmond, 1933.

Blunt, John (pseud.). *Man-Midwifery Dissected: Or the Obstetric Family-Instructor, For the Use of Married Couples, and Single Adults of Both Sexes*. London, 1793.

Boardman, Andrew. *An Essay on the Means of Improving Medical Education and Elevating Medical Character*. Philadelphia, 1840.

Boardman, Henry A. *The Claims of Religion Upon Medical Men*. Philadelphia, 1844.

Boerhaave, Herman. *Dr. Boerhaave's Academical Lectures on the Theory of Physic: Being a Genuine Translation of His Institutes and Explanatory Comment*. 6 vols. London, 1751–57.

Bonner, Thomas N. *American Doctors and German Universities: A Chapter in International Intellectual Relations, 1870–1914*. Lincoln, Neb., 1963.

———. *The Kansas Doctor: A Century of Pioneering*. Lawrence, Kans., 1959.

———. *Medicine in Chicago, 1850–1950: A Chapter in the Social and Scientific Development of a City*. Madison, Wis., 1957.

Boorde, Andrew. *The Breuiary of Helthe, for all maner of syckenesses and diseases which may be in man, or woman doth folowe*. London, 1547.

Bourke, Michael P. *Some Medical Ethical Problems Solved*. Milwaukee, 1921.

Bové, Frank J. *The Story of Ergot*. New York, 1970.

Boyd, Linn J. *A Study of the Simile in Medicine*. Philadelphia, 1936.

Braden, Charles. *Christian Science Today; Power, Policy, Practice*. Dallas, 1958.

Bradford, Thomas L. *The Life and Letters of Dr. Samuel Hahnemann*. Philadelphia, 1895.

Braid, James. *Neurypnology: Or, the Rationale of Nervous Sleep, Considered in Relation with Animal Magnetism*. London, 1843.

Branch, Edward D. *The Sentimental Years, 1836–1860*. New York, 1934.

Brieger, Gert H., ed. *Medical America in the Nineteenth Century: Readings from the Literature*. Baltimore, 1972.

Brim, Charles J. *Medicine in the Bible*. New York, 1936.

Brinton, Daniel G., and George H. Napheys. *The Laws of Health in Relation to the Human Form*. Springfield, Mass., 1870.

Broca, Paul. *Mémoires d'Anthropologie de Paul Broca*. Paris, 1871.

Brock, Arthur J., ed. and trans. *Greek Medicine: Being Abstracts Illustrative of Medical Writers from Hippocrates to Galen*. London, 1929.

Brooks, Stewart M. *Civil War Medicine.* Springfield, Ill., 1966.

Brown, John. *The Elements of Medicine.* London, 1795.

Browne, Edward G. *Arabian Medicine.* Cambridge, 1962.

Brush, Edmund C. *The Place and the Work of the Medical Profession.* Zanesville, O., 1899.

Bryant, Lillian T. *The City Physician.* New York, 1905.

Buchanan, John. *The Centennial Practice of Medicine.* Philadelphia, 1876.

―――. *The Physiological and Therapeutic Uses of Our New Remedies.* Philadelphia, 1873.

Buck, Albert H. *The Dawn of Modern Medicine: An Account of the Revival of the Science and Art of Medicine Which Took Place in Western Europe during the Latter Half of the Eighteenth Century and the First Part of the Nineteenth.* New Haven, 1920.

Buckley, James M. *Faith-Healing, Christian Science, and Kindred Phenomena.* New York, 1892.

Bulloch, William. *The History of Bacteriology.* London, 1938.

Burnet, John. *Early Greek Philosophy.* London, 1930.

Burnham, John C. *Psychoanalysis and American Medicine, 1894–1918: Medicine, Science, and Culture.* New York, 1967.

Burns, John. *The Principles of Midwifery.* London, 1832.

Burr, Colonel B., ed. *Medical History of Michigan.* 2 vols. Minneapolis-St. Paul, 1930.

Burrow, James G. *A M A, Voice of American Medicine.* Baltimore, 1963.

Burton, Clarence H. *The First Homeopathic Physician in Michigan.* Detroit, 1915.

Burton, Robert. *The Anatomy of Melancholy.* New York, 1948.

Bush, George. *Mesmer and Swedenborg: Or, the Relation of the Developments of Mesmerism to the Doctrines and Disclosures of Swedenborg.* New York, 1847.

Butler, Richard, M.D. *An Essay Concerning Bloodletting.* London, 1734.

Butler, Samuel W. *Doctor's Commons: An Ethic Address Delivered before the District Medical Society, for the County of Burlington, January 10, 1854.* Burlington, N.J., 1854.

Butterfield, Herbert. *The Origins of Modern Science, 1300–1800.* London, 1957.

Cabot, Richard C. *Ethical Forces in Practice of Medicine.* Harvard, 1905.

Caldwell, Charles. *Elements of Phrenology.* Lexington, Ky., 1824.

―――. *Thoughts on the Education, Qualifications, and Duties of the Physicians of the United States.* Louisville, Ky., 1849.

Calhoun, Daniel H. *Professional Lives in America: Structure and Aspiration, 1750–1850.* Cambridge, Mass., 1965.

Callcott, George H. *A History of the University of Maryland.* Baltimore, 1966.

Campbell, Donald E. H. *Arabian Medicine and Its Influence on the Middle Ages.* 2 vols. London, 1926.

Campbell, Leslie C. *Two Hundred Years of Pharmacy in Mississippi.* Jackson, Miss., 1974.

Capen, Nahum. *Reminiscences of Dr. Spurzheim and George Combe; and a Review of the Science of Phrenology, from the Period of Its Discovery by Dr. Gall, to the Time of the Visit of George Combe to the United States, 1838, 1840.* New York, 1881.

Carpenter, William B. *The Doctrine of Evolution in Its Relations to Theism.* London, 1882.

————. *Nature and Man: Essays Scientific and Philosophical.* London, 1888.

Carson, Joseph. *History of the Medical Department of the University of Pennsylvania, from Its Foundation in 1765.* Philadelphia, 1869.

Carter, Russell K. *Divine Healing or "Faith-Cure."* New York, 1887.

Cassedy, James H. *Demography in Early America: Beginnings of the Statistical Mind, 1600–1800,* Cambridge, Mass., 1969.

Cassino, Samuel E., ed. *The Naturalists' Director, 1886.* Boston, 1886.

Castiglioni, Arturo. *A History of Medicine.* New York, 1958.

Cathell, Daniel W. *The Physician Himself, and What He Should Add to the Strictly Scientific.* Baltimore, 1882.

Chadwick, French E. *Temperament, Disease and Health.* New York, 1892.

Chaillé, Stanford E. *Origin and Progress of Medical Jurisprudence, 1776–1876.* Philadelphia, 1876.

Channing, Walter. *Remarks on the Employment of Females as Practitioners in Midwifery. By a Physician.* Boston, 1820.

Chapman, Nathaniel. *A Compendium of Lectures on the Theory and Practice of Medicine.* Philadelphia, 1846.

Chase, Heber. *The Medical Student's Guide: Being a Compendious View of the Collegiate and Clinical Medical Schools, the Courses of Private Lectures, the Hospitals, and Almshouses, and Other Institutions Which Contribute Directly or Indirectly to the Great Medical School of Philadelphia.* Philadelphia, 1842.

Chauvois, Louis. *William Harvey: His Life and Times, His Discoveries, His Methods.* London, 1957.

Chew, Samuel. *Lectures on Medical Education: Or, On the Proper Method of Studying Medicine.* Philadelphia, 1864.

Choate, Clara E. *The Unfolding: Or, Mind Understood Healing Power.* Boston, 1885.

Clark, Sir George N. *A History of the Royal College of Physicians of London.* 2 vols. Oxford, 1964–66.

Clark, Paul F. *Pioneer Microbiologists of America.* Madison, Wis., 1961.

————. *The University of Wisconsin Medical School: A Chronicle, 1848–1948*. Madison, Wis., 1967.

Clark, Rufus W. *The Sources of a Physician's Power; An Address Delivered at the Commencement of the Albany Medical College, May 28, 1863*. Albany, 1863.

Clark, Thomas D. *Pills, Petticoats and Plows: the Southern Country Store*. Indianapolis, 1944.

Clarke, Edward H., et al. *A Century of American Medicine, 1776–1876*. Philadelphia, 1876.

Clarke, Erwin L. *American Men of Letters, Their Nature and Nurture*. New York, 1916.

Clemens, Samuel L. *Christian Science; With Notes Containing Corrections to Date*. New York, 1907.

Clendening, Logan. *Source Book of Medical History*. New York, 1942.

Close, Charles W. *Phrenopathy: Or, Rational Mind Cure*. Bangor, Me., 1900.

Cobbett, William, ed. *The Rush Light*. New York, 1800.

Coleman, William R. *Biology in the Nineteenth Century: Problems of Form, Function, and Transformation*. New York, 1971.

Collyer, Robert H. *Lights and Shadows of American Life*. Boston, 1843.

Combe, George. *The Constitution of Man Considered in Relation to External Objects*. Boston, 1833.

————. *Elements of Phrenology*. Boston, 1834.

Comrie, John D. *History of Scottish Medicine*. 2 vols. London, 1932.

Cooke, John E. *Treatise of Pathology and Therapeutics*. 3 vols. Lexington, Ky., 1828.

Coombs, Frederick. *Popular Phrenology*. New York, 1848.

Cope, Edward D. *The Origin of the Fittest: Essays on Evolution*. New York, 1887.

————. *The Primary Factors of Organic Evolution*. Chicago, 1896.

Corner, Betsy C. *William Shippen, Jr.: Pioneer in American Medical Education*. Philadelphia, 1951.

Corner, George W. *Two Centuries of Medicine: A History of the School of Medicine, University of Pennsylvania*. Philadelphia, 1965.

————. *A History of the Rockefeller Institute, 1901–1953*. New York, 1965.

Corwin, Edward H. L. *The American Hospital*. New York, 1946.

Coulter, Harris Livermore. *Divided Legacy: A History of the Schism in Medical Thought*. 3 vols. Washington, D.C., 1973.

————. "Political and Social Aspects of Nineteenth Century Medicine in the United States: Formation of the A.M.A. and Its Struggle with Homeopathic and Eclectic Physicians." Ph.D. diss., Columbia University, 1970.

Cowen, David L. *Medicine and Health in New Jersey: A History*. Princeton, 1964.

Cox, Joseph A. *Practical Paragraphs for Patients and Physicians.* Wheeling, W. Va., 1902.

Cramp, Arthur J., ed. *Nostrums and Quackery and Pseudo-Medicine.* 3 vols. Chicago, 1911–36.

Crawford, S. P. *The Physician and His Profession: An Address to the Graduating Class of the Medical Department of the University of Nashville.* Nashville, 1858.

Cream, Robert C. *Inaugural Dissertation on the Chemical History and Physiological and Therapeutical Action of Tartarized Antimony.* Edinburgh, 1835.

Credé, Karl Siegmund Franz. *Die Verhütung der Augenentzündung der Neugeborenen.* Berlin, 1884.

Crombie, Charles M. *Remarks on Midwifery to Midwives: An Introductory Address.* Aberdeen, 1872.

Crosby, Rev. Howard. *The Ethics of Medical Men.* New York, 1875.

Cullen, William. *First Lines of the Practice of Physic.* 4 vols. Edinburgh, 1796.

Cullingworth, Charles J. *Charles White, F.R.S.: A Great Provincial Surgeon and Obstetrician of the Eighteenth Century.* London, 1904.

Cumston, Charles G. *An Introduction to the History of Medicine, from the Time of the Pharaohs to the End of the Eighteenth Century.* New York, 1926.

Currie, William. *An Historical Account of the Climates and Diseases of the United States of America, and of the Remedies and Methods of Treatment.* Philadelphia, 1792.

Curti, Merle E. *The Growth of American Thought.* New York, 1951.

Cushing, Harvey W. *The Life of Sir William Osler.* New York, 1940.

Cutter, Irving S., and Henry R. Viets. *A Short History of Midwifery.* Philadelphia, 1964.

Da Costa, Jacob M. *The Higher Professional Life: Valedictory Address to the Graduating Class of Jefferson Medical College, April 2, 1883.* Philadelphia, 1883.

———. *Professional Aspirations.* Philadelphia, 1891.

Daniels, George H. *American Science in the Age of Jackson.* New York, 1968.

———. *Science in American Society: A Short History.* New York, 1971.

Darlington, Cyril D. *Darwin's Place in History.* Oxford, 1959.

Darnton, Robert. *Mesmerism, and the End of the Enlightenment in France.* Cambridge, Mass., 1968.

Darwin, Charles R. *The Descent of Man, and Selection in Relation to Sex.* London, 1871.

Davies, John B. M. *Preventive Medicine, Community Health, and Social Services.* London, 1971.

Davies, John D. *Phrenology: Fad and Science; A Nineteenth Century American Crusade.* New Haven, 1955.

Davis, Andrew Jackson. *The Principles of Nature, Her Divine Revelations, and a Voice to Mankind.* New York, 1847.

———. *The Magic Staff: An Autobiography.* New York, 1876.

Davis, Michael M. *America Organizes Medicine.* New York, 1941.

Davis, Nathan S. *Contributions to the History of Medical Education and Medical Institutions in the United States of America, 1776–1876.* Washington, D.C., 1877.

———. *History of Medical Education and Medical Institutions in the United States, from the First Settlement of the British Colonies to the Year 1850.* Chicago, 1851.

———. *History of the American Medical Association from its Organization up to January, 1855.* Philadelphia, 1855.

———. *The New York State Medical Society and Ethics.* New York, n.d.

Debus, Allen G. *The English Paracelsians.* London, 1965.

———, ed. *Science, Medicine and Society in the Renaissance; Essays to Honor Walter Pagel.* 2 vols. New York, 1972.

DeCamp, Lyon S., and Catherine C. DeCamp. *Darwin and His Great Discovery.* New York, 1972.

Deitrick, John E., and Robert C. Berson. *Medical Schools in the United States at Mid-Century.* New York, 1953.

Delacoux, Alexis. *Biographie des sages-femmes célèbres, anciennes, modernes et contemporaines, avec 20 portraits.* Paris, 1834.

Deleuze, Joseph P. F. *Histoire critique du magnétisme animal.* Paris, 1813.

Derbyshire, Robert C. *Medical Licensure and Discipline in the United States.* Baltimore, 1969.

Dewees, William Potts. *Compendious System of Midwifery, Chiefly Designed to Facilitate the Inquiries of Those Who May Be Pursuing This Branch of Study.* Philadelphia, 1824.

———. *A Practice of Physic, Comprising Most of the Diseases Not Treated in* Diseases of Females, *and* Diseases of Children. 2 vols. Philadelphia, 1830.

Dickson, Thomas. *A Treatise on Blood-Letting, with an Introduction, Recommending a Review of the Materia Medica.* London, 1765.

Didama, Henry D. *The Model Physician: A Valedictory Address, Delivered in Wieting Hall, Syracuse, February 19th, 1875.* Syracuse, N.Y., 1875.

Dobbs, Archibald E. *Education and Social Movements, 1700–1850.* London, 1919.

Donald, David H. *An Excess of Democracy: The American Civil War and the Social Process.* Oxford, 1960.

Donnison, Jean. *Midwives and Medical Men: A History of Inter-Professional Rivalries and Women's Rights.* New York, 1977.

Drake, Daniel. *An Inaugural Discourse on Medical Education, Delivered at the Opening of the Medical College of Ohio, in Cinn., November 11, 1820.* Cincinnati, 1820.

————. *Practical Essays on Medical Education, and the Medical Profession in the United States.* Cincinnati, 1832.

————. *Strictures on Some of the Defects and Infirmities of Intellectual and Moral Character in Students of Medicine.* Louisville, Ky., 1847.

Draper, George. *Acute Anterior Poliomyelitis.* Philadelphia, 1917.

————. *Human Constitution: A Consideration of Its Relationship to Disease.* Philadelphia, 1924.

Draper, John W. *The Humors and Shakespeare's Characters.* Durham, N.C., 1945.

Dresser, Annetta G. *The Philosophy of P. P. Quimby, with Selections from His Manuscripts and a Sketch of His Life.* Boston, 1895.

Dudgeon, Robert Ellis. *Lectures on the Theory and Practice of Homeopathy.* Manchester, 1854.

Duffy, John. *Epidemics in Colonial America.* Baton Rouge, 1971.

————. *The Healers: Rise of the Medical Establishment.* New York, 1976.

————. *A History of Public Health in New York City, 1625–1866.* New York, 1968.

————, ed. *The Rudolph Matas History of Medicine in Louisiana.* 2 vols. Baton Rouge, 1958–62.

Dukes, Cuthbert E. *Lord Lister (1827–1912).* London, 1924.

Dunglison, Robley. *On Certain Medical Delusions: An Introductory Lecture to the Course of Institutes of Medicine in Jefferson Medical College of Philadelphia, Delivered November 4, 1842.* Philadelphia, 1842.

————. *The Practice of Medicine: A Treatise on Special Pathology and Therapeutics.* 2 vols. Philadelphia, 1848.

Dunlop, Richard. *Doctors of the American Frontier.* New York, 1965.

Dunn, Leslie C. *A Short History of Genetics: The Development of Some of the Main Lines of Thought, 1864–1939.* New York, 1965.

Dunster, Edward S. *An Argument Made before the American Medical Association at Atlanta, Georgia, May 7, 1879, against the Proposed Amendment to the Code of Ethics Restricting the Teaching of Students of Irregular or Exclusive Systems of Medicine.* Ann Arbor, Mich., 1879.

Dupotet de Sennevoy, Jean, baron. *An Introduction to the Study of Animal Magnetism.* London, 1838.

Dutton, Walton r. *Venesection: A Brief Summary of the Practical Value of Venesection in Disease.* Philadelphia, 1916.

Earle, Arthur S., ed. *Surgery in America, from the Colonial Era to the Twentieth Century: Selected Writings.* Philadelphia, 1965.

Earnest, Ernest P. *S. Weir Mitchell, Novelist and Physician.* Philadelphia, 1950.

Eberle, John. *A Treatise on the Practice of Medicine.* 2 vols. Philadelphia, 1831.

Eddy, Mary Baker. *Christian Healing and the People's Idea of God.* Boston, 1915.

——. *Message to the Mother Church, Boston, Massachusetts, 1901.* Boston, 1901.

——. *The People's Idea of God; Its Effect on Health and Christianity.* Boston, 1912.

——. *Science and Health with Key to the Scriptures.* Boston, 1875.

Ekirch, Arthur A. *Man and Nature in America.* Lincoln, Neb., 1973.

Elliotson, John. *Human Physiology.* London, 1840.

Emerson, Edward W. *Essays, Addresses and Poems.* Cambridge, Mass., 1930.

Emmet, Thomas A. *Incidents of My Life: Professional—Literary—Social, with Services in the Cause of Ireland.* New York, 1911.

Encyclopaedia Britannica: Or, a Dictionary of Arts and Sciences Compiled upon a New Plan. 3 vols. Edinburgh, 1771.

Ernst, Robert. *Immigrant Life in New York City, 1825–1863.* New York, 1949.

Essex Institute, Salem, Mass. *The Naturalist's Director.* Part I–II. *North America and the West Indies.* Salem, 1865.

Evans, Warren Felt. *Esoteric Christianity and Mental Therapeutics.* Boston, 1886.

——. *The Mental-Cure, Illustrating the Influence of the Mind on the Body, Both in Health and Disease, and the Psychological Method of Treatment.* Boston, 1869.

——. *The Primitive Mind-Cure; The Nature and Power of Faith: Or, Elementary Lessons in Christian Philosophy and Transcendental Medicine.* Boston, 1885.

——. *Soul and Body: Or, the Scriptural Science of Health and Disease.* Boston, 1876.

Eustatiev, Aleksiei G. *Homeopathia Revealed: A Brief Exposition of the Whole System Adapted to General Comprehension.* New York, 1846.

Faber, Knud H. *Nosography in Modern Internal Medicine.* New York, 1923.

Falta, Wilhelm. *Endocrine Diseases, Including Their Diagnosis and Treatment.* Philadelphia, 1923.

Faira, José Custodio de. *De la cause du sommeil lucide: ou, étude de la nature de l'homme.* Paris, 1819.

Findley, Palmer. *Priests of Lucina: The Story of Obstetrics.* Boston, 1939.

Fish, Carl R. *A History of American Life: The Rise of the Common Man.* New York, 1927.

Fishbein, Morris. *Fads and Quackery in Healing: An Analysis of the Foibles of the Healing Cults, with Essays on Various Other Peculiar Notions in the Health Field.* New York, 1932.

————. *A History of the American Medical Association from 1847 to 1947.* Philadelphia, 1947.

————. *The Medical Follies: An Analysis of the Foibles of Some Healing Cults.* New York, 1925.

Fiske, John. *Studies in Religion: Being the Destiny of Man; the Idea of God; Through Nature to God; Life Everlasting.* Boston, 1902.

Flack, Isaac H. [Harvey Graham]. *Eternal Eve: The History of Gynaecology and Obstetrics.* Garden City, N.Y., 1951.

————. *Lawson Tait, 1845–1899.* London, 1949.

Flexner, Abraham. *Abraham Flexner: An Autobiography.* New York, 1960.

————. *Daniel Coit Gilman, Creator of the American Type of University.* New York, 1946.

————. *I Remember.* New York, 1940.

————. *Medical Education: A Comparative Study.* New York, 1925.

————. *Medical Education in the United States and Canada: A Report to the Carnegie Foundation for the Advancement of Teaching.* New York, 1910.

Flexner, Simon, and James T. Flexner. *William Henry Welch and the Heroic Age of American Medicine.* New York, 1941.

Flint, Austin. *Essays on Conservative Medicine and Kindred Topics.* Philadelphia, 1874.

————. *Medical Ethics and Etiquette: The Code of Ethics Adopted by the American Medical Association, with Commentaries by Austin Flint.* New York, 1883.

————. *A Treatise on the Principles and Practice of Medicine, Designed for the Use of Practitioners and Students of Medicine.* Philadelphia, 1866.

Forbes, John, ed. *The Cyclopaedia of Practical Medicine.* 4 vols. Philadelphia, 1848.

Forbes, Thomas R. *The Midwife and the Witch.* New Haven, 1966.

Ford, John P. *The Difficulties, Duties, and Rewards of the Physician.* Nashville, 1856.

Forrest, Derek W. *Francis Galton: The Life and Work of a Victorian Genius.* New York, 1974.

Forster, Edward J. *A Sketch of the Medical Profession, from the Professional and Industrial History of Suffolk County.* Boston, 1894.

Fosdick, Raymond B. *The Story of the Rockefeller Foundation.* New York, 1952.

Foster, Sir Michael. *Lectures on the History of Physiology during the Sixteenth, Seventeenth, and Eighteenth Centuries.* New York, 1970.

Fowler, Lorenzo N. *Temperaments: Their Classification and Importance.* London, 1864.

Fowler, Orson S. *Maternity: Or, the Bearing and Nursing of Children.* New York, 1856.

————. *Phrenology Proved, Illustrated and Applied, Accompanied by a Chart.* New York, 1851.

————. *The Practical Phrenologist; And Recorder and Delineator of the Character and Talents . . . : A Compendium of Phreno-Organic Science.* Boston, 1869.

Francesco, Grete de. *The Power of the Charlatan.* New Haven, 1939.

Freud, Sigmund. *New Introductory Lectures on Psychoanalysis.* New York, 1933.

Frothingham, George E. *A Lecture on the Code of Medical Ethics, Delivered before the Students' Medical Social Science Association, December 15, 1885.* Tecumseh, Mich., 1886.

Gall, Franz J. *On the Origin of the Moral Qualities and Intellectual Faculties and the Plurality of the Cerebral Organs.* London, n.d.

Galton, Francis. *A Descriptive List of Anthropometric Apparatus, Consisting of Instruments for Measuring and Testing the Chief Physical Characteristics of the Human Body.* Cambridge, 1887.

————. *Hereditary Genius: An Inquiry into its Laws and Consequences.* New York, 1870.

————. *Inquiries Into Human Faculty and Its Development.* London, 1883.

Galvin, George W. *The Doctor, the Hospital, and the Patient.* Boston, 1898.

Garceau, Oliver. *The Political Life of the American Medical Association.* Cambridge, Mass., 1941.

Garnett, Alexander Y. P. *Exposition of Facts to the Medical Profession of Washington and Georgetown, D.C.* Washington, D.C., 1877.

Garrison, Fielding H. *Contributions to the History of Medicine.* New York, 1966.

————. *An Introduction to the History of Medicine.* Philadelphia, 1929.

————. *John Shaw Billings: A Memoir.* New York, 1915.

Giere, Ronald N., and Richard S. Westfall, eds. *Foundations of Scientific Method: The Nineteenth Century.* Bloomington, Ind., 1973.

Giovanni, Achille de. *Clinical Commentaries Deduced from the Morphology of the Human Body.* London, 1909.

Glaister, John. *Dr. William Smellie and His Contemporaries: A Contribution to the History of Midwifery in the Eighteenth Century.* Glasgow, 1894.

Gliddon, Aurelius J. L. *Faith Cures: Their History and Mystery.* London, 1890.

Glueck, Sheldon. *Five Hundred Criminal Careers.* New York, 1930.

————. *Mental Disorder and Criminal Law: A Study in Medico-Sociological Jurisprudence.* Boston, 1925.

————. *Preventing Crime.* New York, 1936.

————, and Eleanor Glueck. *Juvenile Delinquents Grown Up.* New York, 1940.

Godman, John D. *Contributions to Physiology and Pathologic Anatomy, Containing the Observations Made at the Philadelphia Anatomical Rooms during the Session of 1824–1825.* Philadelphia, 1825.

Goldsmith, Margaret L. *Franz Anton Mesmer: The History of an Idea.* London, 1934.

Goodell, William. *A Sketch of the Life and Writings of Louyse Bourgeois, Midwife to Marie de Medici, the Queen of Henry IV of France.* Philadelphia, 1876.

Goodman, Louis S., and Alfred Gilman. *The Pharmacological Basis of Therapeutics: A Textbook.* New York, 1955.

Goring, Charles B. *The English Convict: A Statistical Study.* London, 1913.

Gorton, David A. *The History of Medicine, Philosophical and Critical, from Its Origin to the Twentieth Century.* 2 vols. London, 1910.

Gottschalk, Stephen. *The Emergence of Christian Science in American Religious Life, 1885–1910.* Berkeley, 1974.

Gouley, John W. S. *Conferences on the Moral Philosophy of Medicine, Prepared by an American Physician.* New York, 1906.

Gradle, Henry. *Bacteria and the Germ Theory of Disease.* Chicago, 1883.

Grande, Francisco, and Maurice B. Visscher, eds. *Claude Bernard and Experimental Medicine: Collected Papers from a Symposium Commemorating the Centenary of the Publication of* An Introduction to the Study of Experimental Medicine. Cambridge, Mass., 1967.

Gray, John F. *The Early Annals of Homeopathy in New York: A Discourse before the Homeopathic Societies of New York and Brooklyn on the 10th of April, 1863.* New York, 1863.

Greeley, Stephen S. N. *The Aims, Duties, Responsibilities, and Elements of Success, in Medical Practice: An Address, Delivered at the 34th Commencement of the Berkshire Medical College, Pittsfield, Massachusetts, November 25, 1856.* Pittsfield, Mass., 1856.

Greg, William R. *Enigmas of Life.* Boston, 1873.

Grier, James. *A History of Pharmacy.* London, 1937.

Grisolle, Augustin. *Traité pratique de la pneumonie aux différents âges, et dans ses rapports . . . maladies aigues et chroniques.* Paris, 1841.

Gross, Samuel D. *Autobiography of Samuel D. Gross, M.D..* 2 vols. Philadelphia, 1893.

———. *History of American Medical Literature from 1776 to the Present Time.* Philadelphia, 1875.

———. *Lives of Eminent American Physicians and Surgeons of the Nineteenth Century.* Philadelphia, 1861.

Guerra, Francisco. *American Medical Bibliography 1639–1783.* New York, 1962.

Guistino, David de. *Conquest of Mind: Phrenology and Victorian Social Thought.* London, 1975.

Gunn, Robert A. *Medical Intolerance.* New York, 1877.

Guthrie, Douglas. *A History of Medicine.* London, 1945.

————. *Lord Lister: His Life and Doctrine.* Edinburgh, 1949.

Hadra, Berthold E. *The Public and the Doctor, By a Regular Physician.* Dallas, 1902.

Haeckel, Ernst H. P. A. *The Evolution of Man: A Popular Exposition of the Principal Points of Human Ontogeny and Phylogeny.* 2 vols. New York, 1876.

Hahnemann, Samuel. *The Chronic Diseases: Their Specific Nature and Homeopathic Treatment.* New York, 1845.

————. *Materia Medica Pura.* New York, 1846.

————. *Organon of Homeopathic Medicine.* New York, 1843.

Hale-White, Sir William. *Great Doctors of the Nineteenth Century.* London, 1935.

Hall, Marshall. *Observations on Bloodletting, Founded upon Researches on the Morbid and Curative Effects of Loss of Blood.* London, 1836.

————. *Practical Observations and Suggestions in Medicine.* 2 vols. London, 1845–46.

————. *Principles of the Theory and Practice of Medicine.* Boston, 1839.

————. *Researches Principally Relative to the Morbid and Curative Effects of Loss of Blood.* Philadelphia, 1830.

Haller, John S. *Outcasts from Evolution: Scientific Attitudes of Racial Inferiority, 1859–1900.* Urbana, 1971.

Haller, John S., and Robin M. Haller. *The Physician and Sexuality in Victorian America.* Urbana, 1974.

Hameed, A., ed. *Theories and Philosophies of Medicine.* New Delhi, 1973.

Hamilton, Frank H. *Conversations between Drs. Warren and Putnam on the Subject of Medical Ethics with an Account of the Medical Empiricisms of Europe and America.* New York, 1884.

Hamilton, William. *The History of Medicine, Surgery, and Anatomy, from the Creation of the World, to the Commencement of the Nineteenth Century.* 2 vols. London, 1831.

Hare, Hobart A., ed. *A System of Practical Therapeutics.* 4 vols. Philadelphia, 1891–97.

Harrington, Thomas F. *The Harvard Medical School: A History, Narrative and Documentary, 1782–1905.* 3 vols. New York, 1905.

Harris, Seale. *Woman's Surgeon: The Life Story of J. Marion Sims.* New York, 1950.

Harris, Seymour E. *The Economics of American Medicine.* New York, 1964.

Harrison, John P. *Lecture on the Responsibilities of the Medical Profession.* Louisville, Ky., 1831.

————. *Medical Ethics: A Lecture, Delivered before the Ohio Medical Lyceum.* Cincinnati, 1844.

———. *Moral Exposures of the Medical Profession: An Introductory Lecture Delivered in the Medical College of Ohio.* Cincinnati, 1842.

Haven, Erastus O. *The Relation of the Medical Profession to Science: An Address before the Graduating Class of the Department of Medicine and Surgery, of the University of Michigan, March 30, 1864.* Ann Arbor, Mich. 1864.

Havens, Lester L. *Approaches to the Mind: Movement of the Psychiatric Schools from Sects Toward Science.* Boston, 1973.

Haymaker, Webb, and Francis Schiller, eds. *The Founders of Neurology: One Hundred and Forty-Six Biographical Sketches by Eighty-Eight Authors.* Springfield, Ill., 1970.

Hazard, Paul. *The European Mind 1680–1715.* Cleveland, 1963.

Hechtlinger, Adelaide, comp. *The Great Patent Medicine Era: Or, Without Benefit of Doctor.* New York, 1970.

Hedderly, Frances. *Phrenology: A Study of Mind.* London, 1970.

Heidel, William A. *Hippocratic Medicine, Its Spirit and Method.* New York, 1941.

Hempel, Charles J., comp. *New Homeopathic Pharmacopoeia and Posology: Or, the Mode of Preparing Homeopathic Medicines, and the Administration of Doses.* New York, 1850.

Hering, Constantin. *The Guiding Symptoms of Our Materia Medica.* 2 vols. Philadelphia, 1879–80.

Hewitt, Henry S. *The Relations and Reciprocal Obligations between the Medical Profession and the Educated and Cultured Classes: An Oration Delivered before the Alumni Association of the Medical Department of the University of the City of New York, February 23, 1869.* New York, 1869.

Hills, Monson. *A Short Treatise on the Operation of Cupping.* London, 1832.

Hinsdale, Burke A. *History of the University of Michigan.* Ann Arbor, Mich., 1906.

Hirsch, Edwin F. *Frank Billings, the Architect of Medical Education, an Apostle of Excellence in Clinical Practice, a Leader in Chicago Medicine.* Chicago, 1966.

Hiss, A. Emil. *Thesaurus of Proprietary Preparations and Pharmaceutical Specialties, Including 'Patent' Medicines, Proprietary Pharmaceuticals, Open-Formula Specialties, Synthetic Remedies, etc.* Chicago, 1898.

A History of the New York Kappa Lambda Conspiracy. New York, 1839.

Hitchcock, Alfred. *Unwritten Studies and Duties of the Physician.* Fitchburg, 1859.

Hitchcock, Edward. *The Need for Anthropometry: A Paper Read before the American Association for the Advancement of Physical Education, at Its Second Annual Meeting in Brooklyn, New York, November 26, 1886.* N.p., 1887.

————, and H. H. Seeyle. *An Anthropometric Manual Giving the Average and Mean Physical Measurements and Tests of Male College Students and Methods of Securing Them: Prepared from the Records of the Department of Physical Education and Hygiene in Amherst College during the Years 1861–1862 and 1887–1888 Inclusive.* Amherst, 1889.

Hoch, A. F. *The Natural Law of Mind Healing and Mind Creating of Sickness, Disease and Deformity.* Los Angeles, 1915.

Hodge, Hugh L. *Foeticide or Criminal Abortion.* Philadelphia, 1872.

————. *On Diseases Peculiar to Women, Including Displacements of the Uterus.* Philadelphia, 1860.

Hofstadter, Richard. *Anti-Intellectualism in American Life.* New York, 1963.

Holbrook, Stewart H. *The Golden Age of Quackery.* New York, 1959.

Holcombe, William H. *How I Became a Homeopath.* Chicago, 1866.

Holmes, Oliver W. *Currents and Counter-Currents in Medical Science, with Other Addresses and Essays.* Boston, 1861.

————. *The Position and Prospects of the Medical Student: An Address Delivered before the Boylston Medical Society of Harvard University, January 12, 1844.* Boston, 1844.

————. *The Writings of Oliver W. Holmes.* 14 vols. Boston, 1911.

Holyoke, Dr. *A Collection of Choice and Safe Remedies.* London, 1712.

Homberger, Julius. *Batpaxomyomaxia: A Fight on "Ethics".* New Orleans, 1869.

Hooker, William. *Physician and Patient: Or, a Practical View of the Mutual Duties, Relations and Interests of the Medical Profession and the Community.* London, 1850.

Hooker, Worthington. *Homeopathy: An Examination of its Doctrines and Evidences.* New York, 1851.

————. *Lessons from the Story of Medical Delusions.* New York, 1850.

————. *The Treatment Due from the Medical Profession to Physicians Who Become Homeopathic Practitioners.* Norwich, Conn., 1852.

Hooton, Earnest A. *The American Criminal: An Anthropological Study.* Cambridge, Mass., 1939.

————. *Crime and the Man.* Cambridge, Mass., 1939.

————. *Why Men Behave Like Apes and Vice Versa: Or, Body and Behavior.* Princeton, 1940.

Hosack, David. *An Introductory Lecture on Medical Education: Delivered at the Commencement of the Annual Course of Lectures on Botany and the Materia Medica.* New York, 1801.

————. *Lectures on the Theory and Practice of Physic, Delivered in the College of Physicians and Surgeons of the University of the State of New York.* Philadelphia, 1838.

Hrdlička, Aleš. *Anthropometry.* Philadelphia, 1920.

Hull, David L. *Darwin and His Critics: The Reception of Darwin's The-*

ory of Evolution by the Scientific Community. Cambridge, Mass., 1973.

Hume, Edgar E. *Max von Pettenkofer, His Theory of the Etiology of Cholera, Typhoid Fever and Other Intestinal Diseases, a Review of His Arguments and Evidence.* New York, 1927.

Hunt, Ezra Mundy. *A Physician's Counsels to His Professional Brethren.* Philadelphia, 1859.

———. *Professional Ethics: An Essay Read before the Medical Society of New Jersey, at the Annual Meeting, May 27, 1873.* Newark, New Jersey, 1873.

Hunter, John. *A Treatise on the Venereal Disease.* Philadelphia, 1818.

Hurley, William R. *The Relation of the Physician to the Public: An Address.* Knoxville, Tenn., 1858.

Hutchinson, Sir Jonathan. *The Pedigree of Disease: Being Six Lectures on Temperament, Idiosyncrasy and Diathesis.* London, 1884.

Ince, Joseph, ed. *Science Papers, Chiefly Pharmacological and Botanical, of Daniel Hanbury.* London, 1876.

Inglis, Brian. *Fringe Medicine.* London, 1964.

———. *A History of Medicine.* Cleveland, 1965.

Jackson, James. *Letters to a Young Physician Just Entering Practice.* Boston, 1855.

Jackson, Samuel. *Address to the Medical Graduates of the University of Pennsylvania.* Philadelphia, 1840.

———. *On the Methods of Acquiring Knowledge: An Introductory Lecture to the Course of the Institutes of Medicine, for the Session of 1838–1839.* Philadelphia, 1838.

Jacoby, George W. *Physician, Pastor and Patient; Problems in Pastoral Medicine.* New York, 1936.

Jacques, Daniel H. *The Temperaments: Or, the Varieties of Physical Constitution in Man, Considered in Their Relations to Mental Character and the Practical Affairs of Life.* New York, 1884.

Jahr, Gottlieb H. G. *New Homeopathic Pharmacopoeia and Poslogy: Or the Preparation of Homeopathic Medicines and the Administration of Doses.* Philadelphia, 1842.

James, William. *The Principles of Psychology.* 2 vols. New York, 1890.

———. *The Varieties of Religious Experience: A Study on Human Nature.* New York, 1961.

Jameson, Eric. *The Natural History of Quackery.* London, 1961.

January, R. W. *Defence against the Attacks of Prof. Eve, and Others, of the Medical Faculty.* Nashville, Tenn., 1854.

Jastrow, Joseph. *Error and Eccentricity in Human Belief.* New York, 1962.

Johnston, James F. W. *The Chemistry of Common Life.* 2 vols. London, 1855.

Johnston, William V. *Before the Age of Miracles: Memoirs of a Country Doctor.* New York, 1972.

Johnstone, Robert W. *William Smellie, the Master of British Midwifery.* Edinburgh, 1952.

Jones, William H. S., trans. *Hippocrates.* 4 vols. Cambridge, Mass., 1939–45.

———. *The Doctor's Oath: An Essay in the History of Medicine.* Cambridge, Mass., 1924.

Kaufman, Martin. *Homeopathy in America: The Rise and Fall of a Medical Heresy.* Baltimore, 1971.

Keith, Sir Arthur. *The Religion of a Darwinist, Delivered at South Place Institute.* London, 1925.

Kelemen, Elisabeth Z. *A Horse-and-Buggy Doctor in Southern Indiana, 1825–1903.* Madison, Ind., 1973.

Kelly, Emerson C. *Encyclopedia of Medical Sources.* Baltimore, 1948.

Kelly, Howard A. *Cyclopedia of American Medical Biography from 1610 to 1910.* 2 vols. Philadelphia, 1912.

Kelly, Howard A., and Walter L. Burrage. *American Medical Biographies.* New York, 1920.

———. *Dictionary of American Medical Biography.* New York, 1928.

Kerr, John M. M., and R. W. Johnstone, and Miles H. Phillips, eds. *Historical Review of British Obstetrics and Gynecology, 1800–1900.* Edinburgh, 1954.

Kershaw, John D. *An Approach to Social Medicine.* Baltimore, 1946.

Kett, Joseph F. *The Formation of the American Medical Profession: The Role of Institutions, 1780–1860.* New Haven, 1968.

Keynes, Sir Geoffrey L. *The Life of William Harvey.* Oxford, 1966.

King, Lester S. *The Growth of Medical Thought.* Chicago, 1963.

———. *Mainstreams of Medicine: Essays on the Social and Intellectual Context of Medical Practice.* Austin, Texas, 1971.

———. *The Medical World of the Eighteenth Century.* Chicago, 1958.

———. *The Road to Medical Enlightenment, 1650–1695.* London, 1970.

King, Marian. *Mary Baker Eddy: Child of Promise.* Englewood Cliffs, N.J., 1968.

King, William Harvey, ed. *History of Homeopathy and Its Institutions in America; Their Founders, Benefactors, Faculties, Officers, Hospitals, Alumni, etc.* 4 vols. New York, 1905.

Klibansky, Raymond, Erwin Panofsky, and Fritz Saxl. *Saturn and Melancholy: Studies in the History of Natural Philosophy, Religion and Art.* New York, 1964.

Knox, George F. *The Art of Cupping: Being a Brief History of the Oper-*

ation, from Its Origin to the Present Time; Its Utility, Minute Rules for Its Performance; A List of the Diseases in Which It Is Most Beneficial; and a Description of the Various Instruments Employed. London, 1836.

Koestler, Arthur. *The Sleepwalkers: A History of Man's Changing Vision of the Universe*. London, 1959.

Konold, Donald E. *A History of American Medical Ethics, 1847–1912*. Madison, Wis., 1962.

Kremers, Edward, and George Urdang. *A History of Pharmacy: A Guide and a Survey*. Philadelphia, 1940.

Kretschmer, Ernst. *Physique and Character: An Investigation of the Nature of Constitution and of the Theory of Temperament*. New York, 1925.

———. *The Psychology of Men and Genius*. London, 1931.

Kuhn, Thomas S. *The Structure of Scientific Revolutions*. Chicago, 1962.

Laënnec, René T. H. *A Treatise on the Diseases of the Chest and on Mediate Auscultation*. New York, 1835.

Lankester, Edwin Ray. *On Comparative Longevity in Man and the Lower Animals*. London, 1870.

Latham, Robert G., trans. *The Works of Thomas Sydenham*. London, 1848–50.

Laufe, Leonard E. *Obstetric Forceps*. New York, 1968.

La Wall, Charles H. *The Curious Lore of Drugs and Medicines: Four Thousand Years of Pharmacy*. Garden City, N.Y., 1927.

Leake, Chauncey D., ed. *Percival's Medical Ethics*. Baltimore, 1927.

LeCanu, Louis-René. *Études chimiques sur le sang humain*. Paris, 1837.

Lechevalier, Hubert A., and Morris Solotorovsky. *Three Centuries of Microbiology*. New York, 1965.

Ledermann, Erich K. *Philosophy and Medicine*. Philadelphia, 1970.

Lee, Edwin. *Animal Magnetism and Homeopathy*. London, 1838.

Leonard, Charles H., ed. *The Code of Medical Ethics, (American Medical Association, American Institute of Homeopathy, Natural Eclectic Society) and Advertiser*. Detroit, 1878.

Leonardo, Richard Anthony. *History of Gynecology*. New York, 1944.

Leven, Maurice. *The Incomes of Physicians: An Economic and Statistical Analysis*. Chicago, 1932.

Lewandowsky, Max H. *Praktische neurologie, für ärzte*. Berlin, 1912.

Lind, James. *An Essay on Diseases Incidental to Europeans in Hot Climates*. London, 1792.

Lindeboom, Gerrit A. *Herman Boerhaave: The Man and His Work*. London, 1968.

Lindsley, Charles A. *The Prescription of Proprietary Medicines for the*

Sick—Its Demoralizing Effects on the Medical Profession. New Haven, Conn., 1882.

Linné, Carl von. *A General System of Nature, through the Three Grand Kingdoms of Animals, Vegetables, and Minerals.* 7 vols. London, 1806.

Litoff, Judy B. *American Midwives: 1860 to the Present.* Connecticut, 1978.

Little, L. Gilbert. *Nervous Christians.* Nebraska, 1956.

Lloyd, Wyndham E. B. *A Hundred Years of Medicine.* London, 1936.

Lobstein, Johann F. D. *Remarks on the Pernicious Effects and Fatal Consequences of Bloodletting.* New York, 1832.

Locke, Frederick J. *Syllabus of Eclectic Materia Medica and Therapeutics.* Cincinnati, 1895.

Lombroso, Cesare. *Crime, Its Causes and Remedies.* Boston, 1911.

———. *The Female Offender.* London, 1895.

Long, Dorothy. *Medicine in North Carolina: Essays in the History of Medical Science and Medical Service, 1524–1960.* 2 vols. Raleigh, N.C., 1972.

Long, Esmond R. *A History of American Pathology.* Springfield, Ill., 1962.

———. *A History of Pathology.* New York, 1928, 1965.

Longmate, Norman. *Alive and Well: Medicine and Public Health, 1830 to the Present Day.* Harmondsworth, 1970.

Ludlum, William S. *Dispensaries, Their Origin, Progress and Efficiency.* New York, 1876.

Lurie, Edward. *Louis Agassiz: A Life in Science.* Chicago, 1960.

Lydston, G. Frank. *Addresses and Essays.* Chicago, 1890.

———. *The Diseases of Society.* Philadelphia, 1904.

———. *Gonorrhoea and Urethritis.* Detroit, 1892.

———. *Over the Hookah: the Tales of a Talkative Doctor.* Chicago, 1896.

———. *The Surgical Diseases of the Genito-Urinary Tract, Venereal and Sexual Diseases.* Philadelphia, 1899.

Lynch, Kathleen M. *Medical Schooling in South Carolina, 1823–1969.* Columbia, S.C., 1970.

MacAuliffe, Leon. *Morphologie médicale: Étude des quatre types humains.* Paris, 1912.

MacDonald, Robert. *Mind, Religion and Health, with an Appreciation of the Emmanuel Movement; How Its Principles Can be Applied in Promoting Health and in the Enriching of Our Daily Life.* New York, 1908.

Mackay, Charles. *Extraordinary Popular Delusions and the Madness of Crowds.* Boston, 1932.

———. *Memoirs of Extraordinary Popular Delusions.* London, 1841.

MacLean, Charles. *Practical Illustrations of the Progress of Medical Improvement for the Last Thirty Years: Or, Histories of Cases of Acute Diseases, as Fevers, Dysentery, Hepatitis, and Plague, Treated According to the Principles of the Doctrine of Excitation.* London, 1818.

McElroy, Zenas C. *On the Dynamics, Principles and Philosophy of Organic Life: An Effort to Obtain Definite Conceptions of How Do Medicines Produce Their Effects?* St. Louis, 1869.

McFaddon, Charles J. *Medical Ethics.* Philadelphia, 1949.

McFerran, Ann. *Elizabeth Blackwell: First Woman Doctor.* New York, 1966.

McGrigor, Sir James. *Medical Sketches of the Expedition to Egypt from India.* London, 1804.

McIntire, Charles. *The Percentage of College-Bred Men in the Medical Profession.* Philadelphia, 1883.

McKay, William J. S. *History of Ancient Gynaecology.* London, 1901.

McKelvey, Blake. *American Prisons: A Study in American Social History Prior to 1915.* Chicago, 1936.

Mabee, Charles R. *The Physicians' Business and Financial Adviser.* Cleveland, 1900.

Major, Ralph H. *A History of Medicine.* 2 vols. Springfield, Ill., 1954.

The Male Mid-Wife and the Female Doctor: The Gynecology Controversy in Nineteenth Century America. New York, 1974.

Mandeville, Bernard. *A Treatise of the Hypochondriack and Hysterick Passions, Vulgarly Call'd the Hypo in Men and Vapours in Women; in Which the Symptoms, Causes, and Cure of Those Diseases are Set Forth after a Method Entirely New.* London, 1711.

Maple, Eric. *Magic, Medicine and Quackery.* London, 1968.

Mapleson, Thomas. *A Treatise of the Art of Cupping: In Which the History of That Operation Is Traced; the Various Diseases in Which It Is Useful Indicated; and the Most Approved Method of Performing It Described.* London, 1813.

Markham, William O. *Bleeding and Change in Type of Diseases.* London, 1866.

Marks, Geoffrey, and William K. Beatty. *Women in White: Their Role as Doctors through the Ages.* New York, 1972.

Marryat, Thomas. *Treatise on Therapeutics.* Bristol, 1758.

Martí Ibáñez, Félix, ed. *History of American Medicine: a Symposium.* New York, 1959.

Mason, Augustus. *Social Ethics as Connected with the Business of the Physician: The Mutual Duties of Physician and Public.* Lowell, 1849.

Mathews, Joseph McDowell. *How to Succeed in the Practice of Medicine.* Philadelphia, 1905.

Maudsley, Henry. *Body and Mind: An Inquiry into Their Connection and Mutual Influence, Specially in Reference to Mental Disorders.* London, 1870.

————. *The Physiology and Pathology of the Mind.* London, 1867.

Mauriceau, François. *The Accomplish'd Midwife, Treating of the Diseases of Women with Child, and in Child-Bed: As Also, the Best Directions How to Help Them in Natural and Unnatural Labours.* London, 1673.

Mead, Kate C. (Hurd). *A History of Women in Medicine.* Connecticut, 1938.

Meade, Richard H. *An Introduction to the History of General Surgery.* Philadelphia, 1968.

Means, James H. *The Association of American Physicians: Its First Seventy-Five Years.* New York, 1961.

Medical Society of the State of New York. *A System of Medical Ethics.* New York, 1823.

————. *A System of Medical Ethics, Reported to and Adopted by the New York State Medical Society and Introduced by the Cayuga County Medical Society, 1833.* Auburn, N.Y., 1838.

Melinsky, Michael A. H. *Healing Miracles: An Examination from History and Experience of the Place of Miracle in Christian Thought and Medical Practice.* London, 1968.

Meredith, L. P. *Examination, Appreciation, and Fees.* Cincinnati, 1874.

Meriam, Horatio C. *Footprints of a Profession, or Ethics in Materials and Methods.* St. Louis, 1887.

Merrill, Ayres P. *A Public Lecture on Medical Ethics, and the Mutual Relations of Patient and Physician.* Memphis, 1857.

Mesmer, Franz Anton. *Mémoire sur la découverte du magnétisme animal.* Paris, 1779.

Mettler, Cecilia C. *History of Medicine: A Correlative Text, Arranged According to Subjects.* Philadelphia, 1947.

Meyer, Donald B. *The Positive Thinkers: A Study of the American Quest for Health and Personal Power from Mary Baker Eddy to Norman Vincent Peale.* Garden City, N.Y., 1965.

Miller, Perry. *The Life of the Mind in America from the Revolution to the Civil War.* New York, 1965.

Milne, John S. *Surgical Instruments in Greek and Roman Times.* Oxford, 1907.

Minot, F. *Hints in Ethics and Hygiene.* Boston, 1878.

Mitchell, John K. *Impediments to the Study of Medicine: A Lecture, Introductory to the Course of Practice of Medicine.* Philadelphia, 1850.

————. *An Oration Delivered before the Philadelphia Medical Society.* Philadelphia, 1825.

————. *On the Usefulness of the Medical Profession beyond the Limits of the Profession: A Lecture Introductory to the Course of Practice of Medicine in Jefferson Medical College of Philadelphia.* Philadelphia, 1842.

Mitchell, Silas W. *Doctor and Patient.* Philadelphia, 1888.

————. *The Early History of Instrumental Precision in Medicine: An Address before the Second Congress of American Physicians and Surgeons, September 23, 1891.* New Haven, 1892.

————. *Lectures on Diseases of the Nervous System, Especially in Women.* Philadelphia, 1885.

————. *Two Lectures on the Conduct of the Medical Life.* Philadelphia, 1893.

Mitchell, Thomas D. *Annual Address to the College of Physicians and Surgeons of Lexington, in Which the Principles and Practice of Medical Ethics are Illustrated and Urged as Essential to the Welfare of the Profession.* Lexington, Ky., 1839.

Mohr, James C. *Abortion in America: The Origins and Evolution of National Policy.* New York, 1978.

Montgomery, Joseph F. *The Ethics of the Medical Profession.* San Francisco, 1871.

Morant, George. *Hints to Husbands: A Revelation of the Man-Midwife's Mysteries.* London, 1857.

Morison, Samuel E. *The Development of Harvard University since the Inauguration of President Eliot, 1869–1929.* Cambridge, Mass., 1930.

Morley, Charles. *Elements of Animal Magnetism: Or, Process and Application for Relieving Human Suffering.* New York, 1847.

Morse, John T. *Life and Letters of Oliver Wendell Holmes.* 2 vols. New York, 1896.

Morten, Honnor. *The Midwives' Pocketbook.* London, 1897.

Mowris, James A. *An Exposé of Surgical Seduction! As Practiced by Physicians Who Specialize on Female Diseases.* Syracuse. N.Y., 1871.

Mumford, James G. *A Narrative of Medicine in America.* Philadelphia, 1903.

Mumey, Nolie. *Silas Weir Mitchell, the Versatile Physician (1829–1914).* Denver, 1934.

Mutual Life Insurance Co. of New York. *Instructions to the Medical Examiners of the Medical Insurance Company of New York.* New York, 1866.

Nebinger, Andrew. *Criminal Abortion: Its Extent and Prevention.* Philadelphia, 1870.

Newsholme, Sir Arthur. *Evolution of Preventive Medicine.* Baltimore, 1927.

Nicolle, Jacques. *Louis Pasteur: A Master of Scientific Inquiry.* London, 1961.

Niederkorn, Joseph S. *The Physician's and Student's Ready Guide to Specific Medication.* Bradford, Ohio, 1892.

Noonan, John S., ed. *The Morality of Abortion: Legal and Historical Perspectives.* Cambridge, Mass., 1970.

Norwood, William F. *Medical Education in the United States before the Civil War.* Philadelphia, 1944.

Olmsted, James. *Francois Magendie: Pioneer in Experimental Physiology and Scientific Medicine in Nineteenth Century France.* New York, 1944.
Olmsted, James, and Evangeline H. Olmsted. *Claude Bernard and the Experimental Method in Me'icine.* New York, 1961.
O'Malley, Charles D., ed. *The History of Medical Education: An International Symposium Held February 5–9, 1968.* Berkeley, 1970.
Osler, William. *An Alabama Student and Other Biographical Essays.* New York, 1909.
———. *The Evolution of Modern Medicine: A Series of Lectures.* New Haven, 1921.
———. *The Principles and Practice of Medicine, Designed for the Use of Practitioners and Students of Medicine.* New York, 1892.

P. B. *The Cheap Doctor.* Norwich, n.d.
Packard, Alpheus Spring. *Lamarck, the Founder of Evolution: His Life and Work, with Translations of His Writings on Organic Evolution.* New York, 1901.
———. *Standard Natural History.* Boston, 1885.
Packard, Francis R. *The History of Medicine in the United States: A Collection of Facts and Documents Relating to the History of Medical Science in This Country.* Philadelphia, 1901.
———. *Some Account of the Pennsylvania Hospital from Its First Rise to the Beginning of the Year 1938.* Philadelphia, 1938.
Pagel, Walter. *Paracelsus: An Introduction to Philosophical Medicine in the Era of the Renaissance.* New York, 1958.
Paine, Martyn. *The Institutes of Medicine.* New York, 1860.
Paine, William. *New School Treatment Reduced to a Science, with Rules and Directions That All Who Can Read Understandingly May Treat Disease with Far Better Success than Physicians of the Sectarian Schools of Physic.* Philadelphia, 1884.
Parker, Gail T. *Mind Cure in New England, from the Civil War to World War I.* Hanover, N.H., 1973.
Parkinson, James. *The Chemical Pocket-Book: Or, Memoranda Chemica, Arranged in a Compendium of Chemistry, with Tables of Attractions, etc.* Philadelphia, 1802.
Pearson, Karl. *Darwinism, Medical Progress and Eugenics.* London, 1912.
———. *A First Study of the Statistics of Pulmonary Tuberculosis.* London, 1907.
———. *National Life from the Standpoint of Science.* London, 1905.
———. *On the Relationship of Health to the Psychical and Physical Characters in School Children.* Cambridge, 1923.

Peel, Robert. *Christian Science: Its Encounter with American Culture.* New York, 1958.

———. *Mary Baker Eddy: The Years of Discovery.* New York, 1966.

Pepper, William. *Higher Medical Education, the True Interest of the Public and of the Profession.* Philadelphia, 1894.

Percival, Thomas. *Extracts from Medical Ethics: Or, a Code of Institutes and Precepts, Adapted to the Professional Conduct of Physicians and Surgeons in Private or General Practice.* Lexington, Ky., 1821.

Pereira, Jonathan. *Elements of the Materia Medica and Therapeutics.* 2 vols. London, 1854–55.

Persons, Stow. *American Minds: A History of Ideas.* New York, 1958.

Peter, Robert. *The History of the Medical Department of Transylvania University.* Louisville, Ky., 1905.

Pickard, Madge E., and Roscoe Carlyle Buley. *The Midwest Pioneer: His Ills, Cures, and Doctors.* Crawfordsville, Ind., 1945.

Pilpoul, Pascal. *La querelle de l'antimonie.* Paris, 1928.

Ploss, Hermann H., Max Bartels, and Paul Bartels. *Woman: An Historical, Gynaecological and Anthropological Compendium.* London, 1935.

Podmore, Frank. *Mesmerism and Christian Science: A Short History of Mental Healing.* Philadelphia, 1909.

Post, Alfred C. *Anniversary Oration, before the New York Academy of Medicine.* New York, 1849.

Post, Alfred C., and William S. Ely, et al. *An Ethical Symposium: Being a Series of Papers Concerning Medical Ethics and Etiquette from the Liberal Standpoint.* New York, 1883.

Powell, Lyman P. *The Emmanuel Movement in a New England Town: A Systematic Account of Experiments and Reflections Designed to Determine the Proper Relationship between the Minister and the Doctor in the Light of Modern Needs.* New York, 1909.

Powell, Thomas S. *A Colloquy on the Duties and Elements of a Physician.* Atlanta, 1860.

Powell, William Byrd. *The Natural History of the Human Temperaments; Their Laws in Relation to Marriage, and the Fatal Consequences of their Violation to Progeny, with Indications of Vigorous Life and Longevity: Followed by a Fugitive Essay on the Protection of Society against Crime.* Cincinnati, 1856.

Poynter, Frederick N., ed. *Medicine and Science in the 1860s.* London, 1968.

Puschmann, Theodor. *A History of Medical Education from the Most Remote to the Most Recent Times.* London, 1891.

Pusey, William A. *A Doctor of the 1870s and 1880s.* Springfield, Ill., 1932.

Quételet, Lambert A. J. *Anthropométrie ou mesure des différentes facultés de l'homme.* Brussels, 1871.

Radcliffe, Walter. *Milestones in Midwifery*. Bristol, 1967.

————. *The Secret Instrument: The Birth of the Midwifery Forceps*. London, 1947.

Rather, Lelland J. *Mind and Body in Eighteenth Century Medicine: A Study Based on Jerome Gaub's* De regimine mentis. Berkeley, 1965.

Rauch, John H. *Report on Medical Education, Medical Colleges and the Regulation of the Practice of Medicine in the United States and Canada, 1765–1889*. Springfield, Ill., 1889.

Ravenel, Mazÿck P., ed. *A Half Century of Public Health: Jubilee Historical Volume of the American Public Health Association, in Commemoration of the 50th Anniversary Celebration of its Foundation*. New York, 1921.

Rayack, Elton. *Professional Power and American Medicine: The Economics of the American Medical Association*. Cleveland, 1967.

Reed, Louis S. *The Healing Cults: A Study of Sectarian Medical Practice, Its Extent, Causes, and Control*. Chicago, 1932.

Rees, George Owen. *On the Analysis of the Blood and Urine, in Health and Disease; with Directions for the Analysis of Urinary Calculi*. London, 1836.

Rees, John T. *Remarks on the Medical Theories of Brown, Cullen, Darwin and Rush*. Philadelphia, 1805.

Renouard, Pierre V. *History of Medicine, from Its Origin to the Nineteenth Century, with Appendix, Containing a Philosophical and Historical Review of Medicine to the Present Time*. Cincinnati, 1856.

Rhodes, Geoffrey. *Mind Cures*. London, 1915.

Ricci, James V. *The Development of Gynaecological Surgery and Instruments: A Comprehensive Review of the Evolution of Surgery and Surgical Instruments from the Hippocratic Age*. Philadelphia, 1949.

————. *The Genealogy of Gynaecology: History of the Development of Gynaecology throughout the Ages, 2000 B.C.–1800 A.D.* Philadelphia, 1950.

————. *One Hundred Years of Gynecology, 1800–1900: Comprehensive Review of the Speciality during Its Greatest Century*. Philadelphia, 1945.

Richardson, Sir Benjamin W. *Lecture On the Poisons of the Spreading Diseases: Their Nature and Mode of Distribution*. London, 1867.

Richmond, Julius B. *Currents in American Medicine: A Developmental View of Medical Core and Education*. Cambridge, Mass., 1969.

Riesman, David. *The Story of Medicine in the Middle Ages*. New York, 1935.

Riley, Frank L. *Spiritual Healing*. Los Angeles, 1917.

Ringer, Sydney. *A Handbook of Therapeutics*. New York, 1875.

Rix, Harriet Hale. *Christian Mind-Healing: A Course of Lessons in the Fundamentals of New Thought*. Los Angeles, 1914.

Riznik, Barnes. *Medicine in New England, 1790–1840*. Sturbridge, Mass., 1965.

Robbins, Christine C. *David Hosack, Citizen of New York.* Philadelphia, 1964.

Roberts, John B. *Modern Medicine and Homeopathy.* Philadelphia, 1895.

Robertson, Charles A. *Medical Ethics and Medical Dissensions: A Paper Read before the Albany County Medical Society.* Albany, 1871.

Robinson, George Canby. *The Patient as a Person: A Study of the Social Aspects of Illness.* New York, 1939.

Robinson, Victor. *The Story of Medicine.* New York, 1943.

Rokitansky, Karl von. *Manual of Pathological Anatomy.* London, 1849–54.

Rooke, Charles. *The Anti-Lancet: Or Invalids' Guide to the Restoration of Health, Showing the Origin of All Diseases, and the Principles of Life and Death.* Leeds, 1860.

———. *Anti-Lancet: Or the Destructive Practice of Bleeding, etc., Exposed and Denounced, Showing the Principles of Life and Death and the Origin of All Diseases.* Scarborough, 1867.

Roosa, Daniel B. St. John. *Christian Scientism.* New York, n.d.

———. *The Coming Medical Man: An Anniversary Discourse.* New York, 1875.

———. *A Doctor's Suggestions to the Community: Being a Series of Papers upon Various Subjects from a Physician's Standpoint.* New York, 1880.

———. *The Relations of the Medical Profession to the State.* New York, 1879.

Root, Julia A. *Healing Power of Mind: A Treatise on Mind-Cure.* Peoria, Ill., 1886.

Rorty, James. *American Medicine Mobilizes.* New York, 1939.

Rosen, George. *Fees and Fee Bills: Some Economic Aspects of Medical Practice in Nineteenth Century America.* Baltimore, 1946.

———. *From Medical Police to Social Medicine: Essays on the History of Health Care.* New York, 1974.

———. *A History of Public Health.* New York, 1958.

———. *Madness in Society: Chapters in the Historical Sociology of Mental Illness.* Chicago, 1968.

———. *The Specialization of Medicine.* New York, 1944.

Ross, James. *The Graft Theory of Disease: Being an Application of Mr. Darwin's Hypothesis of Pangenesis to the Explanation of the Phenomena of the Zymotic Diseases.* London, 1872.

Rothstein, William G. *American Physicians in the Nineteenth Century, from Sects to Science.* Baltimore, 1972.

Rudder, W. *The Complete Physician.* Albany, 1861.

Rush, Benjamin. *Medical Inquiries and Observations.* 4 vols. Philadelphia, 1794–98.

Ryan, Michael. *A Manual of Medical Jurisprudence, Compiled from the Best Medical and Legal Works.* Philadelphia, 1832.

Sarton, George. *Galen of Pergamon.* Lawrence, Kans., 1954.

Schlesinger, Arthur M. *The Rise of the City, 1878–1898.* New York, 1933.

Schwartz, Jozua M. W. *The Healers.* New York, 1906.

Scott, Henry H. *A History of Tropical Medicine, Based on the Fitzpatrick Lectures.* 2 vols. Baltimore, 1939.

Seldes, Gilbert V. *The Stammering Century.* New York, 1928.

Sellers, Charles G. *Jacksonian Democracy.* Washington, D.C., 1958.

Selye, Hans. *The Stress of Life.* New York, 1956.

Semmelweis, Ignác F. *Die Aetiologie, der Begriff und die Prophylaxis des Kindbettfiebers.* Budapest, 1861.

Sergi, Giuseppe. *L'Uomo secondo le origini, l'antichita, le variazioni e la distribuzione geografica.* Turin, 1911.

Sewall, Thomas. *Memoir of Dr. Godman: Being an Introductory Lecture.* New York, 1832.

Shafer, Henry B. *The American Medical Profession, 1783 to 1850.* New York, 1936.

Sheldon, William H. *The Varieties of Human Physique: An Introduction to Constitutional Psychology.* New York, 1940.

————. *The Varieties of Temperament: A Psychology of Constitutional Differences.* New York, 1942.

Shryock, Richard H. *American Medical Research, Past and Present.* New York, 1947.

————. *The Development of Modern Medicine: An Interpretation of the Social and Scientific Factors Involved.* Philadelphia, 1936.

————. *Medical Licensing in America, 1650–1965.* Baltimore, 1967.

————. *Medicine in America: Historical Essays.* Baltimore, 1966.

————. *The Unique Influence of the Johns Hopkins University on American Medicine.* Copenhagen, 1953.

Siegel, Rudolph E. *Galen's System of Physiology and Medicine.* Basel, 1968.

Sigerist, Henry E. *American Medicine.* New York, 1934.

————. *Civilization and Disease.* Ithaca, N.Y., 1943.

————, ed. and trans. *Four Treatises of Theophrastus von Hohenwhem called Paracelsus.* Baltimore, 1941.

————. *The Great Doctors: A Biographical History of Medicine.* New York, 1933.

————. *Man and Medicine: An Introduction to Medical Knowledge.* New York, 1932.

Simmons, J. P. *Origin of Man.* Atlanta, 1875.

Sims, James M. *The Story of My Life.* New York, 1968.

Singer, Charles J. *The Discovery of the Circulation of the Blood.* London, 1922.

————. *A Short History of Anatomy from the Greeks to Harvey.* New York, 1957.

————. *From Magic to Science: Essays on the Scientific Twilight.* New York, 1958.

Smallwood, William M., and Mabel S. C. Smallwood. *Natural History and the American Mind.* New York, 1941.

Smellie, William. *Treatise on the Theory and Practice of Midwifery.* London, 1766.

Smith, Grafton Elliot. *The Old and the New Phrenology.* Edinburgh, 1924.

Smith, Robert W. I. *English-Speaking Students of Medicine at the University of Leyden.* Edinburgh, 1932.

Smith, William. *The History of the Province of New York, from the First Discovery to the Year 1732.* London, 1757.

Smith, Wilson. *Professors and Public Ethics: Studies of Northern Moral Philosophers before the Civil War.* Ithaca, 1956.

Smythe, Gonzalvo C. *Medical Heresies: Historically Considered.* Philadelphia, 1880.

Speert, Harold. *Obstetric and Gynecologic Milestones: Essays in Eponymy.* New York, 1958.

Spencer, Herbert R. *The History of British Midwifery from 1650 to 1800: the Fitz-Patrick Lectures for 1927.* London, 1927.

Spurzheim, Johann G. *Outlines of Phrenology.* Boston, 1834.

Stahl, Georg E. *Neu-verbesserte Lehre von den Temperamenten.* Leipzig, 1723.

Stearns, Raymond P. *Science in the British Colonies of America.* Urbana, 1970.

Stern, Bernard J. *American Medical Practice in the Perspectives of a Century.* New York, 1945.

————. *Society and Medical Progress.* Princeton, 1941.

Stern, Heinrich. *Theory and Practice of Bloodletting.* New York, 1915.

Stern, Madeleine B. *Heads and Headlines: The Phrenological Fowlers.* Norman, Okla., 1971.

Stevens, John. *Man-Midwifery Exposed: Or the Danger and Immorality of Employing Men in Midwifery Proved, and the Remedy for the Evil Found. Addressed to the Society for the Suppression of Vice.* London, 1849.

Stevens, Rosemary. *American Medicine and the Public Interest.* New Haven, 1971.

Stevenson, Lloyd G., and Robert P. Multauf, eds. *Medicine, Science, and Culture: Historical Essays in Honor of Owsei Temkin.* Baltimore, 1968.

Stewart, Alexander. *Our Temperaments: Their Study and Their Teaching.* London, 1887.

Stewart, Alexander P., and Edward Jenkins. *The Medical and Legal Aspects of Sanitary Reform.* Leicester, 1969.

Stewart, Ferdinand C. *Hospitals and Surgeons of Paris: An Historical and Statistical Account of the Civil Hospitals of Paris*. New York, 1843.

Stillé, Alfred. *Medical Education in the United States*. Philadelphia, 1846.

————. *Therapeutics and Materia Medica: A Systematic Treatise on the Action and Uses of Medicinal Agents*. 2 vols. Philadelphia, 1860.

Stillé, Charles J. *History of the United States Sanitary Commission: Being a General Report of Its Work during the War of the Rebellion*. Philadelphia, 1866.

Stokes, William. *Lectures on Fever*. London, 1874.

Stookey, Bryon P. *A History of Colonial Medical Education in the Province of New York, 1767 to 1830*. Springfield, Ill., 1962.

Storer, Horatio R., and Franklin Heard. *Criminal Abortion: Its Nature, Its Evidence, and Its Law*. Boston, 1868.

Struik, Dirk J. *Yankee Science in the Making*. New York, 1962.

Sudhoff, Karl. *Essays in the History of Medicine*. New York, 1926.

Sunderland, La Roy. *Pathetism: Man Considered in Respect to His Form, Life, Sensation, Soul, Mind, Spirit; Giving the Rationale of Those Laws Which Produce the Mysteries, Miseries, Felicities, of Human Nature!* Boston, 1847.

Swan, Samuel. *Catalogue of Morbific Products, Nosodes, and Other Remedies, in High Potencies*. New York, 1886.

Swedenborg, Emanuel. *Angelic Wisdom Concerning the Divine Love and the Divine Wisdom*. New York, 1885.

————. *Angelic Wisdom Concerning the Divine Providence*. New York, 1892.

Symington, A. J. *Of Physicians and Their Fees, with Some Personal Reminiscences*. N.p., n.d.

Tarshis, Jerome. *Claude Bernard: Father of Experimental Medicine*. New York, 1968.

Tax, Sol, ed. *Evolution after Darwin: The University of Chicago Centennial*. 3 vols. Chicago, 1960.

Tayler, John L. *Aspects of Social Evolution: First Series, Temperaments*. London, 1904.

Taylor, Arthur N. *The Law in Its Relations to Physicians*. New York, 1904.

Taylor, J. *The Medical Profession: Its Position and Claims*. Middletown, Conn., 1857.

Taylor, John Jay. *The Physician as a Business Man: Or, How to Obtain the Best Financial Results in the Practice of Medicine*. Philadelphia, 1891.

Taylor, Lloyd C. *The Medical Profession and Social Reform, 1885–1945*. New York, 1974.

Temkin, Owsei. *Galenism: Rise and Decline of a Medical Philosophy.* Ithaca, N.Y., 1973.

———, trans. *Soranus, of Ephesus: Gynecology.* Baltimore, 1956.

Thacher, James. *American Medical Biography: Or, Memoirs of Eminent Physicians Who Have Flourished in America, To Which is Prefixed a Succinct History of Medical Science in the United States from the First Settlement of the Country.* Boston, 1828.

———. *American Modern Practice: Or, A Simple Method of Prevention and Cure of Diseases.* Boston, 1817.

Thomas, A. R. *Evolution of the Earth and Man: A Lecture before the Hahnemannian Institute.* Philadelphia, 1892.

Thoms, Herbert. *Chapters in American Obstetrics.* Springfield, Ill., 1933.

Thomson, Samuel. *A Narrative of the Life and Medical Discoveries of Samuel Thomson, Containing an Account of His System of Practice, and the Manner of Curing Disease with Vegetable Medicine, upon a Plan Entirely New.* St. Clairsville, 1829.

———. *Thomsonian Materia Medica: Or, Botanic Family Physician: Comprising a Philosophical Theory, the Natural Organization and Assumed Principles of Animal and Vegetable Life.* Albany, 1841.

Timbs, John. *Doctors and Patients: Or, Anecdotes of the Medical World and Curiosities of Medicine.* London, 1873.

Tischner, Rudolf. *Franz Anton Mesmer.* Munich, 1928.

Todd, John. *Serpents in the Dove's Nest.* Boston, 1867.

Toner, Joseph M. *Contributions to the Study of Yellow Fever.* Washington, D.C., 1874.

Topinard, Paul. *L'Anthropologie.* Paris, 1877.

Troisvèvre, F. Thomas de. *Division naturelle des tempéramens, tirée de la fonctionomie.* Paris, 1821.

———. *Physiologie des tempéramens ou constitutions; nouvelle doctrine applicable à la médecine—pratique, à l'hygiène, à l'histoire naturelle et à la philosophie; précédée d'un examen des diverses théories des tempéramens.* Paris, 1826.

Tucker, Henry H. *The True Physician: An Address Delivered before the Graduating Class of the Medical College of Georgia, at its Annual Commencement, March 1st, 1867.* Georgia, 1867.

Tuthill, Franklin. *First Years of Practice; An Address to the Graduating Class of the New York Medical College, March, 1854.* New York, 1855.

Underwood, Edgar A. *Science, Medicine and History; Essays on the Evolution of Scientific Thought and Medical Practice Written in Honour of Charles Singer.* New York, 1953.

United States Dispensatory. Philadelphia, 1873.

United States Surgeon-General's Office. *The Medical and Surgi-*

cal History of the War of Rebellion. 3 vols. Washington, D.C., 1870–88.

Van Ingen, Philip. *The New York Academy of Medicine: Its First Hundred Years.* New York, 1949.
Viets, Henry R. *A Brief History of Medicine in Massachusetts.* Boston, 1930.
Viola, Giacinto. *Le Legge de Correlazione Morfologica dei Tippi Individuali.* Padua, 1909.
————. *Le problème de la constitution selon l'école italienne.* Bologna, 1931.
Virchow, Rudolph L. K. *Cellular Pathology as Based upon Physiological and Pathological Histology.* New York, 1860.

Waggett, John M. *Mental, Divine and Faith Healings, Their Explanation and Place.* Boston, 1919.
Wain, Harry. *A History of Preventive Medicine.* Springfield, Ill., 1970.
Wallace, Alfred R. *Contributions to the Theory of Natural Selection.* London, 1870.
Walmsley, Donald M. *Anton Mesmer.* London, 1967.
Walsh, James J. *Cures: The Story of the Cures That Fail.* New York, 1923.
————. *History of Medicine in New York, Three Centuries of Progress.* 5 vols. New York, 1919.
————. *History of the Medical Society of the State of New York.* New York, 1907.
Walter, Richard D. *S. Weir Mitchell, M.D. Neurologist: A Medical Biography.* Springfield, Ill., 1970.
Walton, Alice. *The Cult of Asklepios.* Boston, 1894.
Wardrop, J. *On the Curative Effects of the Abstraction of Blood, with Rules for Employing Both Local and General Blood-Letting in the Treatment of Diseases.* Philadelphia, 1837.
Waring, Joseph I. *A History of Medicine in South Carolina, 1670–1900.* Charleston, S.C., 1967.
Watson, John. *The True Physician: An Anniversary Discourse.* New York, 1860.
Watts, G. *A Dissertation on the Ancient and Noted Doctrine of Revulsion and Derivation; Wherein the Absurdity of the Principles on Which the Notion of Revulsion Was Originally Founded, is Evidently Demonstrated, and the Immediate Consequences of Bloodletting Plainly Prov'd.* London, 1754.
Weatherhead, Leslie D. *Psychology, Religion and Healing.* New York, 1952.
Weiss, Harry B., and Howard R. Kemble. *The Great American Water-*

Cure Craze: A History of Hydropathy in the United States. Trenton, 1967.

Weiss, J. *Directions for Using the Improved Cupping Apparatus: Observations on Cupping.* London, 1829.

Wertz, Richard W., and Dorothy C. Wertz. *Lying-in: A History of Childbirth in America.* New York, 1977.

West, Charles. *Lectures on the Diseases of Infancy and Childhood.* Philadelphia, 1850.

Wheeler, John B. *Memoirs of a Small-Town Surgeon.* New York, 1935.

Whipple, Leander E. *The Philosophy of Mental Healing: A Practical Exposition of Natural Restorative Power.* New York, 1893.

White, Charles. *A Treatise on the Management of Pregnant and Lying-in Women, and the Means of Curing, But More Especially of Preventing the Principal Disorders to Which They Are Liable.* London, 1772.

Whitteridge, Gweneth. *William Harvey and the Circulation of the Blood.* London, 1971.

Widdess, J. D. H. *The Royal College of Surgeons in Ireland and Its Medical School, 1784–1966.* Edinburgh, 1967.

Wiggin, James H. *Christian Science and the Bible, with Reference to Mary B. Eddy's* Science and Health. Boston, 1886.

Wightman, William P. D. *The Emergence of Scientific Medicine.* Edinburgh, 1971.

Wilder, Alexander. *History of Medicine.* Augusta, Me., 1901.

Wilder, Harris H. *A Laboratory Manual of Anthropometry.* Philadelphia, 1920.

Williams, Pierce. *The Purchase of Medical Care through Fixed Periodic Payment.* New York, 1932.

Williams, Ralph C. *The United States Public Health Service, 1798–1950.* Washington, D.C., 1951.

Wilson, Bryon R. *Sects and Society: A Sociological Study of the Elim Tabernacle, Christian Science, and Christadelphians.* Berkeley, 1961.

Wilson, Robert C. *Drugs and Pharmacy in the Life of Georgia, 1733–1959.* Athens, Ga., 1959.

Winbigler, Charles F. *Handbook of Instructions for Healing and Helping Others, Containing Scriptural, Psycho-Therapeutic, Psychological, and Optimistic Principles, Simply Stated and Thoroughly Tested.* Los Angeles, 1916.

Winslow, Charles E. A. *The Conquest of Epidemic Diseases: A Chapter in the History of Ideas.* Princeton, 1943.

Winslow, John H. *Darwin's Victorian Malady: Evidence for Its Medically Induced Origin.* Philadelphia, 1971.

Winter, George. *History of Animal Magnetism; Its Origin, Progress, and Present State; Its Principles and Secrets Displayed, as Delivered by the Late Dr. Demainauduc.* Bristol, 1801.

Wolfe, Bernard, and Raymond Rosenthal. *Hypnotism Comes of Age: Its Progress from Mesmer to Psychoanalysis.* New York, 1949.

Wood, George B. *A Treatise on the Practice of Medicine.* Philadelphia, 1849.

Wood, Horatio C. *Therapeutics: Its Principles and Practice.* Philadelphia, 1888.

———. *A Treatise on Therapeutics, Comprising Materia Medica and Toxicology, with Especial Reference to the Application of the Physiological Action of Drugs to Clinical Medicine.* Philadelphia, 1874.

Wood, Isaac. *An Inaugural Address Delivered before the New York Academy of Medicine.* New York, 1850.

Wood, Nathan E. *Dollars to Doctors: Or, Diplomacy and Prosperity in Medical Practice.* Chicago, 1903.

Woodward, A. *Medical Ethics.* Hartford, 1860.

Wootton, A. C. *Chronicles of Pharmacy.* 2 vols. Boston, 1910.

Worcester, Ellwood; Samuel McComb; and Dr. Isidor H. Coriat. *Religion and Medicine: The Moral Control of Nervous Disorders.* New York, 1908.

Wrench, Guy T. *Lord Lister: His Life and Work.* London, 1913.

Yandell, David W. *Temperament: An Address.* Louisville, 1892.

Yandell, Lunsford Pitts. *A Memoir of the Life and Writings of John Esten Cooke.* Louisville, Ky., 1875.

Young, James Harvey. *The Toadstool Millionaires: A Social History of Patent Medicines in America before Federal Regulation.* Princeton, N.J., 1961.

Zilboorg, Gregory. *The Medical Man and the Witch during the Renaissance.* Baltimore, 1935.

Zincke, Foster B. *Last Winter in the United States.* London, 1868.

Index

Note on the Author

John S. Haller, Jr., received his Ph.D. from the University of Maryland in 1968. His doctoral dissertation, "American Concepts of Race, 1859–1900," developed into his first book, *Outcasts from Evolution: Scientific Attitudes of Racial Inferiority, 1859–1900*. This study won the 1971 Anisfield-Wolf Award in Race Relations. His second book, *The Physician and Sexuality in Victorian America*, was written with his wife Robin M. Haller as coauthor. Haller served as professor of history and associate dean for academic affairs at Indiana University Northwest between 1968 and 1980. He is currently at California State University Long Beach, where he is continuing his research and writing in medical and pharmaceutical history and fulfilling duties as associate vice-president for academic affairs/dean of graduate studies.